What are the psychobiologic functions that make it possible for man to compose, hear, and perform music? Is music a language? How does music move the listener? Why do we like to perform and listen to music? What is the nature of meaning in music? These are some of the questions of concern in this book.

Music, Mind, and Brain is a pioneering book on the scientific approach to the nature of music from a psychobiologic point of view. It does not analyze music merely from the musical score, but is concerned with music in the flesh, as a living entity dwelling within man. From this point of view, a view that places emphasis on the function of the brain and how it processes musical sounds differently from other sounds, we gain new knowledge and insight into the workings of the human mind.

This book offers many illustrations of basic forms of emotional communication through music and of the function of rhythmic pulse. An accompanying soundsheet provides some sound and musical illustrations. Aspects of ethnic, classical, and rock 'n' roll music are covered, and the use of computers in producing and analyzing music is explored.

A work that has many scientific and aesthetic implications, *Music, Mind, and Brain* will be of particular interest to the neuropsychologist, neurophysiologist, and linguist, as well as to the thoughtful musician.

MUSIC, MIND, AND BRAIN

The Neuropsychology of Music

MUSIC, MIND, AND BRAIN
The Neuropsychology of Music

Edited by

MANFRED CLYNES

New South Wales State Conservatorium of Music
Sydney, Australia

91-080

PLENUM PRESS • NEW YORK AND LONDON

Library of Congress Cataloging in Publication Data

Main entry under title:

Music, mind, and brain.

"An expanded version of proceedings from the Third Workshop on the Physical
and Neuropsychological Foundations of Music, held August 8–12, 1980, in Ossiach, Austria"—T.p. verso.
   Includes bibliographical references and index.
   1. Music—Psychology—Congresses. 2. Music—Physiological aspects—Congresses. I. Clynes, Manfred, 1925.   . II. Workshop on the Physical and
Neuropsychological Foundations of Music (3rd: 1980: Ossiach, Austria)
ML3830.M98   781'.15   82-546
ISBN 0-306-40908-9   AACR2

First Printing—June 1982
Second Printing—August 1983

An expanded version of proceedings from the Third Workshop
on the Physical and Neuropsychological Foundations of Music,
held August 8–12, 1980, in Ossiach, Austria

Sound sheet © 1982 Manfred Clynes

© 1982 Plenum Press, New York
A Division of Plenum Publishing Corporation
233 Spring Street, New York, N.Y. 10013

Printed in the United States of America

Music flows and stars
Shine on all
Who hear and see
Yet—music has vision:

The deaf can compose

PREFACE

There is much music in our lives - yet we know little about its function.

Music is one of man's most remarkable inventions - though possibly it may not be his invention at all: like his capacity for language his capacity for music may be a naturally evolved biologic function. All cultures and societies have music.

Music differs from the sounds of speech and from other sounds, but only now do we find ourselves at the threshold of being able to find out how our brain processes musical sounds differently from other sounds. We are going through an exciting time when these questions and the question of how music moves us are being seriously investigated for the first time from the perspective of the co-ordinated functioning of the organism: the perspective of brain function, motor function as well as perception and experience.

There is so much we do not yet know. But the roads to that knowledge are being opened, and the coming years are likely to see much progress towards providing answers and raising new questions. These questions are different from those music theorists have asked themselves: they deal not with the structure of a musical <u>score</u> (although that knowledge is important and necessary) but with music in the flesh: music not outside of man to be looked at from written symbols, but music-man as a living entity or system. From this point of view, progress in understanding what makes meaningful music should help us to understand what makes meaning and beauty in us. Such knowledge of brain function eventually will weigh alongside the knowledge of structure and energy in the universe.

This book, while not claiming comprehensiveness, brings together aspects of new music research from different perspectives and angles of attack that should make it specially useful to acquaint the reader with the current state of the art in this field at this critical time, and its direction for the future.

All of the chapters of the book, except chapters I, VII, XIII, XVII, are based on presentations at the conference on the Physical and Neuropsychological Foundations of Music in Ossiach, August 1980. These conferences have done a great deal to encourage work in this young and growing field. Thanks are due most particularly to Juan Roederer for his continuing efforts on behalf of the conferences, as well as to the Austrian Ministry of Science, the University of Alaska, the Austrian Broadcasting Organisation, and the organizers of the Carinthian Summer Festival. I am especially grateful to Dorothy Capelletto for long hours of painstaking and meticulous work, helping with the editing and preparation of the manuscript. The New South Wales State Conservatorium of Music, its Music Research Center and Sentic Research Laboratories have given continuing support for this undertaking and so have Nigel Nettheim, Janice Walker and Brian McMahon, of the staff of the Music Research Center. The work has also been supported by the Education Research and Development Committee (ERD) of the Commonwealth of Australia.

Chapters I, VII, XIII, XVII are by special invitation, and are gratefully acknowledged.

The first part of the book broadly concerns itself with the theme Music and Language - the questions of what is the nature of the language of music, how does the central nervous system organize musical experience. and how are qualities and feelings communicated.

The second part treats the perception and production of various forms of sound, of rhythm, intervals, and scales.

The third part shows how computers can now contribute to better understanding of musical processes by their ability to produce and analyze sound in known and new ways.

The book is dedicated to all those interested in how music functions. And if this book sparks interest in the reader to make his own contribution towards achieving these goals it will have been especially successful.

Manfred Clynes
Sydney, 1981

FOREWORD

A pioneering event in the international scenario of musicology and musical acoustics took place in 1973 when the first Workshop on the Physical and Neuropsychological Foundations of Music was held in Ossiach, Austria, as part of the Carinthian Summer Music Festival. This event brought together leading musicians, neurobiologists, physicists, engineers, philosophers and psychlogists to appraise a variety of controversial and little-explored subjects related to the understanding of how sound patterns are produced in musical instruments, how they propagate through and interact with the acoustical environment, and how they are perceived by the auditory system and interpreted by the human brain. Similar Workshops followed in 1977 and 1980, and there is every indication that they will indeed become periodic components of the Carinthian Summer Festival.

The serene, majestic surroundings in the heart of the Austrian Alps, the beautiful setting of the old Ossiach Monastery where the Workshop sessions were held, and the presence of internationally renowned artists and ensembles provided a most dignified and attractive atmosphere for the discussions. Each Workshop focused on a limited number of truly inter-disciplinary subjects, on which reviews and contributed papers were presented and 'round table' discussions were held. The first Workshop for instance dwelt mainly on psychoacoustics; the second one centered on three subjects: acoustical features of musical instruments relevant to musical tone quality: psychomotor control of music performance; and neuro-psychological aspects of music performance. The third Workshop, held August 8-12, 1980, had the following subtitles: Music, brain and language: Music, cognition and emotion; and Music, computers and electronics.

This book contains a selection of papers given at the 1980 Workshop. On behalf of the organizers of the Carinthian Summer Festival, I would like to express my gratitude to Professor Manfred Clynes as Editor of this volume. And on behalf of the Workshop participants, I would like to expresss my gratitude to Dr. Gerda Fröhlich, who valiantly and successfully took up the directorship of the Carinthian Summer Festival after the tragic and untimely death of my very dear friend, Professor Helmut Wobisch, founder of the Festival and originator and mentor of our Workshop series. Joint sponsors of the last Workshop were the Austrian Ministry of Science, the Austrian Broadcasting Organization and the University of Alaska. Their support is greatly appreciated by all those who have benefited so much from this informative and edifying event.

February 20, 1981   Juan G Roederer
                                                     University of Alaska
                                                     Workshop Director

CONTENTS

Part 3 Concerning Music and Computers

Chapter 1

MUSIC, MIND, AND MEANING

Marvin Minsky

Artificial Intelligence Center
Massachusetts Institute of Technology
Cambridge, Massachusetts, USA

SUMMARY

Speculating about cognitive aspects of listening to music, this essay discusses: how metric regularity and thematic repetition might involve representation frames and memory structures, how the result of listening might resemble space-models, how phrasing and expression might evoke innate responses and finally, why we like music - or rather, what is the nature of liking itself.

INTRODUCTION

Why do we like Music? Our culture immerses us in it for hours every day, and we all know how it touches our emotions, but no one thinks of how music touches-other kinds of thought. It is astonishing for us to have so little curiosity concerning so pervasive an environ-mental influence. I will speculate here about what we might discover, if we were to study musical thinking.

Have we the tools for such work? Years ago, when Science still feared Meaning. the new field of research on Artificial Intelligence supplied ideas about 'representation of knowledge' which helped out in several fields; I will use them here. But are not such tools too alien for anything so subjective and irrational, aesthetic and emotional as music? Not at all; I think the problems are much the same, and those lines wrongly drawn: only the surface of Reason is rational. [1]*

---

*   Numbers refer to Notes, at the end of this Chapter.

Besides, much of what we now know of the mind emerged, this century, from other subjects once considered just so personal and inaccessible. Freud's work on dreams and jokes uncovered the Unconscious, and Piaget's work on children's talk and play initiated developmental psychology. Why did the work of Freud and Piaget have to wait for modern times? Before them, children seemed too childish, and humor too funny, for science to take them seriously.

Why do we like music? We all are reluctant, in music and art, to examine our sources of pleasure or strength. In part we fear success itself - that Understanding might spoil Enjoyment. And rightly so; Art often loses power when its psychological roots are exposed. No matter: when this happens we will go on, as always to seek more robust illusions!

I feel that Music Theory has gotten stuck at trying too long to find Universals. Of course, we would like to study Mozart's music the way those scientists analyze the spectrum of a distant star. Indeed, we find in every musical era some almost universal practices. But we must view these with suspicion. For, they might show only what those composers felt should be universal; if so, the search for truth in art becomes a travesty in which each era's practice only parodies the theory of its predecessor. (Imagine formulating laws of television screenplay, taking it as natural phenomenon, uninfluenced by custom or constraint of commerce.)

The trouble with the search for universal rules concerning thought is that our memories and thinking processes interact as we grow. We do not just learn about things, we learn ways to think about things; then we learn to think about that, and then about that. Before long, our ways of thought become so complicated that, I suspect, we cannot understand the details of any mind, at any moment, without knowing the principles that guided its growth. The anatomy is too obscure without its embryology. Much of this essay speculates on how listening to music engages previously acquired personal knowledge of the listener.

As for the laws of liking music, it has become taboo for music theorists to ask why we like what we like: our seekers have forgotten what they are searching for. To be sure, "there's no accounting for tastes" - in general. No matter: if different people have different preferences, we must not simply ignore the problem; instead we must try to account for how and why that happens! We must enlarge our aspirations to see that music theory is not only about music, but about how people process it. To understand any Art, we must look below its surface, into the psychological detail of its creation and absorption.

If it sounds harder to explain minds than songs - still, sometimes making problems larger makes them simpler! The theory of Equations' Roots seemed hard for centuries, within its little world of real numbers - but suddenly seemed simple, once Gauss exposed the larger world of (so-called) complex numbers. Music, too, should make more sense once seen through listeners' minds.

SONATA AS TEACHING MACHINE

Music makes things in our minds. but afterwards most fades away. What is it that remains? In that old Mozart story. the wonder child heard a concert. then wrote down the score. I do not believe it; history documents so few such tales that they would seem mere legend. (Though, by that argument, so would seem Mozart, too). In any case, most people do not even remember the themes of an evening's concert - yet, when the tunes are played again, they are recognized. Something must remain in the mind to cause this, and perhaps what we learn is not the music itself but a way to hear it. I will explain.

Compare a sonata to a teacher! He calls attention, either dramaticaly or by the quiet trick of speaking softly. Next comes the careful presentation of the elements: useless to introduce too many ideas, or develop them too far; until the themes are learned, the listeners cannot build on them. So, at first one repeats a lot. Sonatas, too, explain first one idea, then another, and recapitulate it all, just to be sure. [2]

Thus Expositions show the basic stuff, the atoms of impending chemistries, and how to make some simple compounds from those atoms. Then. in Developments, those now familiar compounds, made from bits and threads of beat and tone, can clash or merge, contrast or join together. We find it hard to remember details of things that do not fit easily into familiar frameworks - things that seem meaningless. But I prefer to turn that around: a thing has meaning only to one who already knows some ways to represent and process what is meant - who knows its parts and how they are put together. [10]

That is why sonatas start with simple things - as do the best of talks and texts - repeating basics several times before presenting larger things. No one remembers, word for word, all that was said in any lecture, or played in any piece. But if you understood it once, you now own new networks of knowledge, about each theme and how it changes and relates to others. Thus, no one could remember Beeethoven's Fifth Symphony entire, from single hearing. But neither could one ever hear again those first four notes as just four notes! Once but a tiny scrap of sound; it is now a Known Thing - a locus in the web of all the other things we know, whose meanings and significances depend on one another. [3]

If sonatas are lessons, what are the subjects of those lessons? The answer is in the question! One thing the Fifth Symphony taught our culture is how to hear those first four notes. The surface form is just descending major third, first tone repeated thrice. At first, that pattern can be heard two different ways - as fifth and third in minor mode - or third and first, in major. But once we have heard the symphony, the latter is unthinkable - a strange constraint to plant in all our heads! Let us see how it is taught.

The Fifth declares at once its subject, then its near-identical twin. First comes the theme. Presented in a stark orchestral unison, its minor mode location in tonality is not yet made explicit, nor is its metric frame yet clear: the subject stands alone in time. Next comes it twin. The score itself leaves room to view this transposed counterpart as complement - or as a new beginning. Till now, fermatas hide the basic metric frame, a pair of twinned four-measure halves; so far we have only learned to hear those halves as separate wholes.

The next four-measure metric half-frame shows three versions of the subject, one on each ascending pitch of tonic triad. (Now we are sure the key is minor.) This shows us how the subject can be made to overlap itself, the three short notes packed perfectly inside the long tone's time-space. The second frame-half does the same with copies of the complement ascending the dominant seventh chord. This fits the halves together in a most familiar frame of harmony; in rhythm, too, the halves are so nearly congruent that there is no room to wonder how to match them - and attach them - into one eight-measure unit.

The next eight-measure frame explains some more melodic points: how to smooth the figure's firmness with passing tones, and how to counterpoise the subject's own inversion, inside the long note. (I think that this evokes a sort of sinusoidal motion-frame idea that later helps to represent the second subject). It also shows compression of harmonic time; seen earlier, this would obscure the larger metric unit, but now we know enough to place each metric frame precisely on the after-image of the one before.

(Cadence.) (Silence.) (Almost.) (Total.)

Now it is the second subject-twin's turn to stand alone in time. Conductor must select a symmetry: to answer prior cadence, start anew, or close the brackets opened at the start: can he do all at once and still maintain the metric frame? In any case the student hears a long, long unison F (subdominant?) in which he gets to do his homework: For. underneath that silent surface sound. one hears one's mind rehearsing what was heard.

The next frame shows the theme again, descending now by thirds. (We see it was the dominant ninth, not subdominant at all. Fooled us that time - but never again.) Then, tour de force, the subject sounds ascending every scale degree. This new perspective shows us how to see the four-note theme as an appoggiatura - and then, descending on each tonic chord-note, we are shown how to see it as a fragment of arpeggio. (That last descent completes a set of all four possibilities: harmonic and directional. Is this deliberate didactic thoroughness, or just an accidental outcome of the other symmetries?) Finally, the subject's interval is squeezed to nothing, still surviving - even gaining strength - as single tone.

(It always seemed to me a mystery of art: the impact of those moments in quartets when texture turns to single line. and fortepiano shames sforzando. But think: that very act, by which the surface shows the least, must make the largest difference underneath. Shortly, I will propose a scheme in which such sudden, searching changes wake a lot of Difference-Finders. That very change wakes yet more Difference Finders, and that still more in turn. And that is how sudden silence makes the whole mind come alive.)

We are told all this in just one minute of the lesson. and I have touched but one dimension of its rhetoric; besides explaining. teachers beg and threaten, calm and scare, use gesture, timbre, quaver, sometimes even silence. (Most vital, that, in music, too. In fact, in the Fifth, it is the start of the subject!.) Such 'lessons' must teach us as much about triads and triplets as mathematicians have learned about angles and sides! Think how much we were told about minor second intervals, in Beethoven's treatise (Op. 133).

Why on earth should anyone want to learn such things? Geometry is practical - for building pyramids. for instance - but of what use is music-knowledge? [4] Here is one idea. Each child spends endless days in curious ways; we call it "play". He plays with blocks and boxes, stacking them and packing them; he lines them up and knocks them down. What is that all about? Clearly. he is learning Space! But how, on earth, does one learn Time? Can one Time fit inside another, can two of Them go side by side? In Music we find out!

Many adults retain that play-like fascination with making large structures out of smaller things - and one way to understand music involves building large mind-structures out of smaller music-things. So that drive to build music-structure might be the same one that makes us try to understand the world. (Or is it just an accidental mutant variant; evolution often copies extra needless stuff, and minds so news as ours must still contain some).

Sometimes. though, we use our music as a trick to misdirect our ways to understand the world. When thoughts are hurtful, we have no way to make them stop. We can attempt to turn our minds to other matters, but doing this (some claim) just leaves the bad thoughts gnawing underneath. Perhaps that music some call "background" can tranquilize by turning under-thoughts from bad to neutral - to leave the surface thoughts deprived of affect by diverting the unconscious. The 'meanings' we assemble in that detached kind of listening, could be wholly self-contained in solipsistic networks - webs of meaning-like cross-reference that nowhere touch 'reality'. In such a self-constructed world, one needs no truth or falsehold, good or evil, pain or joy. Music, in this unpleasant view, serves as a fine escape from tiresome thought.

SYNTACTIC THEORIES OF MUSIC

Contrast two answers to: "why do we like certain tunes?"

... because they have certain structural features."
... because they resemble other tunes we like."

The first looks for the laws and rules that make tunes pleasant. In language, we know laws for sentences; that is, we know the forms they need to have to be syntactically acceptable - if not the things they need to make them sensible, or even pleasant to the ear. But as to melody, it seems, we only know some features that can help - we know of none we cannot do without. I do not expect much more to come from searching for the formal rules of musical phrase.

The second seeks significance outside the tune itself, just as to ask "which sentences are meaningful?" takes us outside of shared linguistic practice into each person's own tangled webs of thought. And, there, these preferences feed upon themselves, as in all spheres: we tend to like things that re-mind us of the other things we like. So some of us like music that resembles songs and carols, rhymes and hymns we liked in childhood. But this begs the question: if we like tunes like ones we like, where does this music-liking start? I will come back to that later.

The term resemble begs a question, too: what are the rules of musical resemblance? I am sure that this depends a lot on how melodies are 'represented' in each individual mind. And in each single mind, I am sure, the different mind-parts do this different ways; the same tune seems (at different times) to change its rhythm, mode, or harmony. Beyond that, individuals differ more. Some listeners squirm to symmetries and shapes that others scarcely hear at all; some fine fugue subjects seem banal to those who sense but single line. My guess is that our contrapuntal sensors harmonize each fading after-memory with others yet to play; perhaps Bach's mind could do this several ways at once. (But even one such process might suffice, for choosing what one next should try to play. 'Try' is enough for improvisers, since they - like stage magicians - know enough 'ways out' to keep the music going, when bold experiments fail.)

'Feature-based' explanations can't begin to describe such processes as that. Much better are the 'generative' and 'transformational' (for example, neo-Schenkerian) methods of syntactic analysis - but only for the simplest analytic uses. For, at best, the very aim of syntax oriented theories is misdirected; they aspire to describe the things that minds produce - without attempting to describe how they are produced. This only works on very simple things; for complex ones, taxonomy must yield to causal explanation. Therefore, to really understand how memory and process merge in "listening" we will simply have to use much more "procedural" descriptions - that is, the kinds that can describe how processes proceed. [5]

I do not see why many theorists find this disturbing. It is true that this new power has a price: one can say more, with computational description, but prove less. Yet not so much is lost as many think: for Mathematics never could prove very much about such complicated things. Theorems often tell us complex truths about the simple things, but only rarely tell us simple truths about the complex ones. Believing otherwise is wishful thinking, "mathematics envy".

And for that price. a gain. Many musical problems that resist formal solution will become tractable anyway, in future simulations that grow artificial musical semantic networks - perhaps by 'raising' simulated infants in traditional music cultures. [6] It will be exciting when one of these first shows a hint of real 'talent'.

SPACE AND TUNE

When one enters a room one seems to see it all at once; not so with any symphony. "Naturally," one might declare, for "hearing extends in time while vision extends in space." But it really takes time to see new scenes. though we are usually unaware of this. That Consciousness sees seeing as so instant and immediate, is certainly the strangest of our 'optical' illusions.

Still. music can immerse us in some stable-seeming worlds. I will try to explain this by arguing that hearing music is like seeing scenery. Only, instead of treating this analogy light-heartedly, I will hammer it to death - asserting that good music really makes the mind act very much the way it does when seeing things [7] And no mistake: I meant to say "good" music! This little theory does not apply to every bag of musical tricks, but only to those certain kinds.

Our eyes are always flashing sudden flicks of different pictures to our brains - yet none of that saccadic action leads to any sense of change or motion in the world; each thing reposes calmly in its "place"! What makes those objects seem so stable, when their images jump and jerk so? What makes us such innate Copernicans? I'll first propose how this might work in Vision, and then in Music. But first I have to say some things about the way the mind regards itself!

When we speak about illusion, we always talk in terms of someone being fooled - be it another or oneself. "I know those lines are straight: one says, "but they look bent to Me."

Well - who are the different I's and Me's in that? We are all convinced that somewhere in each person struts a central Self, atomic, indivisible. (And secretly we hope that it is also indestructible.)

Instead, I say, inside each mind work many different 'agents'. I can not describe this theory here in much detail (its sources are described in note [11]) but all we really need is this rough sketch: each agent knows what happens to some others, but little of what happens to the rest. In this view, we can see how little it can mean to say a thing like "Eloise was unaware of X" - unless one says more about which of her mind-agents were uninvolved with X. Thinking itself is mainly making mind-agents work together; the very core of fruitful thought is breaking problems into parts, and then assigning every part to agents good at just that kind of job. Among our most important agents are those that make these management assignments, for they are the agents that embody what each person knows about what he knows. But 'self-awareness' is a luxury, and usually an impractical one, for managers who really manage cannot afford to know everything that their subordinates do.

In that division of labor we call "seeing", I will suppose that one agent of the mind - called "Feature-Finder" - sends messages (about features it finds on the retina) to another agent - "Scene-Analyzer". The latter draws conclusions from the many messages it receives and sends its own, in turn, to other mind-parts. For instance, Finder might inform about some scraps of edge and texture; then Analyzer finds that these might fit some bit of shape.

Perhaps those features emanate from some part of a table-leg, but knowing such a thing is not for agents at this level. What Analyzer can do, though, is broadcast a shape-gram message to that host of other agents specialized for finding Vision, a matter more involved with memory and learning. (There is one such agent, at the least, for every kind of thing this mind has learned to recognize.) Thus, we can hope, this message reaches Table-Maker, an agent specialized to gather evidence for tables in the field of view. After many such stages, descendants of those messages finally reach Space-Builder - the agency that purports to inform yet other agencies about Real Things in real World-Places.

Now we can see one reason why perception seems so effortless: while the messages from Analyzer to Table-Maker are based on evidence that Finder supplied, the messages themselves need say little about Finder itself, or what it did. Partly this is because it would take Analyzer too long to explain all that; but in any case the recipients could make no use of all that information - not being engineers or psychologists, but just little specialized nerve-nets [8], also [11].

Messages. in this scheme, go various ways. Each motion of eye or head or body makes Finder start anew, and such motions are responses (by muscle-moving agents) to messages that Analyzer sends when he needs to resolve ambiguities, or fetch more details. Analyzer himself responds to messages from 'higher up'; for instance, Space-Builder may have asked "is that a table?" of Table-Maker, who replies (to himself) "Perhaps, but it shoud have another leg - there", so he asks Analyzer to verify this for him, and Analyzer gets the job done - by making Eye-Mover look down and to the left. [9]

When you look up, you are never frightened that the ground has disappeared - although it certainly has dis-appeared. This is because Space-Builder remembers all the answers to its questions - and never changes any of those answers without reason; moving eyes or raising head provides no cause to exorcise that floor inside your current spatial model of the room. My paper on "frame-systems" (Minsky, 1975) says more about these concepts, but here we only need these few details.

Now, back to our illusions. While Finder is not instantaneous, it is very, very fast: a highly parallel pattern matcher. Whatever Analyzer asks, Finder answers in an eye-flick, a mere tenth-second or so (or less if we have image-buffers). And still more speed comes from the way we mentioned just above, in which Space-Builder can often tell himself, from his own high-speed model memory, about what has been seen before. I argue that all this speed is another root of our illusion: if answers seem to come as soon as questions asked, they will seem to have been there all along.

The illusion is enhanced another way - by "expectation" or "default". Those agents know good ways to lie and bluff! Aroused by only partial evidence for "table", Table-Maker supplies Builder with fictitious details about some "typical table" whiles its servants find out about the real one! Once so informed, Builder can quickly move and plan ahead, with little risk, ready to make corrections later. This only works, of course, if the prototypes are good - but that is what intelligence is all about.

As for "awareness" of how all such things are done, there simply is not room for that. Space-Builder is too remote and different to understand how Finder does its work of eye-fixation. Each part of mind is unaware of almost all that happens in the others. (That is why we need psychologists; we think we know what happens in our minds - because those agents are so facile with "defaults" - but, actually, we are almost always wrong.) True, each agents needs to know which of its servants can do what - but as to how, that has no place or use inside those tiny minds inside our minds.

Finally, we return to how both music and vision build things in our minds. Eye-motions show us real objects; phrases show us music-objects. We learn a room with body motions; large music-sections show us "music-places". Walks and climbs move us from room to room; so do transitions between sections. Looking back in vision is like recapitulation in music; both give us time, from time to time, to revise or review conceptions of the whole.

So, hearing a theme is like seeing a thing in a room. An allegro is like the room itself, and the whole sonata is like an entire building. I do not mean to say that Music builds just the sorts of thing that Space-Builder does. (I know that is too naive -comparing sound and place like in a little child's poem. Still, truth may lie in simple thoughts.) I do mean to say that composers stimulate coherency by engaging the same sorts of inter-agent coordinations that Vision uses to produces its illusion of a stable world - of course. using different agents. I think the same is true of talk or writing, the way these very paragraphs make sense - or sense of sense - if any.

COMPOSING AND CONDUCTING

In Seeing, we can move our eyes; Lookers can choose where they shall look. and when. In music one must listen here - that is, the part played now, it's simply no use asking Music-Finder to look there - because it isn't then now.

But then, if composer and conductor choose what part you hear does not this ruin our analogy? When Music-Analyzer asks its questions, how can Music-Finder answer them - unless miraculously the music happens to be playing what it wants at just that instant? If so, then how can music paint its scenes - unless composers know exactly what the listeners will ask at every moment? How to ensure, when Analyzer wants something - now, that just that "something" will be playing - now?

Well, that is just the secret of music, one end to the other, of writing, playing. and conducting! Music need not, of course, confirm the listener's every expectation; each plot demands some novelty. Still, whatever the intent, control is required, or novelty will turn to nonsense. And if allowed to think too much himself, the listener will find unanswered questions in any score, about accidents of form and figure. voice and line, temperament and difference-tone.

So, every music artist must anticipate and pre-direct the listener's fixations: he draws attention here, distracting it from there: forcing hearer (again, like a magician) to ask just questions that the composition is about to answer. Only by establishing such pre-established harmony, can music make it seem that something is there.

RHYTHM AND REDUNDANCY

A popular song has a hundred measures, a thousand beats. What must the Martians imagine we mean by those measures and beats, measures and beats! The words themselves reveal an awesome repetiousness. Why isn't music boring?

Is hearing so like seeing, that we need a hundred glances to build each music-image? Some repetitive musical textures might serve to remind us of time-persistent things like wind and stream. But much of sound is one-time: you must hear a pin drop now or seek and search for it; that is why we have no ear-lids. Poetry drops pins - says each thing once. or less. So does some music.

Why, then, do we tolerate music's relentless rhythmic pulse? There is no one answer, for we hear in different ways, on different scales. [10] Some of those ways portray the spans of time directly, but others speak of musical things, in worlds where time folds over on itself. And there, I think, is where we use those beats and measures.

What I mean is this: Music's metric frames are transient templates - used for momentary matching. Its rhythms are 'synchronization pulses' used to match new phrases against old - better to notice Differences and Change. As these are sensed, the rhythmic frames fade from our awareness, their work done; the messages of higher-level agents never speak of them, and that is why music is not boring!

Differences and Change! Good music grows from tiny roots, by careful steps. And see how cautiously we handle novelty, enclose the new - like sandwiches - between repeated sections of familiar stuff! The clearest kind of change is near-identity - in Thought just as in Vision. Slight shifts in view may best reveal an object's form - or even that it is there at all.

When we discussed sonatas, we saw how different metric frames are matched together, making it easy to discern the musical ingredients. Once frames were matched then we could see how what was there a major third was changed to seconds here by adding passing tones; that what was once a seventh-chord is now a dominant ninth. Thus matching lets our minds see different things, from different times, together. Fusing all those matching lines of tone from different measures - like Television's separate lines and frames - that is what lets us make those magic music-pictures on our mind-screens.

How do we make our Music-Agents do this kind of work for us? We must have them organized in some special structure specialized for finding differences between frames. Here is a four-level scheme that might work:

Feature-Finders listen for simple time-events,
like notes. or peaks, or pulses
   Measure-Takers note certain patterns of time-events
   like 3/4, 4/4, 6/8.
      Difference-Finders observe that the figure here is
      same as that one there, except a perfect fifth above.
         Structure-Builders perceive that three phrases
         form an almost regular 'sequence'.

I will not give much detail; that is for the future. But many such ideas are seen already in research on Vision. [11] First, the Feature-Finders search the sound-stream for the simplest sorts of musical significance: entrances and envelopes, the tones themselves, the other little, local things. Then Measure-Takers look for metric patterns in those small events, and put them into groups, thus finding beats and postulating rhythmic regularities. Then the Difference-Finders can begin to sense events of musical importance - imitations and inversions, syncopations and suspensions. Once these are found. the Structure-Builders can start work on a larger scale.

The entire four-level Agency is just one layer of a larger system in which analogous structures are repeated on larger scales. At each scale, another level of order (with its own sorts of Things and Differences) makes larger-scale descriptions, and thus consumes another order of structural form. As a result, notes become figure and those turn to phrase, and those into sequence - and notes become chord, and those make progression, and -

so, on and on. Relations at each level, turn to Thing at next above; more easily remembered and compared. This time-warps things together, changing tone into tonality, and line into polyphony.

The more regular the rhythm, the easier the matching goes, and fewer Difference agents are excited further on. Thus, once used for 'lining up', the metric structure fades from your attention, because it is represented as a fixed and constant object-frame (like the floor of the room you are in) - until some metric alteration makes the measure-takers change their minds. [12]

And so the regularities are hidden from attention while expressive nuances are sensed and emphasized and passed along. Rubato or crescendo, ornament or passing tone - the alterations at each level become the objects for the next. The mystery is solved; the brain is so good at sensing difference at each stage that it forgets the things themselves, whenever they are the same. And as for liking music, that depends on what remains.

SENTIC SIGNIFICANCE

Why do we like any tunes in the first place? Do we simply 'associate' some tunes with pleasant experiences? Should we look back to the tones and patterns of mother's voice or heartbeat? Or, could it be that some themes are innately likable? All these theories could hold truth, and others too - for nothing need be single-cause inside the mind. [13]

Clynes, physiologist and pianist, describes (1977, 1969) certain specific temporal sensory patterns, and claims that each is associated with a certain common emotional state. For example, in his experiments, two particular patterns (that gently rise and fall) are said to suggest states of love and reverence; two others (more abruptly) signify anger and hate. He claims that these and other patterns - he calls them "sentic" - arouse the same effects through different senses - that is, embodied as acoustical intensity, or pitch, or tactile pressure, or even visual motion - and that this is cross-cultural. The time-lengths of these sentic shapes, the order of one second, could correspond to parts of musical phrases.

Clynes studied the muscular details of instrumental performances with this in view, and concluded that music can engage emotions through these sentic signals. Of course, more experiments are needed to verify that such signals have the reported effects. Nevertheless, I would quite expect to find something of the sort for a quite different reason: namely, to serve in the early social development of children. For, sentic signals, if they exist, would be very useful in helping infants to learn about themselves and others.

All learning theories require brains to somehow impose 'values' on events - implicit or explicit in the choice of what to learn to do. Most such theories say that certain special signals are involved in this, called reinforcers. For many goals, it should suffice to use some simple 'primary' physiological stimuli like eating, drinking, relief of physical discomfort. But human infants must learn social signals too. The early learning theorists in this century assumed that social sounds (e.g. of approval) could become reinforcers - by association with innate reinforcers - but real evidence for this was never found. If parents could exploit some innate sentic cues, this might explain that mystery.

This might also touch another, deeper problem: of how an infant forms an image of its own mind. Self-images are important for at least two reasons. First, external reinforcement can be but one part of human learning; the growing infant must eventually learn to learn from inside - to free itself from parent. With Freud, I think that children replace and augment the real one with self-constructed inner parent-image. Second, one needs a self-model simply in order to make realistic plans for solving ordinary problems. For example, one must know enough about one's own disposition to be able to assess which plans are feasible. Pure self-commitment does not work; one simply cannot carry out a plan that one will find too boring to complete, or that is too vulnerable to other, competing interests. Both reasons point to needs for models of one's own behavior. But how could a baby be smart enough to build such a model?

Innate sentic detectors could help, by teaching children about their own affective states. For, if distinct signals arouse specific states, the child can associate those signals with those states. Just knowing that the states exist - that is, having symbols for them - is half the battle. If those signals are the same in others as in oneself then, from social discourse, one can learn some rules about those states' behavior. Thus a child might learn: Conciliatory signal changes Angry to Affectionate. Given that sort of information, a simple learning machine should be able to construct a 'finite-state person-model'. This model would be crude at first, to be sure - but half of that job, too, is getting started. And once the baby has a crude model of some Other, he can copy and adapt it to begin work on making his model of himself.

Returning to music, it seems just barely possible that we conceal, in the innocent songs and settings of our children's musical cultures, some lessons about successions of our own affective states. Sentically encrypted, those ballads could encode instructions about conciliation and affection, aggression and retreat - just the sorts of knowledge of signals and states that we need to get along with othes. In later life, more complex music might illustrate more intricate kinds of conflict and compromise, ways to fit goals together to achieve more than one thing at a time. Finally, for grown-ups our Burgesses and Kubricks fit Beethoven's Ninths to Clockwork Oranges.

If reader finds this all far-fetched, so do I. But before rejecting it entirely, recall the problem: why do we have Music, and let it occupy our lives with no apparent reason? When no idea seems right, the right one must seem wrong.

THEME AND THING

Beethoven's Fifth: what is its subject: is it just those first four notes? Does it include the twin, transposed companion too? What of the other variations, augmentations and inversions? Do they all stem from a single prototype? In this case, yes.

Or do they? For later in the symphony the theme appears in triplet form, to serve as counter-subject of the scherzo. Three notes and one, three notes and one, three notes and one; still they make four. Melody turns into monotone rhythm; meter is converted to two equal beats. Downbeat now falls on an actual note, instead of a rest. With all those changes, the themes are very different, yet still the same. Neither allegro nor scherzo subject alone can be the single prototype; separate and equal, they span across musical time.

Well, then, is there some more abstract idea they both embody? This is like the problem raised by Wittgenstein (1953), of what words like "game" mean. I argue (Minsky, 1975) that for Vision, "chair" can be described by no single prototype; better to use several prototypes, connected in relational networks of samenesses and differences. But I doubt that these serve well to represent musical ideas; there are better tools in contemporary Artificial Intelligence research, like constraint systems. conceptual dependency, frame systems and semantic networks. That is where the action is, today, in dealing with such problems. (Computer Music Journal, 1980 contains good reviews of recent work on musical cognition.)

Still what we really want to know is: "What is a good theme?" Without that bad word "good", I do not think the question is well-formed - because anything is a theme, if everything is music!

Now, let us split that question into (1) what mental conditions or processes do pleasant tunes evoke? and (2) what do we mean by "pleasant"? Both questions are hard, but the first is only hard; to answer it will take much thought and much experiment. Good.

The second question is very different. Philosophers and scientists have struggled mightily to understand what pain and pleasure are. I especially like Dennett's (1978) explanation of why all that has been so difficult. He argues that there simply is not any one such thing as 'pain' at all; instead 'it' works in different ways at different times, and all those ways have too little in common for the usual sorts of definition. He is right, I think, but then - if pain is no single thing - why do we talk and think as though it were, and represent 'it' with such spurious clarity?

I claim this is no accident: illusions of this sort have special uses. They play a role connected with a problem facing any Society (in or outside the mind) that learns from its experience. The problem is how to assign the credit and blame, for each accomplishment or failure of the Society as a whole, among the myriads of agents involved in everything that happens. To the extent that the agents' actions are decided locally, so must also these credit decisions be made locally.

How, for example, can a mother tell that her child has a need (or that one has been satisfied), before she has learned specific signs for each such need? That could be arranged, by evolution gathering together signals from many different internal processes concerned with needs, and providing them with a single, common, output - an infant's sentic signal of discomfort (or contentment). By a genetically pre-established harmony, this would evoke a corresponding central state in the parent. We would feel this as something like distress, as we do when babies cry.

The satisfaction side needs signals, too. Suppose, among the many things a child does, there is one that mother 'likes' - and so she makes approving sounds. The child has just been walking there, and holding this just so; and thinking that, and speaking in some certain way. How can its mind find out which what was 'good'? The trouble is, each thing it did just then, must owe, in turn, to little plans it made before. We cannot 'reward' a going to some certain place: you cannot reward an act. One only can reward the agency that selected that strategy - and the agency who wisely activated that agency - and so on.

To do this, one must propagate, to all those agencies and processes, some message that they all can use to evaluate what they did - the plans they made, their strategies and the things that they constructed. But all these various recipients have so little in common that such a message, to work at all, must express the essence of oversimplification. So 'good' is a centralization that enables a tutor, inside or outside a society, to tell its members that one or more of them has done something good - that satisfies some need - without having to understand which ones, or how, or even why.

Now words like 'satisfies' and 'needs' have many senses, yet we seem to understand that phrase - the same illusion of substantiality that fools us into thinking it tautologous. unworthy of study, to ask "why do we like pleasure"? The social discourse levels where we use such clumsy words as 'like' or 'good' or 'that was fun' must (by that very poverty of word and sign) most coarsely crush together many different meanings. 'Good' is no symbol that means as "table" does. Instead, it names an injunction: "activate all those (unknown) processes that correlate and sift and sort, in learning, to see what changes (in myself) should now be made". 'Like', then, is a name we use for when we send such structure-building signals to ourselves. [14]

And that is another reason we like music. Liking is just how certain mind parts make the others learn the things they need to understand that music. Hence liking (and its relatives) are at the very heart of understanding what we hear. So Affect and Aesthetic do not lie in other academic worlds, that music theories safely can ignore. Those separate worlds are Academic-Self deceptions, used to make our problems seem like someone else s. [15]

NOTES

[1] I do not mean that understanding Emotion is easy, only that understanding Reason is harder. Our culture has a universal myth in which we see emotion as more complex and obscure than intellect. Indeed. emotion might be 'deeper' in some sense of prior evolution, but this need not make it harder to understand; in fact, I think today we actually know much more about emotion than reason.

Now. to be sure, we know a bit about the surface ways of Reason - the ways we organize and represent ideas we get. But whence come those ideas themselves - that so conveniently fill these envelopes of order? A poverty of language shows how little this concerns us: we 'get' ideas: they 'come' to us: we are 'reminded of'. I think this shows that ideas come from processes obscured from us, with which our surface thoughts are almost uninvolved. Instead, we are entranced with our emotions - so easily observed, in others and ourselves. Perhaps the myth persists because emotions (by their nature) draw attention, while the processes of Reason (much more intricate and delicate) must hide themselves in privacy, to work best left alone.

In any case, those old distinctions - Feeling, Reason and Aesthetic - are like the Earth and Air and Fire of an ancient Alchemy. We shall need much better concepts for a working psychic chemistry.

[2]   Music has many forms, and there are many ways to teach. I do not say that Beethoven consciously intended to teach at all. but still, he was a master of inventing forms for exposition - including forms that swarm with more ideas, and work our minds much harder.

[3]   Learning to recognize is not the same as memorizing. A mind might build an agent that can sense a certain stimulus, yet build no agent that can reproduce it. How could such a mind learn that the first half-subject of Beethoven's Fifth - call it "A" - pre-figures the second half - call it "B"? Simple: an agent $\underline{A}$ that recognizes "A" sends a message to another agent $\underline{B}$, built to recognize "B". That message serves to 'lower $\underline{B}$'s threshold' so that after $\underline{A}$ hears "A", $\underline{B}$ will react to smaller hints of "B" than it would otherwise. Result: that mind 'expects' to hear "B" after "A"; for example, it will discern "B", given fewer or more subtle cues, and might complain if it cannot. And yet that mind cannot reproduce either theme, in any generative sense. The point is that inter-agent messages need not be in surface music-languages, but in codes that bias certain other agents to behave in different ways.

Andor Kovach pointed out to me that composers dare not use this simple. four-note motive any more. So memorable was Beethoven's treatment, that now an accidental hint of it can wreck another piece by moving listener's mind into that other, unintended place.

[4]   True or not, it is often said that Mathematicians are unusually involved with music, but not the other way around. Perhaps both share a liking to make simple things more complicated - but Mathematics may be too constrained to satisfy that want entirely. while Music can be rigorous $\underline{or}$ free. The way the Mathematics game is played. most variations lie $\overline{outside}$ the rules. while Music can insist on perfect canon, or tolerate a casual accompaniment. So Mathematics might need Music, too, but not the other way around. A simpler theory: since music engages at earlier ages, some mathematicians $\underline{are}$ those missing mathematical musicians.

[5]   In science one always first explains in terms of what can be observed. (Earth, Water, Fire, Air). But things that come from complicated processes need not show their natures on the surface. (The steady pressure of a gas conceals those countless, abrupt micro-impacts.) To talk of what such things might mean or represent, one has to speak of how they are made.

But one cannot do that, for the mind, without good ways to describe complicated $\underline{processes}$. Before computers came, $\underline{no}$ languages were good for that. Piaget tried algebra and Freud tried diagrams, other psychologists used Markov chains and matrices - none came to much. Behaviorists, quite properly, had ceased to speak at all. Linguists flocked to formal syntax, and made progress for a time, but reached a limit: transformation grammar shows the contents of the registers (so to speak), but has no way to talk of what controls them. This makes it hard to say how surface speech relates to underlying designation and intent - a baby-bath condition. The reason I like ideas from Artificial Intelligence research is that there we tend <u>first</u> to seek procedural description - which seems more right for mental matters.

[6]   We can already write computer programs that write better music than most people can, but still that music is quite 'bad'. I do not know quite what to do about this; our lowest standards are so high that we find it hard to distinguish early progress from worthless noise.

[7]   Edward Fredkin suggested to me the theory that music-listening might exercise some innate 'map-making' mechanism. When I mentioned the puzzle of music's repetitiousness, he compared it to how rodents explore new places: first one way a little, then back to home. Do it again a few times. Go a little further. Try small digressions, but frequently return to base. Both men and mice explore new territories that way, making mental maps lest they get lost. Music might portray this building process, or even exercise those very organs of the mind.

[8]   Only in the past few centuries have painters learned enough technique and trickery to simulate reality. (Once so informed, they often now choose different goals.) Thus, <u>Space-Builder</u>, like an ordinary person, knows nothing of how vision works, nor of perspective, foveae, or blind-spots. We only learn such things in school: millenia of introspection never led to their suspicion - nor meditation, transcendental or mundane. The mind holds tightly to its secrets - not from stinginess, nor shame, but simply that it does not know them.

[9]   Nor is <u>Scene-Understander</u> autonomous; his questions to <u>Analyzer</u> are responses to requests from others. There need be no First Cause, in such a network. See [13].

[10]   What is the difference between merely <u>knowing</u> (or remembering, or memorizing) and <u>understanding</u>? We all agree that to understand something you must know what it means - and that is about as far as we ever get. I think I know why that happens. A thing or idea seems meaningful, only when we have <u>several</u> different ways to represent it - different perspectives and different associations. Then you can turn it around in your mind, so to speak: however it seems at the moment, you can see it another way; you never come to a full stop. In other words. one can <u>think</u> about it. If there's only one way - if it just sits in your mind doing nothing - you wouldn't call it thinking.

So a thing has any real 'meaning' only when it has several; if you understood it just one way, you did not understand at all. That is why the seekers of the 'real' meanings never find them - and this holds true especially of words like "understand" itself!

[11]   The idea of interconnecting Feature-Finders, Difference-Finders and Structure-Builders are well exemplified in Winston's work (1975.) Measure-Takers would be kinds of Frames as described in Minsky (1975.) The idea of 'societies of agents', developed in Minsky (1977, 1980a, b) comes from my work with Seymour Papert.

[12]   Rhythm has other roles, of course. Societies (in minds or lands) with different functions see things different ways. Agents used for dancing do attend to rhythm, while other forms of music demand less steady pulses.

We all experience a phenomenon we might call 'persistence of rhythm' - in which our minds maintain the "beat" through episodes of ambiguity. I presume that this emerges from a basic feature of how agents are usually assembled: at every level, many agents of each kind compete (Minsky, 1980a). Thus, agents for 3/4, 4/4 and 6/8 compete to find best fits. However, once in power, each agent 'cross-inhibits' its competitors. Thus, once 3/4 takes charge of things, 6/8 will find it hard to "get a hearing" - even if the evidence on his side becomes slightly better.

When none of them has any solid evidence for long enough, then agents change at random, or take turns. Thus, anything gets interesting - in a way - if monotonous enough! We all know how, when word or phrase is oft enough repeated, it - or we - begin to change; because the restless Searchers start to amplify minutiae, interpret noise as structure. This happens at all levels: for when things are regular at one, the Difference agents at the next will fail - to be replaced by other, fresh ones that then re-present the sameness different ways. (Thus Meditation, undirected from the higher mental realms, fares well with the most banal of inputs from below.)

[13]   Theories about children need not apply to adults, because (I suspect) human minds do so much self-revising that things can get detached from their origins. One might end up liking both Art of Fugue and Musical Offering, mainly because each one's subject illuminates the other, giving each a richer network of 'significance'. Dependent circularity need be no paradox here, for, in thinking (unlike logic) two things can support each other in mid-air. To be sure, such autonomy is precarious; once detached from origins, might one not drift strangely awry? Indeed so, and many people seem quite mad, to one another.

[14]   Most of the 'uses' of music mentioned here - learning about time, fitting things together, getting along with others, and suppressing

one's troubles - all seem very 'functional' and overlook much larger scales of 'use'. Curt Roads pointed out to me: "every world above bare survival is self-constructed; whole cultures are built around common things people come to appreciate." These appreciations, represented by aesthetic agents. play roles in more and more of our decisions - as what we think is beautiful gets linked to what we think is important. Perhaps, Roads suggests, when groups of mind-agents cannot agree, they tend to cede decisions to those others concerned with what we call aesthetic form and fitness. With small effects at many little points, those cumulative preferences for taste and form can shape a world.

[15] Many readers of a draft of this complained about its narrow view of music - what about Jazz, or 'modern' forms, or songs with real words; or monophonic chant and raga, gong and block. and all those other kinds of sounds? And several claimed not to be so intellectual, to simply hear and feel and not build buildings in their minds. There simply is no room to talk of all those things; besides, no composition can please everyone. I will say just two more things.

First thing - for those who argue music doesn't make them do so much construction: what makes you sure you know your mind so surely? It is ingenuous to think that you can 'just react' to anything a culture works a thousand years to grow. A mind that thinks in terms of direct apprehension has more in its unconscious than it has in its philosophy.

Second: it makes little sense to vilify a view of music as insufficiently comprehensive. For what is 'music' anyway - all things played on all instruments? Fiddlesticks. All structures made of sound? That has a hollow ring. The things I said of the word 'tune' hold true for 'music', too: it does not follow that because a word be public, so must also be the ways it works on minds. Before one seeks the grail that holds the essence of all music, first see the folly of a simpler quest: to grasp the essence of one single noise, that 'music' word itself.

ACKNOWLEDGMENTS

Conversations and/or improvisations with Maryann Amacher, John Amuedo, Betty Dexter, Harlan Ellison, Edward Fredkin, Bernard Greenberg. Danny Hillis. Douglas Hofstadter, William Kornfeld, Andor Kovach, David Levitt, Tod Machover, Charlotte Minsky, Curt Roads, Gloria Rudisch, Frederic Rzewski, Stephen Smoliar. In memory of Irving Fine.

REFERENCES

These ideas have many more antecedents than I have quoted.

Beethoven. L. von, "Grosse Fugue," in E-flat, Op.133.

Clynes, M., 1977, "Sentics: The Touch of Emotions," Doubleday, New York.

Computer Music Journal, Vols. 4(2), Summer 1980, 4(3), Fall 1980.

Dennett, D., 1978, Why a machine can't feel pain, in "Brainstorms: Philosophical Essays on Mind and Psychology," Bradford Books, Montgomery, VE.

Minsky, M., 1974, "A Framework for Representing Knowledge," MIT, Artificial Intelligence Laboratory, AI Memo 306, Cambridge, Ma. Condensed version in "The Psychology of Computer Vision," 1975, P.H. Winston, ed., McGraw-Hill, New York.

Minsky, M., 1977, Plain talk about neurodevelopmental epistemology, Proc. 5th Int. Joint Conf. on Artificial Intelligence, Cambridge, Ma., August 1977. Condensed version in "Artificial Intelligence," 1979, Winston and Brown, eds., Vol. 1, MIT Press.

Minsky, M., 1980a, "Jokes and the Logic of the Cognitive Unconscious," MIT Artificial Intelligence Laboratory, AI Memo 603, Cambridge.

Minsky, M., 1980b, K-lines: A theory of memory, Cog. Sci., 4(2): 117-133.

Winston, P.H., 1975, Learning structural descriptions by examples, in "Psychology of Computer Vision," P.H. Winston, ed., McGraw-Hill, New York.

Wittgenstein, L., 1953, "Philosophical Investigations," Oxford.

Chapter II

BRAIN MECHANISM IN MUSIC
Prolegomena for a Theory of the Meaning of Meaning

Karl H. Pribram

Neuropsychology Laboratories
Stanford University
Stanford, California, USA

INTRODUCTORY REVIEW

Research into the relationship between musical abilities and the brain has benefited from a series of recent technical innovations. These have made possible two basic approaches: One involves the use of dichotic listening techniques and infers hemispheric specialization on the basis of comparing performance between the left and right ears. A second approach is to construct musical tasks which are similar to those in classical experimental psychology and where brain-behavioral correlates have been demonstrated in animal models. Thus by delineating similarities and differences in processing between musical and non-musical tasks, models or theories of brain function can be attempted.

Recent research results, bearing almost exclusively on the problem of hemispheric specialization, have been collected into a volume entitled "Music and the Brain" edited by MacDonald Critchley and R.A. Henson (1977). I will very briefly summarize the findings reported in this volume. Though basic to the purpose of this paper which is to understand the manner in which musical meaning is generated, many of these studies appear as isolated reports whose only reason for being seems to be that they do relate brain function to one or another aspect of musical experience and expression.

1. <u>Musical rhythm</u> is apparently a deep-seated function since unilateral injection of intracarotid barbiturates (the Wada test) fails to interfere with rhythm even though injection of the right carotid (producing a reversible right hemispherectomy) produces severe melodic distortion and injection of the left carotid produces difficulties in singing words that might accompany these melodies (Bogen and Gordon, 1971). When the temporal sequences become more complex, however, the number of correct identifications made by the right ear (and therefore the left hemisphere) in a dichotic listening experiment were significantly greater than those made with the left ear (Robinson and Solomon, 1974).

2.   Musical competence is an important determinant of the pattern of cerebral organization.   There   is   a   relationship   between   musical sophistication and pitch discrimination (McGuinness, 1974), and left ear (right   hemisphere)   superiority   has   been   demonstrated   for   pure   tone discrimination   in   dichotic   listening   experiments   (Haydon   and   Spellacy, 1973).   Timbre, as examined by a musical chord test, is similarly represented (Gordon,   1970;   Kallman   and   Corballis,   1975).   In   general,   the   greater   the musical   sophistication   of   the   subject,   the   more   the   left   hemisphere   is brought into play.   Thus, as noted above, melodic line is represented in the right hemisphere as is the processing of single musical notes presented in a brief visual display to naive subjects.   When, however, these same displays were   shown   to   sophisticated   subjects   they   processed   the   notes   equally   well in both the right and left visual fields (Oscar-Berman et al., 1974).

3.   Musical   memory   appears   to   involve   interacting   hierarchies   of representations of sequences of pitch, melodies, timbre and harmonies, as well as contextual considerations such as overall phrase interval and scale thus involving both cerebral hemispheres.   A review of what is known, much of it her own work, is presented by Diana Deutsch (1977) in the Music and the Brain volume.

4.   Musical   attention   is   reviewed   in   the   same   chapter.   Deutsch distinguishes attentional 'channels' for spatial location, frequency range and timbre.   In addition, Efron and Yund (1975) have demonstrated a dissociation in the processing of the frequency and intensity dimensions of sounds by the auditory system   The   experimental   studies   on   musical   attention   have   in general   focused   on   identifying   such   separations   of   processing   'channels' which must not be confused with separations of processing hemispheres. The   experiments   reviewed   above   (paragraph   2)   noted   that   often   such channels   are   modified   by   experience   to   become   more   complex   and competent to process musical input.   When that input is discriminated into attended alternatives it becomes appropriate and useful to describe it as musical information.   Pribram and McGuinness (1975) have defined channel competence   as   the   inverse   of   its   equivocation   (the   sum   of   internal redundancy   -   the   complement   of   information   -   plus   noise).   Channel organization   and   therefore   musical   attention   is   thus   dependent   on   the competence to process musical information.   Thus competence is, in turn, dependent on the organization of musical memory.

NEW DEPARTURES

Nowhere in the volume on Music and the Brain is there an attempt at providing a neurological theory of musical competence or of the meaning which music generates.   Without such a theory, the findings reported become fragments of little concern to either the brain scientist or the musician interested in how he came to his current state.   Theory, especially when it essays into a new domain, is perforce sketchy and may be proved wanting by subsequent test.   But the essence of theory is that it is testable and that modifications of a theory on the basis of fact are possible.   With these caveats before us, I shall venture a neurological theory of musical competence and some experimental tests that address this theory.

A brain theory of musical competence and musical meaning must be compatible with known facts about brain function, with known facts about psychological processes and with known facts about the physics, i.e. the tools, of music. These facts are most easily encompassed by taking seriously the analogy of music to language. In a sense, music is a language-like form by which humans express themselves and communicate with each other. Musical competence and meaning are not dependent on the tongue (lingua) as is verbal language but neither are gestural languages (such as American Sign Language), nor is the written word.

The study of natural languages is encompassed by the discipline of semiotics, the study of signs. Semiotics is customarily divided into semantics, pragmatics, and syntactics (see e.g. Websters 3rd International Dictionary; Charles Peirce, 1934; Morris, 1946). Semantics deals with the meaning of signs, i.e. what they refer to, indicate, denote, or connote; pragmatics with their use, i.e. how signs relate to their user; and syntactics with the rules of relationships among signs per se.

I have elsewhere identified, on the basis of neuropsychological data, brain mechanisms responsible for the semantic, pragmatic and syntactic organization of languages (see e.g. Pribram, 1971, 1976, 1979). The proposal can be summarized as follows:

1. Sensory input is initially processed into images (icons) and information. Iconic images have wholistic "Gestalt" properties; information, as noted above, is based on the discrimination of differences between alternatives in the input. There is now a considerable body of evidence that the right hemisphere of the brain (of right handed persons) is somewhat more specialized for image processing while the left hemisphere is more adept at processing information.

2. In man, image and information undergo further processing: Indicants (deictic pointers, icons) become derived from images; symbols from information. The process of derivation is a complex one which involves a stepwise interaction between brain competence and cultural invention (Pribram, 1976, 1978). For instance, a gestural sign will come to indicate an image through repetitive consensual validation. The indicant (an iconic gesture) will then become discriminated from others, thus providing information about what is indicated. Once this information processing competence has become sufficiently developed, the information is encoded in memory and when communicated tells as much about the use of the information as about what the information indicates. If, for instance, a routine gesture is under certain circumstances accompanied by a vocalization, that vocalization may initially convey urgency. When the vocalization becomes more and more regularly associated with the gesture because it is found useful over distances, the vocalization can become an arbitrary token, a symbol of the information. However, the communicative value of the symbol depends as much on the history of its usage as on what it refers to because there is nothing intrinsic in the vocalization which indicates

that to which it refers. This historical aspect of symbols makes them especially amenable to two separate types of processing: Semantic which establishes their original referential meaning, and pragmatic which deals with the historical and current use to which the user puts the symbols. Also, because of this arbitrary nature of symbols, and their historicity, i.e. dependency on their historical development, rules of usage, syntactical structures of arrangement of symbols become especially effective.

3.   Semantic processing, which relates indicant and symbol to the sensory input from which they derive, is carried out by systems which involve the posterior cortical convexity of the brain, especially in the intrinsic "association" areas that surround the cortex which initially receives the input (the primary sensory projection areas).

4.   Pragmatic processing which relates sign and symbol to their user is carried out by systems which involve the frontolimbic cortical formations of the brain. These systems intimately interconnect the core portions of the brain such as the mesencephalic reticular formation and hypothalamus with the frontal lobes of the cerebral cortex.

5.   Syntactic processing, the arrangement of indicants and symbols, is carried out by the motor systems of the brain to which both posterior and frontal cortical formations project. Since the motor systems carry out the computations of both the posterior cortical convexity and the frontolimbic formations, the problems of syntax are on the one hand similar to those that characterize motor behavior of any kind (see e.g. Reynolds, 1970 for such communicative behavior as play, assertive and sexual interactions) and on the other hand these problems are dependent on the particular computations that determine semantic and pragmatic processing.

To return to brain and music a theory of musical competence and musical meaning can be outlined on the basis of this theory of semiotics. Such a neurological theory of music would specify a distinction between indicants of musical images and symbols of musical alternatives and between musical semantics, pragmatics and syntactics. Experimental tests of the theory would involve showing that processing of musical indicants such as melody and harmony are predominantly right hemisphere related and that processing of musical symbols such as hierarchically arranged phrase structures predominantly involve the left hemisphere. Further, such tests would be directed at relating the posterior cortical convexity to the processing of sensory input into musical indicants and symbols while showing that the frontal (and limbic) portions of the brain involve the user in musical experience and expression. A grammar of music should, according to the theory, be related to the motor systems of the brain.

As reviewed in the introductory section of this essay, there is a considerable data base which indicates that indeed musical image processing is predominantly a right hemisphere and musical information processing a left hemisphere function. Furthermore, there is some evidence (reviewed in the Introduction) that brain lesions (or intracarotid barbiturate injections) which interfere with grammatical constructions of spoken language also interfere with the ordering of any but the simplest melodic structures in music.

There is also a body of evidence which relates the motor aspects of syntactic structure of music to that of verbal languages, notably the detailed analysis of Leonard Bernstein (1976) and the even more detailed and sophisticated elaborations of a Chomskian approach by Lerdahl and Jackendoff (1977) and Jackendoff and Lerdahl (1979). However, these scholars fail to emphasize sufficiently that the syntactic structure of music is more dependent on pragmatic processing while that of natural language is more dependent on semantic processing, a difference which provides a point of entry into examining some persistent problems that have plagued linguists as well as those interested in music for several decades.

REFERENCE AND MEANING

In this last section I wish therefore to explore to somewhat greater depth the similarities and differences between musical and linguistic communication by developing further the insights on this topic provided by Leonard Bernstein (1976). Bernstein brings to this work his prodigious and deep knowledge of music and considerable analytic skills. He is excited by Chomsky's "Language and Mind" (1972) and presents the case for considering music in the same terms as those in which Chomsky considers natural language. Chomsky, himself, has responded to this attempt by insisting on the uniqueness of the language system (1980), while others (for example, Lerdahl and Jackendoff, 1977) have been more overtly critical of some of the technical details of Bernstein's position. I will here emphasize the positive aspects of Bernstein's overall approach by showing that in addition to providing a more universal framework for understanding music, it is at the same time extremely valuable in illuminating some hitherto difficult reaches of linguistic analysis. Any such approach must, however, (as Chomsky rightly emphasizes) also account for the major differences between natural language and musical systems.

Bernstein begins with phonology. He suggests that the first communicative uses of sounds were sung. His conjecture is supported by the fact that the vocalizations of non-human primates consist almost entirely of changes in pitch and duration - articulations appear to be characteristically human to such an extent that early attempts at eliciting communicative competencies in apes foundered on just this point. Such observations would suggest that at the phonological level music and speech begin in phylogeny and ontogeny with a common expressive mode.

As noted above, this common expressive phonology apparently was brought into the service of gestural communication in situations where vision had become restricted. The course of events allowed a distinction to arise between a categorical expression and one based on the more continuous aspects of phonology sensitive to octaval relationships. The categorical expressions became useful phonemic tokens representing gestures which in turn represented occurrences. This hierarchical representational system gave reference to the phonemic tokens - words had been developed.

The study of the reference of words is thus a legitimate central concern of linguistics. A great deal of this concern becomes transferred to the more encompassing study of the semantics of natural languages. The obvious direction of inquiry is to ascertain the referential roots of the indicants and symbols that constitute utterances in the natural languages.

But philosophers* have long held that there is an important distinction to be made between reference and meaning. Meaning in any non-referential sense has, however, eluded precise definition.

I have elsewhere (Pribram, 1973a, 1975) attempted such a definition in terms of the structure of redundancy. Following the lead of information - theoretic formulations which take up the philosopher's distinction - I equated information with reference (correlations between input and output, between sender and receiver) and meaning with the structure of redundancy in the sense that Garner (1962) uses this phrase. Whereas information processing reduces redundancy, meaning enhances it by innumerable variations on the structure of a theme. In subsequent publications a case was made for relating competence to information processing and meaning: As noted earlier, competence was defined as the reciprocal of equivocation where equivocation is the sum of noise and redundancy in an information transmission channel (Pribram and McGuinness, 1975; Pribram, 1976).

What this definition of meaning means for utterances is that meanings are conveyed by patterns of repetitions of referents, repetitions of the information to which the elements of the utterances (phonemes. words) refer. The information conveyed by a literary masterpiece may be encapsulated in an abstract or digest - what makes the original exercise a masterpiece is the meaning generated by slight variations on the informative theme, a theme that is perhaps endlessly repeated as in the repetitions of behavior that characterize the tragic hero in Greek drama. The very variations themselves assume some basic repetitive pattern so that variation can be assessed.

Recently, Zajonc (1968) has performed a series of experiments which resulted in data of central concern to this issue of the effect of repetition. Zajonc showed that subjects would express a liking or dislike for a verbal or geometric pattern simply on the basis of how often that pattern had been repetitiously experienced and that this liking or dislike appeared to be relatively independent of what the pattern referred to in cognitive consiousness. Furthermore, reaction times in expressing the feelings were shorter than those expressing recognition.

---

*   For example, Rudolf Carnap in <u>Meaning and Necessity</u> (947, p.126): "In traditional logic we often find two correlated concepts: on the one hand, what was called the "extension" or "detonation" (in the sense of J.S. Mill) of a term or a concept; on the other hand what was called its "intention", "comprehension", "meaning" or "connotation".

In another series of experiments performed in my laboratory (Pribram, Lim. Poppen and Bagshaw. 1966; Pribram and Tubbs, 1967; Pribram, Plotkin, Anderson and Leong, 1977) it was shown that the amygdala of the limbic systems and the related frontal cortex are critically involved in processing redundancy. In still other experiments also carried out in my laboratory (Schwartzbaum and Pribram, 1960; Schwartzbaum, Wilson and Morrissette. 1961; Kimble, Bagshaw and Pribram, 1965; Bagshaw, Kimble and Primbram, 1965 Bagshaw and Benzies, 1968; Luria, Pribram and Homskaya, 1964) these frontolimbic formations were shown to be involved in habituation to novelty. The major finding in these experiments was that while repetition produces behavioral habituation in normal human and non human primates, subjects with frontolimbic lesions failed to habituate. Further, this loss of behavioral habituation is accompanied by loss of visceroautonomic responses to dishabituation (orienting) when the repititious stimulus is varied, i.e. made novel. These results were interpreted to suggest that behavioral habituation was dependent on the visceroautonomic components of the orienting reaction. Loss of habituation and visceroautonomic reactions did not, however, preclude repetition from producing discrimination learning (Douglas and Pribram, 1966). On the other hand, lesions of the posterior cortical convexity result in severe disturbances of discrimination learning and performance (see reviews by Pribram, 1954, 1960, 1971, 1974).

Thus the neurobehavioral and psychophysiological data obtained in these experiments are in consonance with the distinction resulting from the Zajonc experiments that repetition is processed by two separate mechanisms. What is added by the Zajonc results is that liking (and disliking) are produced by habituation. Clinically, lesions in the region of the amygdala produce a syndrome of "deja or jamais vu", an inappropriate feeling of familiarity or unfamiliarity. The neurobehavioral and psychophysiological data had always been interpreted in the context of these clinical observations in terms of a novelty-familiarity dimension. The new evidence suggests that this reading of the clinical data was in error. It is the feeling of familiarity (or unfamiliarity) that should have been emphasized. The fact that the feeling was inappropriate to the circumstance (as indicated by a recognition measure) clearly supports the newer conceptualization.

To summarize these findings: Repetition results in habituation and recognition. Variations on a repetitive pattern (novelties) evoke dishabituation (orienting) which is felt and the feeling is generated independently of recognition of the variation. The thesis to be pursued here is that while the aesthetics of music is a function of the recognition of variations, musical meaning results from the generation of feelings produced by these same variations on patterns of repetition. Clynes (1977; this volume) has a considerable body of research on this issue: He has demonstrated which patterns (essentic forms) evoke which feelings in a variety of different peoples and cultures.

MUSICAL MEANING

Bernstein struggles with these very same ideas in his analysis of musical meaning (pp 119-122): "Ah Meaning. There's the rub." In the next paragraph he begins an analysis of ambiguities of meaning which he claims to be neither exclusively phonological nor syntactic but both. He uses Chomsky's ambiguous sentence, "The whole town was populated by old men and women". The ambiguity stems, of course, from the fact that "old" could modify only "men" or both "men and women". Bernstein points out that the ambiguity in meaning has been produced by a deletion which produces a figure of speech known as "zeugma", meaning in this case two nouns yoked to one adjective.

He goes on to draw the musical analogy: "Try to think of all that melodic material on top as a series of nouns. Now think of the harmonic support underneath as verbal adjective. Put it all together, and what have we got? A zeugma; with the same unchanging adjective modifying all those different nouns."

Bernstein goes on to suggest that by reapplying the transformation rule of deletion to the sentence "The whole town was populated by old men and women", this already ambiguous sentence can be turned into an even more ambiguous sentence: "The whole town was old men and women", which could be a line of poetry. a poetic statement. He defines poetry in terms of its potential to evoke multiple meanings (see also Jakobson and Halle, 1956).

What is lacking in Bernstein's analysis is the recognition of a branch of linguistics (and cognitive science as a whole) which Charles Peirce called Pragmatics (1934). Bernstein does emphasize the historicity involved in making the deletions which result in ambiguity and therefore allow what Peirce calls abductive, metaphorical meanings to emerge. But the centrality of use, the pragmatics of the constructions, have not been as clearly recognized as they might have been - either by Bernstein or Chomsky or for that matter any other linguist. Philosophers, on the other hand, have joined the issue in terms of the distinction between intension and extension (Searle, 1979).

What Bernstein does provide is a framework for understanding the structure of pragmatics of use. He clearly distinguishes this form of meaning from reference although reference must underly it. He notes, for instance, that in musical metaphor the computations that are needed to unravel linguistic reference (which he calls semantic weights: my dog, your dog, all dogs etc.) are totally absent (pp 126-127).

Nor are references to the feelings of the composer or performer to be mistaken for musical meaning: "Music has intrinsic meanings of its own which are not to be confused with specific feelings or moods and certainly not with pictorial expressions or stories" (p 131).

No, meanings are derived from the intrinsic organization of the music, its structure. This structure intends and evokes feelings rather than referencing them. As noted above, this evocation derives from repetition and variations on these repetitions. As also noted, the most pervasive generative transformations (in the Chomskian sense) that evoke such feelings are deletions: "we delete all those logical but unnecessary steps that are built into the deep structure of any comparison and wind up with our conclusive simile" (p 124). Note that the logic of the structure (its deep or underlying structure) has a repetitive familiar core before deletion can be used effectively: "In other words variation cannot exist without the previously assumed idea of repetition. This assumption explains the deletion we heard at the beginning of the symphony" (p 161).

Repetition, redundancy, is therefore the key to the problem of meaning in music. "How many times have I repeated the word "repeat" in this short development?" (p 161). But as Bernstein and others (Garner, 1962; Pribram, 1976) have emphasized, redundancy can be structured and variations can be made on that structure. In terms of the experimental data reviewed above and by Clynes (this volume), such structured variation generates feelings and it is these feelings which give meaning to music.

In fact, as noted earlier, there is ample evidence that semantic reference and pragmatic meaning are processed separately, that the back and front parts of the brain work differently and that in this difference lies the distinction between semantic reference and pragmatic generative meaning as it has been pursued here (Pribram, 1954, 1958a, b, 1960, 1971, 1973, 1976, 1979). The frontolimbic portions of the forebrain have been shown by experiment to be involved in the generation and control of feelings produced by repetition (see above paragraph and review by Pribram and McGuinness, 1975). Furthermore, the processing of variations on repetition, especially temporal variations, has been demonstrated to be a function of the frontolimbic formations of the forebrain (Milner, 1954; Pribram and Tubbs, 1967; Pribram, Lim, Poppen and Bagshaw, 1966).

By contrast, the posterior cortical convexity is involved in image and information processing - the processing (recognition) of the invariances that can be extracted from sensory input to the brain (reviewed by Pribram, 1954, 1958a, b, 1960). These posterior cortical systems operate to reduce redundancy(by correlation, not deletion) , acting much as an editor searching for novelty (Barlow, 1961). Redundancy reduction, the processing of information, constitutes the aesthetics of music (Pribram, 1969a, 1979b) but does not provide "meaning" in the sense that this concept has been pursued here.

In short, neurobehavioral evidence clearly supports the distinction between referential information and meaning generated, as in Bernstein's analysis, by variations on repetitions - the structure of redundancy. What remains to be accomplished is some agreement as to what to call the distinction. Cognitive psychologists use the term semantic store or lexicon to deal with the organization of indicants (derived from images) and symbols (derived from information, i.e., categorical alternatives). They apply the term "episodic" or episode specific to constructions that cluster about some specific incident or context. I have followed the usage of computer scientists and termed image and information processing (of indicants and symbols) "context-free" and episodic processing "context dependent" or "context sensitive" (Pribram, 1971, 1977). These terms were meant to convey the fact that processing by the posterior cortical convexity proceeds hierarchically while processing by the frontolimbic mechanisms has a more web-like "associative" organization. The emphasis by Bernstein on deletion which is also found in Chomsky's work (1980) makes me wonder whether a web-like structure (Quillian, 1967) is secondarily derived from a more hierarchical logical structure by deletion or whether associative structures form independently of logical ones.

MUSIC AND LANGUAGE

The answer to this question may come from an examination of the types of grammar that have been found useful in analyzing linguistic performances. The simplest of these are the stochastic and state dependent grammars in which any particular utterance falls out, as it were, of the probabilities set up by previous utterances. Flesch counts of the incidence of usage of words in the English language are based on such a model and have been found wanting in explaining not only natural speech (Miller, Galanter, and Pribram, 1960) but also language disabilities due to brain damage (Howes, 1957a, b, 1964). A more effective though still limited model has been phrase structure grammar in which the hierarchic relationships between groupings of utterances are mapped. One of Chomsky's major contributions has been to demonstrate the limitations of the phrase structure grammar and to suggest:

(1)   that transformations occur in language;

(2)   that these transformations are rule governed by rules which transcend the hierarchical organizations of phrase structures; and

(3)   that these rules evoke meaning.

What has occupied Chomskian linguistics for the past twenty years is the attempt to specify clearly what such rules might look like.

Meanwhile, computer scientists have been developing organizations of programs that can make them function more usefully. These organizations have departed from simpler hierarchical organizations of list structures which characterized earlier attempts in enhancing artificial intelligence. The new developments go under such names as procedures (Winograd, 1977), scripts (Schank and Abelson, 1977). They are eminently pragmatic in that they group together in a cluster those routines (parts of programs) that are repeatedly used, mark the cluster and call up that marked cluster whenever it is needed. The advantage of such procedures is that computation can simultaneously proceed in several clusters and the results of the computation flexible addressed in response to some overarching "executive" program.

I have elsewhere (Pribram, 1973b) drawn the comparison between the functions of the frontal cortex of primates and such flexible noticing orders and executive programs. The neurobehavioral evidence thus suggests that a procedural pragmatics is the basis for transformational rules. Bernstein has identified in his pursuit of a linguistic analysis of music one very powerful set of procedures for us:

(a   repetition
(b)   variation in repetitions that generate novelty (note that invention and inventory share the same root), and
(c)   deletions of repetitions which generate potential meanings through ambiguity.

My neurobehavioral results obtained on non human primates suggest that this set of procedures is generally applicable to the problem of specifying the nature of transformations and of a generative grammar. It is for this reason that I found Bernstein's contribution exciting and valuable.

The analysis, should it prove viable, has an interesting consequence for understanding music and natural language, especially as used in poetry. These consequences are that the evocative aspects of cognitive competencies are not so much due to transformational rules as they are to transformational procedures. The search for hierarchically organized rule-structures leads in every instance to a phrase-structure grammar. Transformations on these phrase structures are episode specific, involve a large amount of historicity, occur within the context of phrase structures and are extremely context sensitive. Whether one wishes to call such relatively arbitrary (i.e., context dependent) procedures 'rule' governed remains an open question. The resemblance is more to a case than to a phrase structure as has been emphasized by Fillmore (1968). The important point is that the structure of transformational procedures is distinct from a hierarchically organized phrase structure grammar and that different brain systems are involved in organizing the hierarchical and transformational structures.

I believe that comparing music with natural language has been most rewarding: Despite the severely limited information processing and resulting referential semantics, music is rich in meaning. This meaning is derived from pragmatic procedures which also enrich natural languages especially in their poetic usages. Pragmatic procedures are based on repetition, on variations of repetitions and on deletions of expected repetitions. It is processes such as these which have been shown to be functions of the frontolimbic formations of the forebrain which can therefore be considered to construct the long sought-after principles of transformations which are the cornerstone of Chomskian generative grammar. Transformations are shown, however, to be procedural in that they are episode and context specific rather than hierarchically organized: case structural rather than phrase structural. Pragmatic variations on repetitions, deletions of expected phrases, associative clusterings involving a large amount of historicity can be sharply distinguished from hierarchically organized rule structures. This analysis based on the study of music has thus proved a fascinating and unsuspectedly fruitful foray into cognitive science.

SUMMARY

This chapter reviews experiments that relate brain function to musical ability. The results of these experiments are then related to others on natural language in order to construct a theory of how the brain functions when music is created and appreciated. On the level of music the theory involves the work of Chomsky, Bernstein and that of Lerdahl and Jackendoff. On the level of brain function evidence is reviewed to show that different neural systems are involved in syntactic, semantic and pragmatic processing.

The suggestion is made that music and natural language share syntactic structuring. However, music and natural language differ in that natural language is primarily referential (i.e. semantic) while music is primarily evocative (i.e. pragmatic). These suggestions are applied to a theory of meaning which distinguishes reference and evocation not only on logical but also on neurological grounds.

REFERENCES

Bagshaw, M.H., and Benzies, S., 1968, Multiple measures of the orienting reaction and their dissociation after amygdalectomy in monkeys, Exp. Neurol. 29:175-187.

Bagshaw, M.H., Kimble, D.P., and Pribram, K.H., 1965, The GSR of monkeys during orienting and habituation and after ablation of the amygdala, hippocampus and inferotemporal cortex. Neuropsychologia, 3:111.

Barlow, H.B., 1961, Possible principles underlying the transformations of sensory messages, in: "Sensory Communication," W. Rosenblith, ed., MIT Press, Cambridge, Ma.

Bernstein, L., 1976, "The Unanswered Question: Six Talks at Harvard," Harvard University Press, Cambridge, Ma.

Bogen, J.E., and Gordon, H.W., 1971, Musical tests for functional lateralization with intracarotid amobarbital, Nature, 230:524.

Chomsky, N., 1972, "Language and Mind," Harcourt, Brace & Jovanovich, New York.

Chomsky, N., 1980, "Rules and Representations," Columbia University Press, New York.

Clynes, M., 1977, "Sentics: The Touch of Emotions," Doubleday, Garden City, N.J.

Critchley, M., and Henson, R.A., 1977, "Music and the Brain," eds. W. Heinemann Medical Books, Ltd., London.

Deutsch, D., 1977, Memory and attention in music, in: "Music and the Brain," M. Critchley, and R.A. Henson, eds., W. Heinemann Medical Books, Ltd., London.

Douglas, R.J., and Pribram, K.H., 1966, Learning and limbic lesions, Neuropsychologia, 4:197-220.

Efron, R., and Yund, E.W., 1975, Dichotic competition of simultaneous tone bursts of different frequency. III: The effect of stimulus parameters on suppression and ear dominance functions, Neuropsychologia. 13:151-161.

Fillmore, C.J., 1968, The case for case, in: "Universals of Liguistic Theory," Holt, Rinehart & Winston, New York.

Garner, W.R., 1962, "Uncertainty and Structure as Psychological Concepts," John Wiley, New York.

Gordon, H.W , 1970, Hemispheric asymmetries in the perception of musical chords, Cortex, 6:387-398.

Haydon, S.P., and Spellacy, F.J., 1973, Monaural reaction time asymmetries for speech and non speech sounds, Cortex, 9:288-294.

Howes, D.H., 1957(a), On the relation between the intelligibility and frequency of occurrence of English words, J. Acoust. Soc. Am., 29:296-305.

Howes, D.H., 1957(b), On the relation between the probability of a word as an association and in general linguistic usage, J. Abnorm. Soc. Psychol., 54:75-85

Howes, D.H., 1964, Application of the word-frequency concept to aphasia, in: "Ciba Foundation Symposium on Disorders of Language," Churchill, London.

Jackendoff, R., and Lerdahl, F., 1979, Generative music theory and its relation to psychology, (unpublished manuscript).

Jakobson, R., 1956, Two aspects of language and two types of aphasic disturbances, in: "Fundamentals of Language," R. Jakobson, and M. Halle, eds., Mouton, The Hague.

Kallman, H.J., and Corballis, M.C., 1975, Ear asymmetry in reaction time to musical sounds, Perc. Psychophys., 17:368-370.

Kimble, D.P., Bagshaw, M.H., and Pribram, K.H., 1965, The GSR of monkeys during orienting and habituation after selective partial ablations of the cingulate and frontal cortex, Neuropsychologia, 3:121-128.

Lerdahl. F., and Jackendoff, R., 1977, Toward a formal theory of tonal music, J. Mus. Theory, 21(1):111-172.

Luria, A.R., Primbram, K.H., and Homskaya, E.D., 1964, An experimental analysis of the behavioral disturbance produced by a left frontal arachnoidal endothelloma (memingioma), Neuropsychologia, 2:257-280.

McGuinness, D., 1974, Equating individual differences for auditory input, Psychophysiol., 11:113-120.

Miller, G.A., Galanter, E., and Pribram, K.H., 1960, "Plans and the Structure of Behavior," Henry Holt & Co., New York.

Milner, B., 1954, Intellectual function of the temporal lobe, Psychol. Bull., 51:42-62.

Morris, C., 1946, "Signs, Language and Behavior," Prentice Hall, New York.

Oscar-Berman, M., Blumstein, S., and DeLuca, D., 1974, Iconic recognition of musical symbols in lateral visual field. Paper presented at the American Psychological Association Annual Meeting, New Orleans, La.

Peirce, C.S., 1934, "Collected Papers," Harvard University Press, Cambridge, Ma.

Pribram, K.H., 1954, Toward a science of neuropsychology (method and data), in: "Current Trends in Psychology and the Behavioral Sciences, "R.A. Patton, ed., Univ. of Pittsburgh Press, Pittsburgh.

Pribram, K.H., 1958(a), Comparative neurology and the evolution of behavior, in: "Behaviour and Evolution," A. Roe, and G.G. Simpson, eds., Yale University Press, New Haven, Conn.

Pribram K.H., 1958(b), Neocortical function in behavior, in: Biological and Biochemical Bases of Behavior," H.F. Harlow and C.N. Woolsey, eds., University of Wisconsin Press, Madison, Wis.

Pribram, K.H., 1959, On the neurology of thinking, Behav. Sci., 4:265-284.

Pribram, K.H., 1960, The intrinsic systems of the forebrain, in: "Handbook of Physiology, Neurophysiology, II," J. Field, H.W. Magoun, and V.E. Hall, eds., American Physiological Society, Washington, D.C.

Pribram, K.H., 1969, Neural servosystems and the structure of personality, J. Nerv. Men. Dis., 140:30-39.

Pribram, K.H., 1971, "Languages of the Brain," Prentice-Hall, Englewood Cliffs. N.J., (2nd ed., 1977, Brooks/Cole, Monterey, (Ca.)

Pribram, K.H., 1973(a), The comparative psychology of communication: The issue of grammar and meaning, Annals New York Acad. Sci. 223:135-143.

Pribram, K.H., 1973(b), The primate frontal cortex-executive of the brain, in: "Frontal Lobes and the Regulation of Behavior," A.R. Luria, and K.H. Pribram, eds., Academic Press, New York.

Pribram, K.H., 1974, How is it that sensing so much, we can do so little?, in: "The Neurosciences Third Study Volume," G. Schmitt, and F. Worden, eds., MIT Press, Cambridge, Ma.

Pribram. K.H., 1975, Neurolinguistics: The study of brain organization in grammar and meaning, Totus Homo, 6:20-30.

Pribram, K.H., 1976, Language in a sociobiological frame, in "Origins and Evolution of Language and Speech," Academy of Science, New York.

Pribram. K.H., 1977, Modes of central processing in human learning and remembering, in: "Brain and Learning," T.J. Teyler, ed., Greylock Press, Stamford, Conn.

Pribram, K.H., 1978, The linguistic act, in: "Psychiatry and the Humanities, Vol. 3: Psychoanalysis and Language," J.H. Smith, ed., Yale University Press, New Haven, Conn.

Pribram, K.H., 1979(a), The place of pragmatics in the syntactic and semantic organization of language, in: "Temporal Variables in Speech, Studies in Honour of Freida Goldman/Eisler," Mouton, Paris.

Pribram, K.H., 1979(b), Emotions, in: "Handbook of Clinical Neuropsychology," S.B. Filskoy, and T.J. Boll, eds., Wiley & Sons, New York.

Pribram, K.H., Lim, H., Poppen. R., and Bagshaw, M.H., 1966, Limbic lesions and the temporal structure of redundancy, J. Comp. Physiol. Psychol., 61:365-373.

Pribram. K.H., and McGuinness, D. 1975, Arousal, activation and effort in the control of attention, Psych. Rev. 82(2):116-149.

Pribram. K.H., Plotkin, H.C., Anderson, R.M., and Leong, D., 1977, Information sources in the delayed alternation task for normal and 'frontal' monkeys, Neuropsychologia, 15:329-340.

Pribram, K.H., and Tubbs, W.E., 1967, Short-term memory, parsing, and the primate frontal cortex, Science, 156:1765-1767.

Quillian, M.R., 1967, Word concepts: A theory simulation of some basic semantic capabilities, Behav. Sci., 12:410-430.

Reynolds, P.C., 1970, Social communication in the chimpanzee: A review, The Chimpanzee, 3:369-394.

Robinson, G., and Solomon, D.J., 1974, Rhythm is processed by the speech hemisphere, J. Exp. Psychol., 102:508.

Schank, R.C., and Abelson, R.P., 1977, "Scripts, Plans, Goals and Understanding," Erlbaum, Hillsdale, N.J.

Schwartzbaum. J.S., and Pribram, K.H., 1960, The effects of amygdalectomy in monkeys on transposition along a brightness continuum, J. Comp. Physiol. Psychol., 53:396-399.

Schwartzbaum, J.S., Wilson, W.A., Jr., and Morrissette, J.R., 1961, The effects of amygdalectomy on locomotor activity in monkeys, J. Comp. Physiol. Psychol., 54(3):334-336.

Searle, J.R., 1979, "Expression and Meaning," Cambridge University Press, Cambridge, Eng.
Winograd, T., 1977 Framework for understanding discourse, Stanford Univ. Intelligence Monograph, Stanford, (Ca.)
Zajonc, R.B., 1968, Attitudinal effects of mere exposure, J. Personal. Soc. Psychol., 9(2):2.

Chapter III

PHYSICAL AND NEUROPSYCHOLOGICAL FOUNDATIONS OF MUSIC
The Basic Questions

Juan G. Roederer

Geophysical Institute
University of Alaska
Fairbanks, Alaska, USA

INTRODUCTION

The study of the perception of music is a paramount example of interdisciplinary research. in which musicians, physicists, neurobiologists, engineers and psychologists must communicate and work together. The potential spin-off is impressive, though perhaps not yet fully recognized. Musicians can incorporate insights gleaned from the study of music perception into new frontiers of composition and electronic and digital tone generation. They can use new knowledge in brain function, particularly in the area of linguistic processing, to attempt a better understanding of the evolution of musical cultures from primitive rhythmic and melodic patterns to elaborate holistic expressions. And they can combine latest research results in both sensory perception and skilled motor control to formulate better strategies in music pedagogy. Finally, the study of music perception can help dispel many of the fallacies that abound in the musical world, related to piano touch, the role of perfect pitch, the question of tone 'colors' the question of 'playability' vs. 'likeability' of musical instruments, and so on. Engineers can profit from a better knowledge of the workings of the human auditory system to develop better electroacoustical equipment and better concert halls. Instrument builders can improve or simplify their work by focusing on what the study of music perception can yield in terms of understanding why a great instrument sounds great. Neuropsychologists can use the relatively simple sound patterns of music to study basic information-processing mechanisms relevant to speech. Psychologists can benefit from a quantitative understanding of music perception in their studies of aesthetic motivation appreciation. and emotional response, and the application of the results to music therapy.

The study of music perception comprises three broad problem areas pertaining to the fields of psychoacoustics. neuropsychology, and psychology respectively, (Roederer, 1979a): (1) perception of musical tones; (2) interpretation of acoustical information relevant to music; and (3) emotional response to musical messages. At a first glance, each problem area can be linked to a particular processing stage in the auditory system: tone perception to the peripheral sensory system, afferent channels and primary auditory areas in the cerebral cortex; musical message perception to the association areas, the frontal lobes and to the differences in information-processing strategy between the two cortical hemispheres; and emotional response to the interaction between cortical functions and the limbic system of the brain.

In recent years, however, a considerable mutual integration of these three problem areas has taken place (Roederer, 1979b). This is partly due to the scientific results per se. which show that even an elementary percept such as the subjective pitch of a single musical tone is the result of a complex context-dependent pattern recognition process involving higher operations in the cognitive system. On the other hand, this problem area integration is also due to recent progress in the understanding of general human brain functions, and the recognition that in the conscious state even the simplest perceptual events are bound to trigger operations that involve the brain as a whole.

There are three central questions, as fundamental yet mutually interrelated as the above problem areas to which they relate (Roederer, 1979a). Let me consider the third area first. The following seems to me to be the ultimate question of music: "Why do we respond emotionally to music, when the messages therein seem to be of no obvious survival value?" In other words, why are humans motivated to create or register musical messages when such messages seem to convey no such biologically relevant information as do speech, other animal utterancs and environmental sounds? A second central question is: "What in music can be explained in terms of physiological neuropsychological properties, and what has emerged haphazardly through the development of individual cultures?". In other words, can the 'universals' in music be explained on neurophysiological grounds? And finally the interrelated trio of psychoacoustical questions: 'Why do we perceive a complex tone, made up of a superposition of many harmonics, as one single whole of one pitch, one timbre, one loudness?"; 'Why do we call all notes differing by one or more octaves by the same name?' and "Why are all meaningful musical messages made up of a relatively limited repertoire of discrete pitch transitions, with preferred sequences or superpositions thereof, and clearly defined rhythmic struc-tures?'

MUSIC AND THE HOLOLOGIC MODE OF BRAIN FUNCTION

In the last 10-15 years great progress has been made in the under-standing of the brain. Much of it has been achieved in piece-meal fashion and put together in what still resembles more a framework of scientific speculation and modelling rather than an iron-cast integrated theory of brain function. Yet indirect evidence for some crucial modes of brain operations is impressive, though not free from controversy (for example, Roederer, 1979c).

Most germane to the question of perception and processing of information is the way in which the animal brain handles the operations of environmental representation and short-term prediction of environmental events. A mental or cerebral representation of an environmental object, scene, or event is physically defined as the specific spatiotemporal distribution of electrical signals in the neural network of the cerebral cortex that appears in a causal, one-to-one correspondence with the specific features sensed during the presentation or occurrence of that environmental object, scene, or event. According to this definition, 'cognition' is nothing else but the occurrence of a spatial and temporal display of neural activity in the brain that is in one-to-one correspondence with the object, event, or concept being recognized. For instance, the spatiotemporal distributions of neural activity displayed on intervening cortical centers by the perception (or the recall) of the following things - a big red apple, a pile of small green apples, an apple pie, and orchard of apple trees - though widely different, would all bear some subset of neural activity distribution in common, namely the one that appears in correspondence with, and defines the cognition of 'apple'. Even in 'simplest' neural representation engages millions of cortical neurons at the same time, and there is no spatial continuity in the corresponding neural activity distribution.

The act of remembering, or memory recall, of an environmental scene or a sensory event consists of the re-elicitation or 'replay' aspects of that particular spatiotemporal distribution of neural signals which was specific to the original sensory event. In this process it is irrelevant whether the replay was triggered by direct sensory input, by associative recall (see below), by hallucinatory process during a dream, or by electrophysiological stimulation of the brain during neurosurgery. Long-term memory storge is believed to consist of appropriate modifications in the neural tissue, such as changes in electric connectivity (synapses) among cortical neurons.

Since higher organisms had to rely more and more on the information acquired during their own lifetime and stored in the brain, the need for an adequately protected and quickly accessible information storage arose from the very beginning. This led to a distributed memory and the mode of holologic representation (Pribram, 1971) rather than 'photographic' coding and imaging of environmental scenes. A 'photographic' representation would be one in which there is a 'point-to-point' correspondence between features of the stimulus (object) and features of the neural activity distribution (image). A holographic, or in this case 'holologic', representation is one in which information on each feature (point) of the object stimulus is mapped onto the whole domain of the image (as in an optical hologram, where information on one point is spread over the whole domain of the photographic film).

For instance, in the peripheral stages of the auditory tract there is a 'tonotopical organization' of neural signals, in spatial (and temporal) correspondence with the regions of excitation on the basilar membrane of the cochlea (for example. the distinct resonance regions elicited by the first 7-8 harmonics of a musical tone). But, as we move up toward the cortical area, this 'photographic' point-to-point representation is gradually lost (it only remains preserved in the unconscious animal), and the neural representation becomes holologic, with the activity from one point of the basilar membrane mapped onto a large and diffuse ensemble of neurons.

A formidable bonus of the holological mode of storage is the process of associative recall (for example, Kohonen, 1977). Indeed the replay of a specific neural activity can be triggered by causes or cues other than the full sensorial reenactment of the original event - a partial reenactment of the neural activity that occurred during the storage act suffices to release the full specific activity display. For instance, all common information storage systems. such as books. magnetic tapes, phonographic records, films, and the like represent what we called a 'photographic' mode of memory storage, and to retrieve a specific piece of information we must know its address, or else scan through the entire storage register. But with a hologic memory system of recorded music say (which does not yet exist in practice) you would be able to play in the famous four notes ta-ta-ta-taah and retrieve the whole Fifth Symphony of Beethoven!

Hologic information processing and storage are fundamental ingredients for pattern recognition. This is how they relate to music perception: Let us focus on one example: the perception of subjective pitch of complex harmonic tones. For years a battle has been raging between adherents of the so called 'place theory of pitch' (pitch signal encoded in the spatial position of the auditory ne ve fibers activiated by a tone stimulus) and adherents of the 'periodicity pitch theory' (pitch signal encoded in the temporal sequence of neural spikes in fibers activated by a tone). As in so many biological systems, both theories are probably correct under certain circumstances - that is, both mechanisms cooperate in pitch determination. But for complex multi-harmonic tones the pitch mechanism cannot be described by a simple signal-encoding model. The phenomenon of 'fundamental tracking' (pitch perception of a tone with suppressed fundamental), the proven context-dependence of the pitch of inharmonic tones, and the ambiguous or multiple pitches of tones with suppresed lower harmonics all convincingly show that subjective pitch perception requires the operation of a pattern recognition mechanism, just like higher-order perceptual processes in the visual system do.

In a nutshell, this theory of subjective pitch, spearheaded by Terhardt (1972), is as follows. Natural sounds of human and animal acoustic communications contain an important proportion of harmonic tones (vowels, bird song, animal cries). Such tones share a common property - they are made up of a superposition of harmonics, of frequencies that are integer multiples of a fundamental. These tones elicit a complicated resonance pattern on the basilar membrane, with multiple amplitude peaks, one for each harmonic. In spite of its complexity, this pattern preserves the particular distance relationship between neighbouring resonance maxima, even when the fundamental frequency of the tone changes (for higher order harmonics beyond the seventh or eighth, this relationship loses its physical definition because of mutual resonance overlaps). We either learn at an early age, or we have a built-in mechanism, to recognize this invariant characteristic as belonging to 'one and the same thing'. The result is a unique pitch sensation - in spite of the many concurrent harmonics and the ensuing complexity of the primary excitation pattern. The unique pitch sensation corresponds to that of the fundamental, which in 'natural' sounds is usually the most prominent one (with respect to intensity).

If instead of a 'natural' complex sound we are exposed to one in which some normally expected elements are suppressed (a missing fundamental, for example), the partially truncated excitation pattern on the basilar membrane fed into the pitch recognition mechanism can still be matched, within certain limitations, and a pitch is perceived. It is here that the hologic function of the brain comes in. As stated above, one of the fundamental properties of a hologic system is that only a partial reenactment of neural activity (for example, a complex tone with a missing fundamental) suffices to release the full specific activity display (the subjective pitch sensation corresponding to the missing fundamental!). If, however the truncated pattern is lacking too many lower harmonics or is too distorted (for example, inharmonicities of the overtones) and equivocal match is made, and ambiguous or multiple pitch sensations result.

A most interesting by-product of this pattern-recognition theory of pitch is that it leads most naturally to a neuropsychological foundation of harmony (Terhardt, 1974). In this theory it is postulated that tonal music is based essentially upon the pattern recognition mechanism that operates in the auditory system responsible for the extraction of a single pitch sensation from the complicated neural activity distribution elicited by a musical tone. As stated above, this mechanism acquires knowledge of the specific relations that exist between the resonance maxima evoked on the basilar membrane by the lower six to eight harmonics of such a tone. The corresponding primary intervals (octave, fifth, fourth, major third, minor third) thus become 'familiar' to the auditory system, and convey tonal meanings to all external stimuli whose (fundamental) frequencies bear such relationships. Note that in this view the 'familiarity' is physical-physiological, imprinted in the neural circuitry of the auditory system. Even the unique role played by the octave emerges quite naturally as a result of the hologic mode of brain function. The octave is the only interval (besides unison) whose component tones, when sounded together or in succession, do not introduce new resonance regions in activation pattern of the basilar membrane, since the harmonics of the upper tone coincide with the even harmonics of the lower tone. Therefore, a certain signal of similarity of identity is evoked - that pertaining to all notes differing by one or more octaves!

The study of the hologic function of the brain can be expanded to include other fundamental 'intellectual' aspects of music perception such as musical memory, timbre recognition, and musical imaging in composition (for example, Roederer, 1979b).

MUSIC, LANGUAGE, MOTIVATION AND EMOTION

Pitch probably is perceived by higher animals in nearly the same way as by humans. But animals are not spontaneously motivated to listen to abstract pitch successions and superpositions, nor do they respond emotionally to such events. These exclusively human responses - bird song is song to humans but not to the birds, for which is may be merely a means of behaviourally induced or genetically preprogrammed information transmission!

The human brain does not appear to contain many new or drastically different processing centers when compared with the brains of any of our primate ancestors. The only significant quantitative differences lie in the total number of neurons in cortical association areas, particularly the frontal lobes, the proportion of interneurons therein, and the total number of intracortical fibers, all being highest in the human brain. If the neurophysiological differences are of degree only. what makes a human brain human? An animal can recall an environmental representation and display it as an image for use during the course of a behavioral act. It can recall this representation with a varying degree of detail, according to momentary needs. But there is little evidence that an animal can alter a representation without the external input of new information.

Perhaps the most fundamentally distinct operation that the human and only the human brain can perform is to recall images or representations, change them, and store modified or amended versions thereof without any concurrent external input. We call these acts of internal image recall, analysis, correction or alteration without new external inputs 'the human thinking process'. This process involves the generation of new information.

Most likely in parallel with, or as the point of departure for the evolution of a thinking capability in hominids, correlations between complex mental images and simple symbols such as gestures and vocal utterances were established systematically and human language emerged. With the emergence of language, besides fantastically widening the communciation capability with other humans, the thinking process (always as defined above) could be expedited and organized substantially through the mental use of symbolic and hierarchical representations of complex objects, scenes, and situations, thus avoiding the need for slow, full-fledged multisensorial mental imaging during this process. Words and word sequences thus became conditioned stimuli for the associative recall of representations of objects, concepts. and environmental events. Most importantly, the hominid brain started to utilize in a decisive way the neural network responsible for linguistic encoding during the acts of internal information processing and generation (thinking).

Now we can try to speculate on how music could have emerged in relation to the human language capability. With language, cortical areas emerged specializing in linguistic information processing. Language per se is. of course, a learned ability; it is not inborn. What is inborn are the neural networks capable of handling this task and the motivational drive to acquire language. (Like a cat is genetically programmed, or instinctively motivated to train in skilled movements for the purpose of hunting). Now, sound patterns in human speech are extremely complex. Could it be that inborn in humans is a genetic motivation to train the language-handling network in the processing of simple, organized, but otherwise biologically irrelevant sound patterns--as they indeed occur in music? And could this be seen as comparable to a cat instinctively training itself by chasing biologically irrelevant objects? A crying baby being pacified by the song of the mother may be following dictates of its limbic system to pay attention to simple sounds as a prelude to training in speech perception. You or I, overwhelmed by the sounds of Bach's "Kyrie" of the Mass in B Minor may be following an ancestral command to keep up training in acoustical information processing of increasing complexity. In short, I suggest that the human brain is instinctively geared toward exercising or entertaining itself with sound-processing operations even if they are of no immediate need or of no current survival value (but crucial to overall human performance).

The preceding argument deals with the motivation of humans to pay attention to musical sound forms. What about the emotion elicited by musical sound forms? One of the most profound consequences of the evolution of human brain functions has been the emergence of systematic postponement of behavioral goals and rearrangement of behavioral priorities: the body started serving the brain instead of the other way around. This led to conflicts between cortical functions and those of the limbic system. This latter is a phylogenetically old part of the brain, which comprises several structures (hippocampus, amygdala, several thalamic nuclei, and others). In conjunction with the hypothalamus (the part of the brain that integrates the functions of the autonomic nervous system and regulates the endocrine system), the limbic system polices sensorial input, selectively directs memory storage according to the relevance of the information, and mobilizes motor output with the specific function of ensuring a response that is most beneficial for the self-preservation of the organism in a complex environment.

As opposed to the cortical networks controlling intelligent behavior, the limbic system has no learning capability: its neural circuitry is 'prewired' at birth, with functions programmed during the slow course of phylogenetic evolution. (In higher vertebrates, though, the limbic system is able to 'consult' information stored in the cortex, and acquired during the organism's lifetime, before it issues behavioral directives). Motivation and emotion are integral manifestations of limbic function, manifestations of the limbic system's guiding principle of assuring that all cortical processes are carried out so as to be of maximum benefit to the organism.

In animals the limbic system is mostly activated by environmental and somatic input. In humans it can also respond to internally evoked images displayed on the cortex during the process of thinking. In other words, motivation and emotion in man can be triggered with no relationship to the instantaneous state of the environment and the actual response of the organism to it. It is along this line that we must seek a lead toward understanding the emotional response to music (and to art in general). (See also Clynes, 1973; Clynes and Nettheim, this volume.)

All this, of course, is over-simplified 'first-approximation' reasoning. For instance, it does not explain why I respond with goose-pimples to Bach's "Kyrie" every time I listen to it! It does not explain why I definitely prefer the repetitive phrases of Vivaldi to the repetitive phrases of rock music! No doubt training and early exposure to a certain musical culture play a crucial role in shaping an individual's emotional response to music. No doubt the association of music with the nature's sound environment plays a role. No doubt associative recall of the emotional state experienced during the first listening of a given piece or passage plays a role. No doubt that there is a survival value attached to musical forms as a powerful means to congregate and behaviorally uniformize or even control masses of people. But the basis of it all seems to remain: the elicitation of limbic function by the abstract sounds of music somehow in relation to the human brain's capability of language information processing.

MUSIC AND HEMISPHERIC SPECIALIZATION

In the evolution of the human brain, it seems that the immense requirements of information-processing that came with the development of verbal communication resulted in the emergence of hemispheric specialization. In this division of tasks, the analytic and sequential functions of language became the target of the 'dominant' hemisphere (on the left side in about 97% of the subjects). The minor hemisphere emerged as being more adapted for the perception of synthetic, holistic relations. That the speech centers are located in one hemisphere has been known for over 100 years, mainly as the result of autopsy studies conducted on decreased patients with speech and language defects acquired after cerebral hemorrhage (strokes) in one given hemisphere. On the other hand, tests on patients with lesions of the minor (right-side) hemisphere have revealed that visual and auditory pattern recognition is impaired. Generally, all nonverbal auditory tasks are impaired in these patients. This supports the indication that the central mechanisms relevant to the perception of music are located fundamentally in the minor hemisphere (the temporal lobe thereof). This has been confirmed through experiments involving normal, healthy subjects, with the technique of dichotic listening tests, and, very recently and most convincingly, through the technique of brain activity localization with positron-emission tomography. We should point out that hemisphere specialization is not absolute. It has been shown (for instance, with spilt-brain patients) that in adult persons the minor hemisphere seems to cooperate in normal speech, handling the 'musical' contents of speech (vowels, tone of voice. inflections). (For a review, see Roederer, 1979b)

The specialization of the cerebral hemispheres is really of a much more basic nature. involving two quite different operational modes. One mode involves sequential analysis of single-channel information such as required in language processing. The other involves spatial integration or synthesis of the state of activity in many different channels to accomplish the determination of holistic qualities of input stimuli. However, both modes must coexist and cooperate in order to process information about the environment, and program the organism's response to it.

Holistic pattern recognition is a most fundamental requirement for animal survival in an environment in which many correlated events occur at the same time in different spatial locations. In contrast, sequential analysis became the fundamental mode for processing language and for controlling speech and thought processes - wherein the 'events' follow one another serially in time. Indeed, communicating and thinking are brain operations based on short-term time sequencing. Animal communication capabilities: even those of dolphins or sign-language trained primates, appear to be infinitesimal compared to human linguistic capabilities; animals do not think like humans do - and animals do not show any hemisphere specialization.

If music is preferentially handled by the minor hemisphere, does this mean that music mainly involves synthetic operations of holistic quality recognition? This indeed seems to be in agreement with the recent theories of pitch perception the holistic quantity in a musical stimulus is the momentaneous distribution of neural activity corresponding to the vibration-resonance maxima on the basilar membrane (see above). However, an apparent paradox emerges when we consider melodies and the time dependence of musical messages. Wouldn't they require sequencing; i.e. dominant hemisphere operations? It seems to me this is not necessarily so. Speech (and thinking) involves short-term sequencing that mainly engages the short term memory in all auxiliary subroutine operations. Melodies and musical messages on the other hand mostly would seem to exceed the storage time and the capacity of the short term memory and associated information transmission channels. This leads me to the generally accepted idea that prima facie our brain recognizes the typical musical messages as being of holistic nature, long term patterns in time, rather than short term sequences. The phenomenon of melodic fission is a most convincing example of this. Expressed in other words, music seems to be recognized by our brain as the representation of integral, holistic auditory images (the harmonic structure), whose (long term) succession in time bears in itself a holistic Gestalt value (the melodic contours). (For hemispheric function in music, see also Borchgrevink, Pribram, this volume.)

All this is quite germane to the understanding of the evolution of Western music. In a broad sense, we may depict this evolution as a gradual transition between two extreme configurations. At one extreme we find highly structured, clearly defined, emphatically repeated, spatial (harmonic) and temporal (melodic) sound patterns. each one of which bears a value as an unanalyzed whole (for example, a given chord, and a given voice or chord progression respectively). At the other extreme (to which we are now heading), we identify tonal forms whose fundamental value is recognized in the momentary state of the short-term temporal sound signatures, such as rapidly varying noise components, sweeping pitches, speech-like sounds, etc. In the light of what we have said about hemispheric specialization, we may speculate that these two extreme configurations are intimately related to the two distinct processing strategies of the human brain, namely holistic analysis in the minor hemisphere and sequential processing in the language hemisphere. The evolution of western music thus would point to a gradual shift of the 'focal point' of musical processing from the minor hemisphere in, say, baroque of classical music, to the dominant hemisphere in today's avant garde music. Only the future will tell whether the current trends in music merely represent a more or less random effort to break away from traditional forms (which had emerged in part quite naturally as the result of physical properties of the human auditory system), or whether these trends can be channeled into a premeditated exploration and exploitation of vast, still untested processing capabilities of the central nervous system.

SUMMARY

The relationship between some universal features of music perception and relevant basic functions of the human brain is reviewed. Several fundamental questions are formulated, and answers are attempted based on current knowledge and assumptions about the human brain. Particular attention is given to the brain's hologic mode of information-processing, storage and associative recall, to the role of the limbic system, and to hemispheric specialization of certain brain functions. In this context. a possible link between the human capability to acquire language and the motivation to listen to and create musical sounds is discussed.

ACKNOWLEDGMENT

I wish to pay a posthumous tribute to Professor Helmut Wobisch, creator of the Carinthian Summer Festival and its director since 1969 until his untimely death in early 1980. He sparked the idea of the Workshops on the Physical and Neuropsychological Foundations of Music which I had the privilege to direct, and it was only through his constant encouragement and support that these Workshops have become regular and expected events in the world of musicology and musical acoustics.

REFERENCES

Clynes, M., 1973 Sentics: biocybernetics of emotion communication, Annals, New York Acad. of Sc., Vol. 220, 3; 55-131.

Kohonen, T., 1977, "Associatative Memory," Springer-Verlag, Berlin and New York

Pribram. K.H., 1971, "Languages of the Brain", Prentice-Hall, Englewood Cliffs, N.J.

Roederer, J.G., 1979a, The perception of music by the human brain, Human. Assoc. Rev., 30:11-23.

Roederer, J.G., 1979b. "Physics and Psychophysics of Music," 2nd ed., Springer-Verlag, New York

Roederer, J.G., 1979c, Human brain functions and the foundations of science, Endeavour 3:99.

Terhardt, E., 1972, Zur Tonhöhenwahrnehmung von Klangen, I, II. Acoustica 26:173-199.

Terhardt, E., 1974, Pitch, consonance and harmony, J. Acoust. Soc. Am. 55:1061-1069.

Chapter IV

THE LIVING QUALITY OF MUSIC
Neurobiologic Patterns of
Communicating Feeling

Manfred Clynes and Nigel Nettheim

Music Research Center
New South Wales State Conservatorium of Music
Sydney, Australia

This chapter is concerned with the nature of the language of expressive qualities in music. Its three sections consist of (I) Theoretical introduction; (II) Experimental work in the study of dynamic expressive form; (III) Applications to music.

I. THE MEANING AND FUNCTION OF ESSENTIC FORM

The ability of an expressive sound to communicate its quality can be easily lost by changing its dynamic character. One can study what kind of distortions will be most effective or least effective in destroying the essential quality. But little is known about what precisely makes for that quality in a particular dynamic expression that enables it to communicate itself with power and clarity. And practically nothing is understood about a central fact of musical meaning, of communicating power and of delight: how it comes about that a single phrase of music when performed by a great performing artist can move and transform the state of listeners, penetrate their defences and make them glad to be alive - while the performance of the same phrase by a lesser artist, only slightly different in form, does not have this power.

To what extent is this kind of enjoyment of 'livingness' (to use Susan Langer's term, 1953) based on biologic programs? Are there dynamic forms that have an innate meaning, forms that can act upon the nervous system not in arbitrary ways but like keys in a lock, activating thereby specific brain processes to which we react in some sense emotionally? Are we drawn, in composing and listening, to phrases that (among other things) evoke such biologically determined forms? We have answered these questions affirmatively (as have ethologists mainly for animal communication, eg. Eibl-Eibesfeldt, 1973, 1980) through experimental studies (Clynes, 1969, 1975, 1977) and present further evidence concerning this question in this chapter.

47

The dynamic expressive form, however, is only one way music communicates qualities and shades of feeling, although a very important one. Tone color (timbre), harmonic progression, and the subtle stretching or compression of intervals called expressive intonation by Casals (see also Makeig, this volume) are some others.

Tone color provides expressive quality directly on hearing, in contrast to the dynamic expressive form which necessarily has a beginning, middle and end, and takes a number of seconds. In a superior performance tone color and dynamic form complement one another, and subtle changes of timbre occur during the course of expression that enhance the communicative power. Little is known systematically about the expressive power of such timbre changes, and one must anticipate future research on this. In this chapter we shall be concerned with the expressive power of dynamic form, and in particular with the characteristic dynamic expressive forms of specific qualities which we have called essentic forms (Clynes 1968, 1969a).

The use of musical expression related to gesture, dance, and various forms of muscular effort, and breathing such as sighing, gasping, laughing has a long tradition in music theory (Cooke, 1959; Schweitzer, 1905). In the 17th and 18th centuries its study was called 'Affektenlehre' and composers and performers were instructed how to express various affects by specific shapes of phrase. New generations of composers re-invented ways of transducing analog patterns in their own authentic ways.

Leopold Mozart (1756) writes as follows:

It is to be seen, as clear as sunlight, that every effort must be made to put the player in the mood which reigns in the piece itself; in order thereby to penetrate the souls of the listeners and to excite their emotions... That bowing can greatly vary a phrase we have already become in some measure aware... The present chapter will convince us entirely that the bowing gives life to the notes; that it produces now a modest, now an impertinent, now a serious or playful tone, now coaxing, or grave and sublime, now a sad or merry melody; and is therefore the medium by the reasonable use of which we are able to rouse in the hearers the aforesaid emotions. I mean that this can be done if the composer makes a reasonable choice; if he selects melodies to match every emotion,... or if a well-skilled violinist himself possess sound judgment in the playing of, so to speak, quite unadorned notes with common sense, and if he strives to find the desired emotion...

In relation to these comments we can add that ambiguity itself in music is not a virtue, nor, except when deliberately made so, of the essence of music*. It should not be confused with richness of association, and power of suggestion, nor with experiencing at various levels. The clearer a musical expression is, the more powerfully does it act in scanning our whole being and experience for its likeness. And a clearly expressed musical idea is one that is true to its essentic form.

---

* Ambiguity of the score, generally a consequence of the limitation of

MUSICAL THOUGHT

Of course, it is not in the printed score that music lives. The score necessarily is merely a skeleton that needs to be fleshed out; in thought, or in performance. Even in thought, the details, the proportions and subtle inflections can and do exist; and as a musical mind reads the score the mind supplies these, just as in reading a line of poetry the words form their own music in the mind.

Thought provides the quality of sound, the timbre as well as the durations, rise and decay, and loudness envelopes of the musical elements. Further, it thinks the relationship of the sounds with each other (cf. Deutsch, Jackendoff and Lerdahl, this volume), forming phrases, periods and larger units in the mind, silently, yet ringing with inner sound.

We find that many such expressive units appear to correspond in temporal form to essentic forms, the biologic patterns of expressing specific emotions and qualities.

In a sense these essentic form units are elements of musical language. They are elements because they have meaning only when complete - a fraction of an essentic form is empty of its meaning.

The meaning of essentic form in music presents itself directly as the idea of its quality. One may fill oneself with that quality; or consider it; experience it as an element of an unfolding story; use it to scan memory associatively; or not hear its presence. Different musics, different composers and hearers relate differently to it at different times. Our aim is to obtain an understanding of how a quality of emotion is implicit in musical experience, of the points of view of the mind, and how this may be different for different music. And as we learn more about the properties and function of essentic forms, we also learn more about how music can move and enlighten us.

AMPLITUDE RELATIONSHIPS

Music is distinguished from most other sounds - much of the time - in that it uses steady frequencies. The amplitude of musical sound varies continuously as for natural sounds, but discrete frequency steps are used to allow relationship between tones to develop. (It is known that frequency should not be absolutely held constant during a musical tone - small fluctuations give it a quality through which we sense a living originator; see Hartmann, McAdams, this volume. But this is of the nature of a second order effect.) The relationship between musical tones on the basis of peak amplitudes is also known to contribute substantially to expressive communication, and to musical structure, although it is treated by theories of music with less discrimination. Varied and specific amplitude contours of individual tones, however, as an important and integral part of

---

notation, should be distinguished from ambiguity in a particular performance.

expressiveness, and their contribution to relationship, have been kept highly subordinate to that of frequency relationships. This is due to a considerable extent to the musical notation system where amplitude contours of individual tones are specified, if at all, only in crude terms (even in avant-garde music notation, generally). It is left to the performer to supply these forms. Performers on traditional real time instruments would be hard put to shape individual tone envelopes according to precise prescription - knowing yet well their pronounced effect on the quality of performance. Moreover, room acoustics would modify the results, so that to obtain a particular prescribed transient characteristic, the room transfer function would have to be taken into account. Such moment to moment estimations of amplitude are not feasible according to prescription, in the way the estimations of the slower changing moment to moment frequencies are possible. Yet the performing musician independently does in fact estimate just this, in shaping the sound envelope of tones and their relationship in musical phrases! He does this like a cyclist adjusts the bicycle from moment to moment not by prescription, but by 'feel', which represents feedback.

In music this 'feel' for the phrase as also the execution of a bicycle rider's movements has an idea as its guide. For the bicycle rider it is the direction and speed of where he wants to go - for the musician it is the meaningful form of the phrase. Both know when they depart from true form. The resolution with which this is possible depends on skill and discrimination - execution and perception - and both are subject to training. For the musician the form of each phrase, the form of each feeling, is chained to the next by the itinerary of the piece, posed together by the com-poser. The way in which the enchainment (in its 'ideal' form) takes place, as well as the choice of form for each phrase, is determined by the concept that the musician has of the particular piece he is performing (cf. Schnabel, 1942).

The concept springs from the total empathic knowledge of the musician, as does the concept of his dream, and guides the unfolding of the chain. It is thus also that the listener becomes more aware of a missing link in a faulty performance - sound without essentic form.

In shaping the detailed amplitude envelope of each single tone the performer has virtually complete freedom, within the capability of the instrument. We know that Casals, for example, used this freedom - as do great singers - creatively with especially high resolution; in the production of single tones with specific expressive functions in appropriate relationship with frequency and amplitude contours of neighboring and more distant tones.

Using electronic means of generating sounds with or without a computer one has the potential to control such shapes in great detail. Relatively little work is being done, however, to heighten and concentrate true artistic expression in this way - a way that in the past was sought by years of dedicated artistic concentration, study and application. Rather, efforts have been mainly spent in obtaining verisimilitudes to the sounds of existing instruments. (cf. Hartmann, this volume.) Yet it should be possible to obtain expressive performances of existing works that surpass most or all real time performances, not by imitating existing performances or by rule reproduction of musical scores, but by the artistic shaping of detail beyond that possible in real time performance - thus, like a painter or sculptor gaining time as an ally.

Theories of music concern themselves almost exclusively with relationship based on frequency - pitch - and not on amplitude. Amplitude within a phrase, in the theories, apart from general indications of overall loudness, is represented mainly by accent, two valued functions of weak - strong, modified at times by a short - long antithesis. How poorly this compares with the richness of musical possibilities provided by essentic forms!

SUGGESTIVE POWER AND EMOTIONAL CONTAGION OF ESSENTIC FORM

Words denoting specific emotions, like the word joy or anger for example, may induce the mind to imagine aspects of joy or of anger to a various and controllable extent. The dynamic expressive sound forms for specific emotions have more direct power to induce this; and this so to the extent to which they precisely express that particular dynamic shape, i.e. one can say, the more 'pure' and expression of joy or anger they are. In their pure form they require a special effort, a mental screen, to be ignored: it is difficult to remain unaffected in the presence of a true, authentic expression of grief, or of joy, as it indeed also can be in the presence of very sad or joyful music. Such gripping dynamic emotional 'words', or essentic forms, are a means of emotional contagion in daily life, which may be used with a sense of putative power by demagogues and commercial advertisers, or as mutual emotional communication between persons; or in an autocommunicative way as in music and art where the communicative power creates its own rewards.

Essentic form by itself appears to act directly to communicate its quality - no symbolic transformation is required, according to our theory and findings (cf. Langer, 1953, 1973; Piechowski, 1979; Ostwald, 1974).

As will be seen, there is increasing evidence that there appears to be a single common brain algorithm for the various sensory modes underlying the production and recognition of dynamic expression of specific qualities. (Dynamic qualities of expression should be distinguished from aspects of postural or facial expression, which have been extensively studied by Ekman and Friesen (1976) and others. Dynamic qualities in sound are communicated across the telephone for example, without any knowledge of facial expression or of posture, and of course, in music.)

Sundberg in this volume has summarized work (Fonagy, 1976; Fonagy and Magdics, 1963; and Kotlyar and Morozov, 1976) describing the relationship of vocal expression to affect, which is pertinent to this question.

In previous work (Clynes, 1969a, 1969b, 1970, 1973, 1975, 1977, 1980) functional characteristics of essentic form were delineated from extensive studies of expressive voluntary dynamic finger pressure, a uniquely measurable type of expression. The theory of emotion communication which evolved from these studies has direct application to the way music functions. A number of biologic principles of expressive communication that appear to hold were detailed. These properties may be stated as follows:

1.   Exclusivity
Communicating an emotion, or sentic state*, is a single-channel system; only one state can be expressed at any one time (although this can be a compound one).

2.   Equivalence
A sentic state may be expressed by any of a number of different motor output modalities.

3.   Coherence
Regardless of the particular motor output chosen to express a sentic state, its dynamic expression is governed by a brain program or algorithm specific for that state, called essentic form. There is innate coherence between the essentic form and the emotion state seeking expression (e.g. the feeling of a yawn and its expressive form).

4.   Complementarity
The production and recognition of essentic forms are governed by inherent data-processing programs of the central nervous system, biologically coordinated so that a precisely produced form is correspondingly recognized. The recognized form in turn generates a sentic state in the perceiver.

5.   Self-Generation
The intensity of a sentic state is increased, within limits, by the repeated, arrhythmic generation of essentic form.

6.   Generalized Emotion
Sentic states may be experienced and expressed (as in music) as pure qualities or identities, without reference to specific auxiliary relationships to generate or receive these qualities (e.g. one can experience and express joy or sadness in music without any external real life reason).

7.   Communicative Power as a Form Function
The power of essentic form in communicating and generating a sentic state is greater the more closely the form approaches the pure or ideal essentic form for that state.

Applying these principles to music, it is our endeavor to show empirically how a given musical phrase may portray in a specific transformation or musical realization the biologic dynamic form of a particular emotional expression, such as joy or grief for example, and that the more closely that form is approximated the more powerfully does the musical phrase convey the quality. Different means may be employed by different composers to construct these musical analogs, and learning their language involves becoming sensitive to their particular transform.

————————

* To avoid confusion between the term emotion and feeling, the latter often considered a less intense emotion, 'sentic state' is used to denote specific emotion regardless of its intensity (Plutchik and Kellerman, 1980).

It seems that in these transformations, certain essential features of the time-forms are preserved, and thus we are able to use the keys given to us by the composers in place of those fashioned by our biologic nature: gifts of nature become gifts of the muse.

II. EXPERIMENTAL INVESTIGATION OF THE LANGUAGE OF ESSENTIC FORM

We shall describe the following series of experimental studies of the nature of essentic forms as elements of communication. A number of these bear on the question of the common origin of essentic form in sound, touch movement form, and its visual recognition:

1.   Recognition of motor expression of essentic form.

2.   Recognition of visual dynamic essentic form.

3.   Method of finding the transformation of touch expression to sound expressing the same quality.

4.   Recognition of emotionally expressive sounds transformed from touch.

5.   Recognition by Central Australian Aborigines of emotionally expressive sounds generated from white urban touch.

6.   Recognition of combined visual and auditory essentic forms when auditory forms derived from touch are superimposed on the visual forms.

1. Recognition of Motor Expression of Essentic Form

The specific question asked in the first study described here is:

Would a person who was specifically taught these expressive finger pressure patterns of particular emotions as motor skills only, without being told that they had any relation to emotional expression, be able to identify them?

Transient pressure forms of the finger corresponding to the form for anger, hate, grief, love, sex, joy, reverence learned by imitation are carried out by the subject without being told that they express these qualities (having learnt to produce them by mechanical imitation): would a subject be able to identify them as expressing those emotions when given a choice?
The above emotions provide an opportunity for both gross and subtle differentiation (Osgood et al, 1975). Subjects could differentiate between anger and hate, and between love and reverence, as well as between the more contrasting qualities. The study could thus be helpful to elucidate aspects of the linguistics of dynamic expression.
It also seemed that the results would be likely to have application to expressive motion using other parts of the body instead of finger pressure.

Method. Fifty subjects - 25 male, 25 female, drawn from staff and students of the University of New South Wales and Sydney University, Australia, were taught the dynamic form of the finger pressure expression previously identified (Clynes, 1973, 1980) as corresponding to anger, hate, grief, love, sex, joy, reverence (see Fig. 1). Subjects had no previous knowledge of this work and related work involving these expressive forms.

Subjects were seated on a chair opposite the experimenter who was likewise seated, and a curtain was placed between the subject and the experimenter so that only the hand and forearm were visible. The subjects were instructed to place their hands on a finger rest touching it with the 3rd finger, and the experimenter did likewise, with his finger rest. The subjects were told the experiment was a test of motor skills in learning seven different motor patterns. They were asked to learn these patterns as well as possible, paying particular attention to its precise form.

The experimenter demonstrated each motor pattern in turn a number of times, asking the subject to imitate it as well as possible. Each pattern was given an identifying number and the subject was told the number. The experimenter ran through the sequence of seven emotions three or four times in the course of instruction, repeating each expression 10 to 15 times before going on to the next. The teaching process continued till the subject could perform any of the patterns on demand when asked to perform a given numbered pattern. 30 to 40 minutes of instruction were sufficient for subjects to acquire a good working knowledge of these motor patterns, judged visually by the experimenter and two observers assisting in the experiment.

The order of teaching the motor patterns was changed from subject to subject according to a Latin square design.

Subjects were then given a list of the names of seven emotions. They were instructed specifically as follows:

Think of these patterns you have learnt as expressions of emotions. Choose which ones would go with each of the names of emotions on this list. Also score a confidence level for each choice made, on a scale from 1 to 7 (7 being most confident). You may make any changes in your choices as you go along; and you can place each pattern in one category only.

Subjects were told that love was meant as motherly or brotherly love, and that reverence was meant as a feeling for nature or God, but not for a specific person.

Since the paradigm was a forced choice (one of 7 categories) this meant that if 6 choices were correct, the 7th one would be automatically correct; and also that if one mistake was made, two mistakes would necessarily ensue.

Since the finger rest was immobile (having only 0.5 mm of give with moderate pressure) all movements were on a small scale and were related to the production of pressure. For most expressions of emotions the finger remained in about the same position on the finger rest, but for love there was also a slight horizontal movement of approximately 0.5 cm, and for se:: a somewhat more pronounced horizontal movement, about 1 cm. Anger had a jabbing character, without shift of the tip of the finger. Hate had a twist

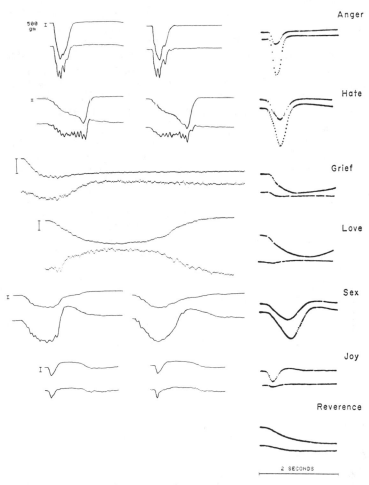

Fig. 1   Examples of sentograms of the essentic forms of emotions. The upper trace for each emotion is the vertical component of transient finger pressure; the lower trace is the horizontal component (shown at ~3x magnified pressure scale). On the <u>right</u>, each form is an average of fifty expressions, reproduced from Clynes, 1969. On the <u>left</u>, recent recordings of single expressions are shown. An approx. 10 Hz tremor is notable to a various extent in specific portions of the forms, particularly in the <u>horizontal</u> components of hate, anger, and sex. These and some other characteristic details are hidden by the averaging process; the latter however gives quite a good measure of the specific form for most emotions. Subtle differences in forms (e.g. between love and grief) may be as significant as more obvious ones. Coherence between the expressive form, and the quality of the feeling that can be producing it voluntarily, appears to be biologically given in terms of CNS programs.

of about 10° with the final part of the expression. Apart from this no twisting movements took place. The character of the expression of joy was first a short downward pressure followed by a rebound (bounce) which then 'floated' back down to the initial state (without at any time losing contact with the finger rest). Grief consisted of a collapse-like production of pressure in which the weight of the arm ended up resting passively on the tip of the finger, accompanied by a slight outward drop of the wrist. For reverence the pressure increased initially accompanied by a slight rise in the wrist, ending in a steady pressure and position. The total times for the expression of each emotion were approximately as follows: anger 0.7 sec, hate 1.6 sec, grief 9.0 sec, love 5.2 sec, joy 1.1 sec, reverence 9.8 sec. Structure of the specific dynamic forms was generally similar to those measured in Clynes (1977) (Fig. 1).

Results. Figure 2 shows the number of correct choices made by the 50 subjects. It may be seen that more subjects (15) scored all seven choices correct than any other score. 14 subjects scored five correct choices. thus 58% of subjects got all choices correct or only one pair of choices wrong. By the nature of the task a score of 4 means that three emotions are mutually confused. Three correct indicates confusion of two pairs, or of all four mutually. Chance expectancy of obtaining seven correct choices is 1 in 5040 and the chance of obtaining a score as good as or better than that obtained is greater than 1 in 10,000,000.

Comparing the actual distribution with that expected by chance, Chi square is > 20,000 and the level of significance p < .000001.

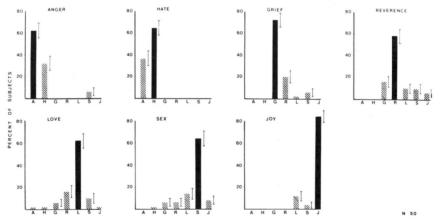

Fig. 2   Identification of expressive motor patterns using finger pressure taught as 'motor skills' without knowledge of what these patterns might represent. A H G R L S and J stand for the names of emotions. 'Correct' identification is shown in solid bars. Shaded bars show errors made. Thus the shaded bar in the graph for Anger shows the percentage of 50 subjects who chose Hate in place of Anger. Standard deviations are drawn with each bar (+). Note the high degree of correct choice.

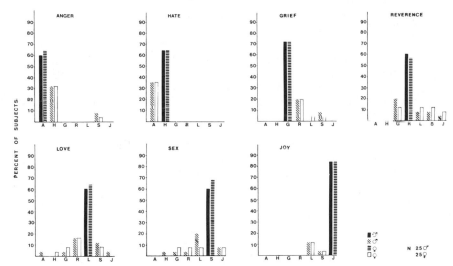

Fig.3   As in Fig. 2. Performance of 25 male and 25 female subjects -
             'correct' (black and horizontally shaded) and 'incorrect' (diagonally
             shaded and white). There was no significant difference in
             performance between males and females. The instructor was male.

The errors in identifying anger were predominantly mistaking it for
hate, and vice versa. No subjects mistook hate for anything else except
anger. Grief was mistaken for reverence by 20% of subjects, and joy for
love by 12%. The correct choice and these switched pairs of qualities
accounted for 94% of the results in anger, 100% for hate, 92% in grief and
96% in joy. The majority of errors were a mutually mistaken pair.

The least well identified were reverence and love, but even those
showed a statistically very high degree of correct identification (p<.0001).

A comparison of male and female scoring is given in Figure 3 - this
shows great similarity in performance throughout. The instructor was male
and yet no significant differences are evident in the scoring of males and
females on this test.

Confidence levels showed a trend of having lower scores when errors
were made. Of those subjects who made some errors (35), 28 subjects had
lower mean confidence levels when making incorrect choices than when
making correct choices, compared with only six who had higher scores.
The mean confidence level for each emotion, as well as the overall mean of
confidence levels (considering all emotions together) were lower for
incorrect choices than for correct choices.

In learning the motor patterns the subjects had opportunity for visual
recognition as well as the kinesthetic experience since they were copying a
motor pattern which they saw being executed. Thus the results imply
contributions both by the kinesthetic and visual sense.

The motor patterns associated with finger pressure expressions of these
seven emotions were correctly recognized by a majority of naive subjects
who learnt them without any hint of their supposed nature.

2. Recognition of Visual Dynamic Essentic Form

In the previous study learning the patterns also involved visual observation of the dynamic form. To what extent does visual perception, apart from the kinesthetic experience, contribute to the ability to recognize these qualities? In this study we ask the question: how well can these finger pressure expressions be recognized, just by visually observing the hand and forearm?

Method. The hand and portion of the forearm of the experimenter were shown as they produced the voluntary dynamic expressions of specific emotions through finger pressure, as described in the previous study. A film and videotape were made of ten expressions of each of the seven emotions, anger, hate, grief, love, sex, joy, reverence, showing only the hand up to the middle of the forearm. There was a 3 to 6 second pause between the completion of one expression and the beginning of the next, and a pause of about 20 seconds between each series of ten expressions. The finger remained in contact with the finger rest throughout. The seven groups of ten expressions were identified by a number from 1 to 7 on the screen. The duration of the film and videotape was 10 minutes. Subjects were shown the film and videotape twice during the measurement session, and scored only on the second viewing. Scoring consisted of identifying each group of expressions by writing a number from 1 to 7 opposite the names of the seven emotions (given in a different order from the presentation). As in the first study subjects were also asked to assign confidence ratings to each choice (from 1 to 7, 7 being the most confident). The 232 subjects (116 male and female) were students of the University of New South Wales, nurses and staff members in the 18 to 25 age group.

Results. Results show an even higher degree of recognition of the expressive qualities (Figs. 4, 5). The greatest number of errors were in discriminating between love and reverence. Anger and hate were confused less often than in the motor skill recognition experiment.

The high degree of recognition observed implies that

(1)   the expressive forms on the film were apparently quite well expressed;

(2)   That a common code prevails within this cultural group for their recognition.

The confidence ratings, moreover, show a highly significant correlation between 'correct' choice and confidence levels ($p < .001$). See Table 2.

Clearly, seeing the forearm and hand producing transient finger pressure in expressing these emotions was sufficient to characterize even the subtle differences between anger and hate, love and reverence, as well as the less subtle differences between sex and love.

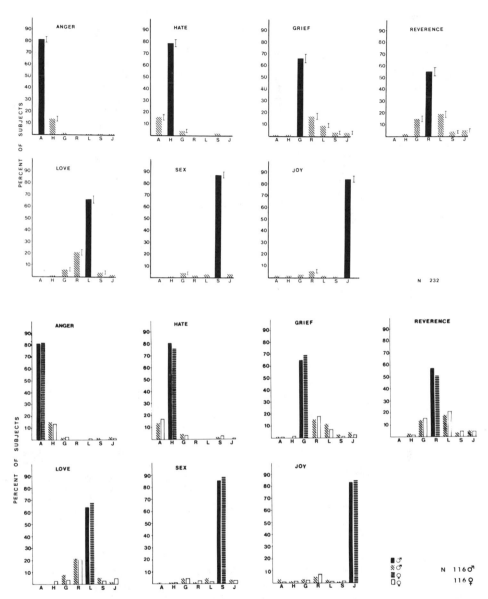

Fig. 4   Recognition by 232 subjects of visual expressions of finger pressure, seen on film (or videotape) showing the hand and forearm only. (As in Figs. 2 and 3). Note the even higher degree of correct recognition. Male and female results are highly similar, even in the distribution of errors.

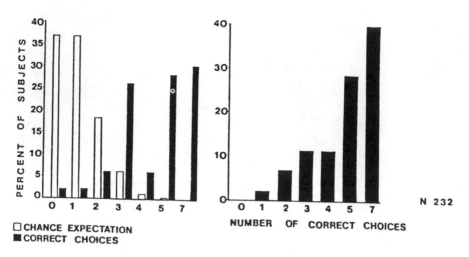

Number of Correct Choices							
	0	1	2	3	4	5	7
Chance Expectation	36.78%	36.81%	18.33%	6.25%	1.39%	0.42%	0.02%
Motor Expt (N 50)	2.0%	2.0%	6.0%	26.0%	6.0%	28.0%	30.0%
Visual Expt (N 232)	0.0%	2.1%	7.3%	10.8%	10.8%	28.9%	40.1%

Fig. 5   (Right) 'Correct' choices among seven emotions by the 232 subjects for the visual recognition of expressions of finger pressure from film (and videotape) as in Fig. 4. More subjects got all 7 'correct' than any other score. A score of 6 correct is not possible since one error necessarily leads to a second error as all 7 listed names of emotions have to be chosen. (Left) Similar tabulation for the motor expression recognition experiment 1 (see Figs. 3 and 4), together with chance expected score distribution (white). Table gives actual and chance expected scores.

Visual observations alone thus produced even better results than the motor skill experiment of Experiment 1. It is likely that the movements executed by the subjects in that study represented the specific dynamic form somewhat imperfectly, and this would have contributed to a slightly higher degree of confusion.*

---

* Analogously, it is easier to recognize a well shaped musical phrase than to play it!

TRANSFORMATION OF TOUCH EXPRESSION TO SOUND THAT EXPRESSES THE SAME QUALITIES

Having achieved a degree of confidence that expressive touch forms used in Experiments 1 and 2 do in fact communicate the intended qualities, we may now investigate whether expressive forms in touch and in sound share a common dynamic form.

In the production of essentic form muscular outputs are used in touch, in movement, and in the articulation of the voice. If the manner of using the motor outputs were programmed by a particular brain algorithm for a specific emotion, one might expect a degree of correspondence between these various outputs (Sundberg, this volume), and possibly in the representation by the visual artist of dynamic form as well.

This in itself however would not ensure that perceiving (quite a different process for each sensory mode) the form in the various sensory modes could lead to recognizing the same originating quality. That is, we need to investigate both the production transform, and its inverse, the perception transform for the various sensory modalities.

If we are to investigate the touch-to-sound transform, we can ask, what is the simplest representation in sound of the touch expressive form?

Of the acoustic parameters which can vary in the course of expressive sound (Williams and Stevens, 1972; Brown et al, 1974; Brown and Lambert, 1976; Scherer, 1979), we limit ourselves to vary only two, amplitude and frequency of a sinusoidal signal. (A recent extensive study by Dillon, 1979, documents that for the perceptual character of onset of sounds, these envelopes are the most critical.) We ask ourselves, can we discover what the constraints are on these parameters that will make the expressive quality of the expression similar to that of the touch expression? And how do the constraints differ for different emotions?

Method of Finding the Transforms

In order to arrive at answers, we chose a number of specific touch expressions, measured sentographically, which had been tape recorded using a PFM modulated data tape recorder. We used the forms of the vertical pressure component only, and did not use the angle of pressure information. The forms were played back repeatedly into an EAI analog computer. Outputs from the computer were fed as envelopes to a VCO and VCA. The output of the VCO was one of the inputs to the VCA. The output of the VCA was fed to a speaker.

Thus the analog computer outputs controlled the frequency and the amplitude envelopes of a sinusoidal sound.

The parameters were varied until the sound produced appeared to have the appropriate quality to the experimenter.

(a) Frequency Envelope

It was found that no change was required in the touch form to produce the frequency envelope, other than scaling. The nature of the scaling has special interest and will be described further.

(b) Amplitude Envelope

The amplitude envelope a priori has the constraint that the sound must begin from zero amplitude and end in zero amplitude - it must begin from silence and end in silence. The pressure trace of the touch form does not necessarily have the same constraint; it does not invariably start and end with zero pressure. To allow for that, the touch form was passed through an imperfect differentiator, of the form,

$$\frac{Ts}{1 + Ts}$$

where s is the Laplace transform and T a time constant. With a time constant of the order of 3 secs this transfer function allowed the faster portions of the form to be well preserved and provided a gradual extinction of the amplitude for the longer expressions of reverence and grief. This end-diminuendo was found to be an important requirement for the longer forms. T corresponds biologically to an adaptation time constant, with a similar transfer function.

With such an adaptation time constant for the long expressions, the touch form also provided the appropriate amplitude envelope.

For the shorter forms (e.g. anger, hate) the adaptation time constant made no noticeable difference, and the amplitude envelope too may be regarded to be largely the unchanged dynamic touch form.

Frequency Envelope Scaling

For the frequency envelope, one needed to choose

(1) The initial frequency - the frequency for zero pressure.
(2) The polarity of modulation: does increasing pressure cause the frequency to go up or down?
(3) The depth scaling - how much frequency deviation should correspond to the maximum pressure exerted? (modulation depth index)

It turned out that these choices were specific for each emotion.

Starting frequencies were chosen lower for anger and for hate, and a medium level for the other emotions. Choices are not critical. (The forms can be transposed over a moderately wide range.)

Polarity needed to be positive for anger, sex, joy, reverence, and negative for hate, grief and love (positive means increasing frequency for increasing (downward) finger pressure). Choices are highly critical.

Modulation depth was very different for different emotions:

Love had only a small modulation; the sound has a steady secure quality. The downward modulation range though quite small (less than a semitone) was essential to the expression of this quality.

Anger an upward modulation range of approximately a minor sixth.

Hate a very small downward modulation - the quality of its hard containment not permitting more modulation.

Grief a downward modulation range of about four semitones.

Sex an upward modulation range of approximately three semitones.

Table 1   Transforms of dynamic forms to sound forms of like expression, as amplitude and frequency modulated sinusoids (see Fig. 6): specific scaling parameters.

EMOTION	Sinusoidal base frequency Hz	FREQUENCY MODULATION Depth and Sign	AMPLITUDE MODULATION		
			Propor- tional	Diff. time constant τ (seconds)	A
ANGER	110	+ 59%	Prop.		
HATE	106	- 5%	Prop.	1.2	0.05
GRIEF	406	- 21%		3.1	1
LOVE	205	- 2.4%	Prop.		
SEX	228	+ 14%		1.0	
JOY	480	-, one octave: biphasic 20% down then 61% up	Prop.	0.32	0.20
REVERENCE	298	+ 9%		4.0	1

+ means : frequency↑as pressure↑   Differentiation time constant
- means : frequency↑as pressure↓   refers to transfer function
\ $\dfrac{A\tau s}{1+\tau s}$ for ampl. mod. where s is the Laplace Transform.

PARAMETERS FOR TRANSFORMING
TOUCH FORMS TO SOUND FORMS OF LIKE EXPRESSION

Joy   initially a downward modulation followed by a swing upwards, which then subsides to the starting point. Total perceived modulation range - one octave - a third down, an octave up and a sixth down.

Reverence an upward modulation of approximately 2 to 4 semitones.

Choices were rather critical: for joy it was especially important to have an octave range, neither more nor less, for it to have a joyful character, even with the appropriate dynamic form. For the other emotions the character is changed if the frequency deviation is altered. Thus a strong expression of anger can assume either a 'weakened' or 'hysterically exaggerated' character for example.

Table 1 shows the parameter values found to be optimal in this first formulation of the transforms.

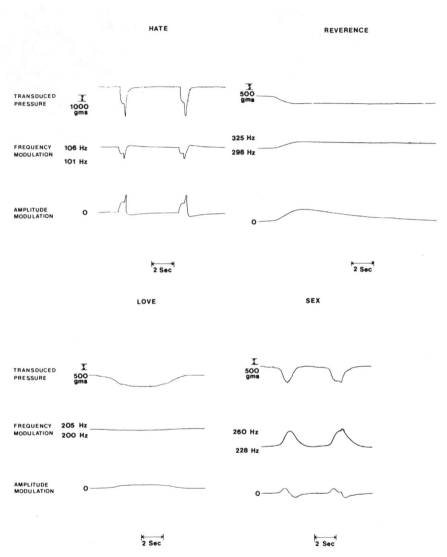

Fig. 6   Examples of transformation of expressive forms of touch to sound
            that expresses the same feeling. The top trace shows expressive
            finger pressure (vertical component); the middle the frequency
            modulation envelope; and the lower trace the amplitude

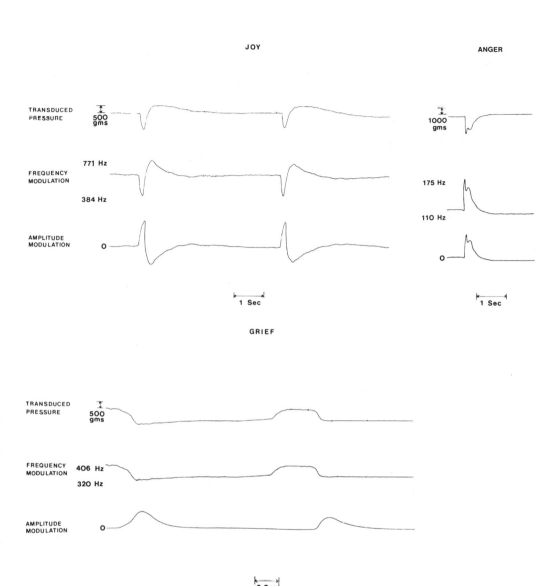

module envelope (time scale is doubled for Joy and Anger). The frequency envelope is the same as the pressure form apart from a vertical scale factor (except for Joy, where the wide dynamic range requires an approximately logarithmic scaling).

Amplitude Envelope Scaling

The scaling of the amplitude generally corresponded to the pressure amplitude used. This was corrected by appropriately increasing the sound amplitude for low starting frequencies and decreasing it for high starting frequencies in order to compensate for the hearing intensity curve. Anger, hate and joy were louder than grief and sex, and reverence and love were softer in that order. For joy, where the pressure curve is biphasic, the amplitude envelope was treated as if it were rectified about an initial zero axis, thus producing an effect that suited the joy expression well - giving somewhat of a 'jump' effect - although it was not resolved by the ear into two separate impulses, being too close together in time. (Fig. 6 and Table 1 show the transforms arrived at.)

3. Recognition of Emotionally Expressive Sounds Tranformed from Touch

Having transformed the selected touch expressions to our own satisfaction, they were tested on a number of subjects in an analogous manner to the visual expressions studied in the previous experiment. Subjects were presented ten expressions of each sound played through a single speaker. The entire sequence of sounds was ten minutes long and was repeated a second time. During the second presentation subjects were instructed to score themselves as in Experiment 2, that is, a forced choice of the seven emotions together with a confidence level for each choice. There were two groups of subjects, one consisting of 80 students and staff members of Massachusetts Institute of Technology and of the University of California, Berkeley, and the second group (109) were medical students of the University of New South Wales. Results (Fig. 7) showed that all emotions were well recognized except for love and reverence between which the choices were indiscriminate. The sounds for anger, grief and joy were chosen best.

Both the groups did equally well; there were no significant differences between them. The same held for males and females. Many of the errors tended to be between pairs - anger and hate, and love and reverence - however there was a considerably greater number of errors involving other pair combinations than in the visual experiment.

Confidence Levels

Confidence level ratings are given in Table 2. These showed that for the well recognized emotions the confidence levels were all significantly greater with the correct choice than with the incorrect choice. For love, however, which was not well distinguished from reverence, confidence levels for the correct choice were actually lower than for the incorrect choice.

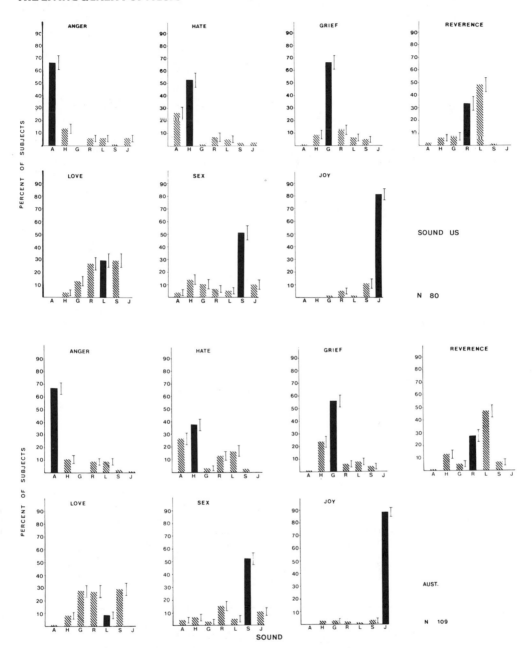

Fig. 7   Recognition of sound expressions transformed from expressive touch. This figure shows that recognition of emotions was high for all emotions except for Love and Reverence which were largely confused with each other. Top group - subjects were students of M.I.T. and University of California, Berkeley. Bottom group - subjects were medical students of the University of New South Wales.

Table 2   ANALYSIS OF CONFIDENCE RATINGS OF RECOGNITION

Emotion	Recognition <u>Correct</u>			Recognition <u>Incorrect</u>			Signif. of Difference between confidence ratings for correct and incorrect choice	
	N	Ave. Conf. Rat.	Stand. Dev.	N	Ave. Conf. Rat.	Stand. Dev.	t	p
1) VISUAL RECOGNITION EXPERIMENT							(t_{230})	
A	187	5.59	1.39	45	5.11	1.65	1.80	< .05
H	181	5.61	1.46	51	4.43	1.96	4.00	< .0005
G	156	4.51	1.67	76	4.45	1.70	0.25	.5
L	155	4.74	1.64	77	3.77	1.84	3.92	< .0005
S	200	5.65	1.64	32	3.97	1.80	4.95	< .0005
J	193	4.95	1.78	39	3.18	1.55	6.33	< .0005
R	129	4.04	1.95	103	4.02	1.70	0.08	.5
All Emotions	1201	5.08	1.73	423	4.13	1.92	(t_{1622}) 8.97	< .00005
2) SOUND RECOGNITION EXPERIMENT							(t_{187})	
A	126	4.93	1.51	63	4.22	1.70	2.80	< .005
H	83	3.54	1.57	106	3.76	1.69	-0.92	
G	114	5.16	1.60	74	3.80	1.70	5.46	< .0005
L	31	3.48	1.49	158	3.87	1.70	-1.30	
S	97	3.84	1.81	92	3.61	1.57	.93	.2
J	161	6.30	1.13	28	5.07	1.95	3.25	< .001
R	57	4.16	1.76	132	3.25	1.90	3.19	< .001
All Emotions	669	4.84	1.81	654	3.77	1.76	(t_{1321}) 10.91	< .00005

Thus for both groups the sound expressions transformed from the touch expressions of anger, hate, grief, sex and joy were well recognized, while the sound transformed from the touch expression for love was largely confused with that transformed from reverence.

4. Recognition of Emotionally Expressive Sounds Generated from White Urban Touch by Central Australian Aborigines

To test whether the ability to recognize these sounds obtained from touch expression was largely cultural, or based on biologic foundations, in the next study we tested these sounds with a group of Central Australian Aborigines. The Aboriginal settlement Yuendumu 200 miles north west of Alice Springs, a settlement of about 800 members of the Warlbiri Tribe, was selected for this study. The same equipment was used to present the sound as in Experiment 3. Sounds were presented to two or three subjects at a time. Males and females were tested separately, and both male and female interpreters were used as most Aboriginals spoke very little English. The names of the emotions were translated into the Warlbiri language, appropriately except possibly for reverence, the word for which was known mainly by the older members of the tribe. This Aboriginal tribe, in common with others, has the custom of initiating younger members of their group into the various mysteries of their tradition at appropriate ages. It became clear that the term reverence took on different significance to them at various stages of their life (not so differently as for many of us!) The subjects were highly attentive to the sounds and rather enjoyed the test. The expression of their faces intently listening to these qualites of sound was most memorable, and suggested a high degree of awareness; they appeared more attentive to the sounds than most urban concert-goers seem to be. As in all tests precautions were taken that the choices of one subject did not influence the choices of others. To simplify the procedure no confidence ratings were taken. For those subjects who could not write, the translator acted as scribe in scoring their choices.

These Aboriginal subjects live under indescribably squalid conditions. For the most part they have no electricity nor running water and live in three feet high hovels under inhuman conditions, for which no words seem adequate. Yet these ill-treated and despised people maintained a shining dignity and at times pride as they performed our tests, the beauty of some of their expressions leaving a deep impression on the experimenters. The expedition to this remote settlement was of eight days duration. Exposure to Western culture of this group was fairly limited, there was no television, no local radio station, hardly any short wave radio sets; but films are shown from time to time. Corroborees are held regularly. Only about one third of the children go to the local school where they are taught English.

The results of 40 Aboriginals, 20 male and 20 female, are shown in Fig. 8. It will be seen that they performed similarly to the other two groups, doing somewhat better with joy (88% correct). In place of the confusion between love and reverence there was a statistically significant switch between the two so that love was significantly recognized as reverence and

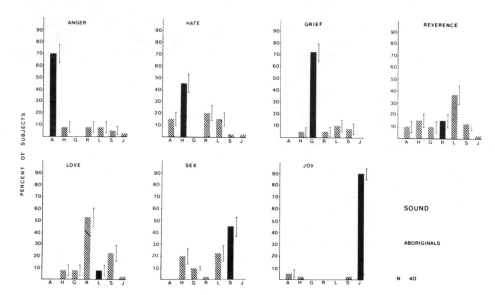

Fig. 8   Recognition by a group of 40 Australian Aborigines, of the
         Warlbiri Tribe in Central Australia, of sounds produced from
         white urban touch expression of finger pressure. Performance is
         very similar to the high recognition shown by the M.I.T. and
         Berkeley students, and by the medical students of the University
         of New South Wales. They did somewhat better than those groups
         in identifying Joy, Anger and Grief, although differences between
         groups were not statistically significant. Instead of confusing
         Reverence and Love they chose more clearly, but the choice was
         opposite of that intended: Love was chosen for Reverence, and
         vice versa. This may have been due to subtleties of translation.
         Differences between male and female scores were not significant
         in this group.

vice versa. Males and females also did equally well, with no statistically significant difference between their recognition scores.

Emotions were recognized as follows: Hate, p .00001; Anger, p .00001; Love, NS; Grief, p .00001; Joy, p .00001; Sex, p .00001; Reverence, NS.

The high degree of similarity in the degree of 'correct' recognition between the Aboriginal and the white student group despite their widely different educational and cultural backgrounds is surprising even in the context of our theory. The results show not only a statistically significant recognition but the relative percentages of errors are generally similar for the five best recognized emotions. Thus it seems that not only are the qualities of the sounds recognized but it would seem that certain of our sounds are more easily recognized than others across all groups. This advantage could be a property of the sounds regardless of their 'purity' i.e. the degree of faithfulness to a hypothetical idealized form; or it could be due to a better realization of some of the forms than others. The latter in turn could be due either to a better touch expression used originally in making the sounds or to a better realized transform for some emotions than for others. To test these questions further, two further studies were conducted.

5. Recognition of Combined Visual and Auditory Essentic Form: Auditory Forms Derived from Touch are Superimposed on the Visual Forms

In order to test the relative contributions to perceived quality by the transformed sound as compared with the touch expressions from which they were made, we superimposed transformed sound expression on the original film of the touch expressions, so that they occurred together with the touch expressions. In this way the subject could see and hear the expressions simultaneously. The film was presented to a group of 75 subjects who scored the test as in the previous studies. The results are shown in Fig. 9 . Clearly, for those emotions which were best recognized separately in the visual presentation and as sound transform, the presentation of both together enhanced the result. Thus for joy we now obtained 100% 'correct' recognition. For love, however, the addition of the sound resulted in a poorer result than had the visual expression alone in Experiment 2. Other emotions showed a result intermediate between the two extremes. Thus it seems likely that our sound transform for love and reverence were not sufficiently distinctive and gave rise to greater confusion. We are thus induced to try to obtain a better transform which could be tested further.

Tests with what is believed to be an improved version are being conducted presently.

By iterating this process, together with a gradually improved sculpturing of the forms independently of the touch expression, using the digital computer, we hope to gradually come nearer to realizing essentic forms of very considerable purity and communicative power. We should expect this gradual progress not to be uniform for all the emotions studied. At present we appear to be nearest for joy, anger and grief. It will be

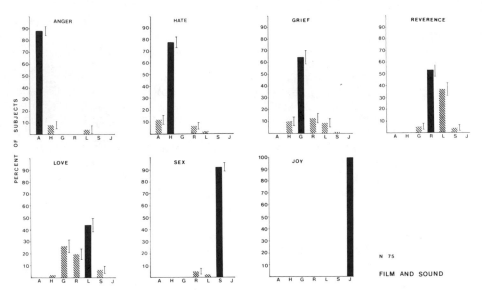

Fig. 9   Recognition for combined visual and sound expression: sounds created from touch expression were superimposed synchronously on the filmed touch expressions. The film was the same as that used in Experiment 2 (Figs. 4 and 5). Combined presentation increased recognition scores further for emotions for which the sound recognition was highest. For Reverence and Love, however, the sounds caused greater confusion. Joy was recognized correctly by 100% of the 75 subjects.

intriguing to see whether by improving the other forms we can obtain a more even recognition score.

III. APPLICATIONS TO MUSIC

Having described some new experiments concerned with the nature of essentic forms, and aspects of their function in Section II, we may now consider how this function is manifest in music. We shall consider the following:

1.   The action of essentic form on the formation of melodies.
2.   Recording of essentic form as a method of analysis of a composition.

We shall briefly summarize:

3.   Sentographic recording as a means of improvising.
4.   Performing music and awareness of essentic form.
5.   Essentic form as a tool for the modern composer.

THE ACTION OF ESSENTIC FORM ON THE FORMATION OF MELODIES

All the expressive sounds we have considered so far display a continuously varying frequency. Melodies however largely use stepwise changing frequencies. How are the two related?

Although the frequency moves in discrete steps in a melody the same is
not generally required of the amplitude envelope. Consider what happens
when we convert the essentic form for the frequency envelope into discrete
steps, while retaining the continuous amplitude envelope. A computer
program to do this has been created.* Fig. 10 shows an example of the
essentic form of grief converted to melody whose frequency outline is
derived from the essentic form by the simple constraint of permitting only
the semitones of a 12 tone scale to be sounded. Each successive tone is
begun when the frequency envelope reaches the frequency of that particular
tone. Such a melody derived from the grief expression does indeed sound sad.
The time values of the individual tones follow the outline of the essentic
form so that they are shorter with increased slope and longer when it
flattens out. Alternate melodic expressions may be obtained by not
permitting every semitone but only other selected tone steps (Table 3.)
Depending on the size of the steps chosen the duration of the tones will be
different in order to correspond to the contour of the essentic form. There
is thus a trade-off between the timing of tones and the interval choice for
the melodic expression of a given essentic form. Given this relationship
alternate melodic versions (using the same amplitude contour) are
compatible with and suggest different harmonic implications. Thus the
theory predicts how, depending on the steps used melodically, the temporal
form of the melody is shaped differently in order to express similar quality.
The above example is shown for a rather slow essentic form.** Forms
like anger or joy which have a rapid rate of change of frequency exhibit the
property that if small steps are used to delineate the melodic outline these
tend to sound almost like continuously changing frequencies or glissandos
(or portamento as it is called in singing). Such 'rolling' effects are often
portrayed in music by fast groups of notes as in ornaments, 'grunt-like'
sounds in basses and so on. A single interval combined with a rapid slide
can often adequately represent such an expression.

When a number of melodic tones succeed one another fairly rapidly one
should consider that initially the new frequency step provides an illusion of
increased loudness. This effect can be compensated for by providing a
slight appropriate initial drop in amplitude at the beginning of each new
frequency

---

*   The program permits us also to delay the sounding of the new tone by an
    amount to compensate for the auditory property that a frequency slide
    of finite size has occured in recognizing an initial frequency with a
    sliding frequency.
** The amplitude envelope is not always unimodal. Thus in joy, for
    example, it has a double peak, the first corresponding to the lowest
    frequencies and the second to the highest.

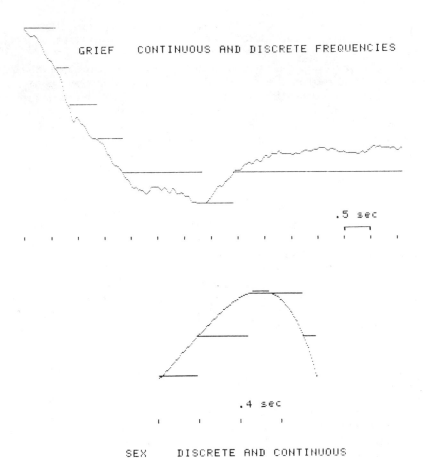

Fig. 10   'Continuous' and 'discrete' frequency contours for a Grief sound
           expression. The discrete steps are semitones that fit the contour
           of the continuous form. Other discrete step combinations are
           derived likewise from the continous form. Durations of the
           melodic tones in the 'discrete' versions are governed by the shape
           of the continuous form.   The set of all 28 possible melodic
           combinations (eliminating 3 combinations using the first two
           semitone steps or less where these semitones steps fall very close
           to the beginning of the form, making them in effect appogiaturas)
           are shown in Table 3.   A similar illustration is shown for
           continuous and discrete frequency contours of sexually expressive
           sounds (at a different time scale), (generated by computer, and
           has no tremor, which is found prominently in single expressions of
           hate, grief and sex).

Table 3   Set of 28 alternate melodies expressing Grief (shown in the range from C to G). Each melody is one horizontal row. The numbers give the timings of the tones listed at the head of the column. These melodies constitute all the possible combinations of scale steps derived from the essentic form of Grief, as given in Fig. 10. The amplitude envelope contour needs to be that of Grief for all these melodies, as shown in Fig. 6. They can be transposed over a range of about an octave without marked loss of expressive quality.

c^1	b	b flat	a	a flat	g	a flat
0.81	0.23	0.53	0.48	1.49	0.58	3.88
0.81	0.23	0.53	0.48	5.94		
0.81	0.23	0.53	1.97		4.45	
0.81	0.23	1.02		1.49	0.58	3.88
0.81	0.77		0.48	1.49	0.58	3.88
1.05		0.53	0.48	1.49	0.58	3.88
0.81	0.23	0.53	6.42			
0.81	0.23	1.02		5.94		
0.81	0.23	2.50			4.45	
0.81	0.77		0.48	5.94		
0.81	0.77		1.97		4.45	
0.81	1.25			1.49	0.58	3.88
1.05		0.53	0.48	5.94		
1.05		0.53	1.97		4.45	
1.05		1.02		1.49	0.58	3.88
1.58			0.48	1.49	0.58	3.88
0.81	0.77		6.42			
0.81	1.25			5.94		
0.81	2.73				4.45	
1.05		0.53	6.42			
1.05		1.02		5.94		
1.05		2.50			4.45	
1.58			0.48	5.94		
1.58			1.97		4.45	
2.06				1.49	0.58	3.88
1.58			6.42			
2.06				5.94		
3.55					4.45	

step, within the general contour of the amplitude envelope. (This compensates for loudness adaptation at constant frequency.)

Further considerations of staccato versus legato and the many shades in between relate also to the rhythmic functions (see Clynes and Walker, this volume; and Gabrielsson, 1979) and will need to be considered at a future stage.

SENTIC ANALYSIS OF MUSICAL COMPOSITIONS

The analysis of musical structures has been largely carried out by methods like those developed by Schenker (1935) and their elaborations, for tonal music. Such methods do not address themselves to emotional significance and the communication of qualities. They are concerned only with relationships between tones of the score and not their detailed execution other than to emphasize the relative importance of certain tones within the structure. (In performace one would in some manner emphasize the structurally important tones; the analysis says nothing however about the manner of the emphasis.) Schenkerian analysis also is largely time independent: it does not concern itself with the precise timing of phrase components or rhythmic functions. It can deal neither with the vast number of shades of expression made possible through dynamic form and their various qualities, nor with the range of rhythmic energies.

Similarly for atonal, serial music, analysis concerns itself with serial structural aspects of the work.

Sentic analysis consists of recording the essentic forms of the work studied along with its pulse (for aspects of the pulse see Clynes and Walker, this volume). Like the other forms of analysis cited sentic analysis makes use of the printed score, and is not an analysis of an existing performance. It does, however, effectively include the full musical thought of the person carrying out the analysis, unlike Schenkerian analysis. He or she is required to think the music in real time and to record sentographically the essentic forms and pulse of the music as it unfolds. This is done by expressing simultaneously on two sentographs; with the left hand (for right-handed subjects) the essentic form, with the right hand, the pulse.

Two examples of expressive phrases are shown in Fig. 11. The opening of Ballade No 3 in A flat, Op. 47 by Chopin, and the other from Mozart's Sonata in C Minor, K.457. In the first example the left hand expression comprises longing and ecstasy, in the second example qualities of hope and love. The expressive forms recorded are more precisely expressive than the words we can use to describe them. A more detailed analysis of this and other examples is to be found in Clynes, 1977, Appendix III.

IMPROVISATION AND SENTOGRAPHIC RECORDING

An interesting application consists of using two sentographs for improvisation of music thought mentally, expressing the musical pulse with

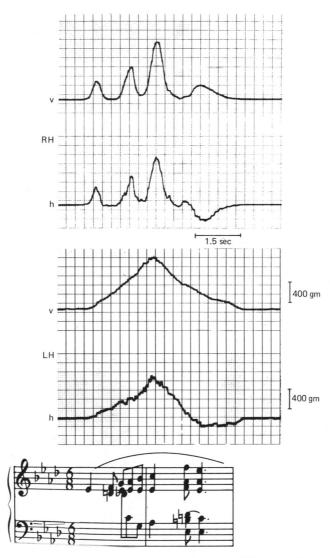

Fig. 11a Chopin, Ballade No. 3 in A Flat Op.47. Sentic analysis of a
musical phrase showing both the dynamic expressive forms (LH),
and pulse (RH); obtained by using two Sentographs, each providing
vertical and horizontal components. The shapes of the forms
correspond to the nuances of expressed feeling.

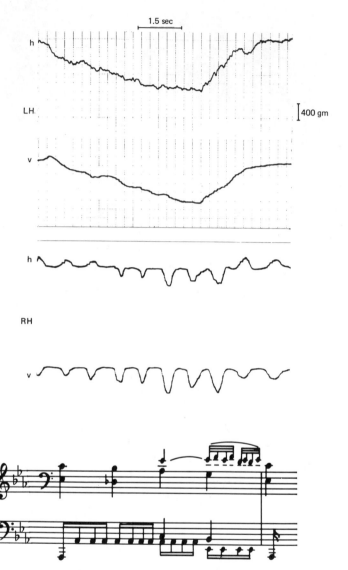

Fig 11b   Mozart, Sonata in C Minor K.457, 2nd Movement. Sentic analysis
           of a musical phrase showing both the dynamic expressive forms
           (LH), and pulse (RH); obtained by using two Sentographs, each
           providing vertical and horizontal components. The shapes of the
           forms correspond to the nuances of expressed feeling.

the right hand and the essentic forms with the left hand, as in sentic music analysis. The mental flow of musical ideas can be sustained naturally in this way and the subject records his own pulse form. (See Clynes and Walker, this volume, for pulse form analysis.) In this way a musician is able to record his own pulse form and to become aware of what it feels like to him, and to experience the significance of being true to one's own pulse form. The spontaneous flow of musical ideas is enhanced under the guidance of one's own pulse form.

APPLICATIONS TO MUSIC PERFORMANCE

A natural application of the study of essentic forms is to the performance of music. Apart from the choice of particular essentic forms constituting a particular interpretation (with freedom of choice of myriad different combinations and shades of forms) the following significant functions result from the awareness by the performer of essentic form. (1) The duration of each essentic form determines the number of expressive entities with which the performer is concerned in a given phrase, or piece of music. Being aware of this prevents trying to express inappropriately with too many separate expressions. (2) The enchainment of essentic forms provides natural continuity of meaningful music realization. (3) Being faithful to a particular essentic form assures musical communication: the performer can have confidence that his meaning is understandable, and temptation for exaggeration is in effect largely eliminated.

COMPOSING WITH ESSENTIC FORMS

Since it is now possible to create essentic forms through computer programs both with continuous and discrete frequency, the composer now has at his disposal a powerful method of evoking various emotions in his discourse and to combine them in ways that he chooses. We have recently developed a computer program which composes pieces based on essentic forms. Considering essentic forms as elements of language, creating poetic statements in sound takes on a new aspect, one which liberates composers and also potentially gives them greater responsibilities and scope. They can be free from the considerations of musical notation and yet not without guiding order - giving the sound proportions of living eloquence. This liberation can also be of value to many who study music in various degrees of seriousness.

Such a computer program makes it possible to provide true expressive forms in a similar way by which harmonies, timbres and other musical parameters are readily formed by digital or analog synthesizers. The dangers of the manipulative use of this should be surpassed by the benefits that will accrue as the user is able to experience for himself the many shades and immense range of feeling that are possible by the subtle realization of expressive dynamic form. He does not produce each form directly himself as with traditional instruments. But in choosing like a painter who mixes colors, his sense of discrimination is sharpened, he can make choices which may prove to be artistic, selecting and combining essentic forms to create musical pieces.

SUMMARY

Common brain programs of biological time forms of expression called 'essentic forms' underlie specific dynamic expressive communication in various sensory modes, it is suggested, both in production and recognition of these elements of language. Experiments in tactile (motoric), sound and visual modes bearing on this are described. A transform that converts a dynamic touch expression form to a sound form of the same expressive quality has been found. The sound transform was tested with 304 subjects, including 40 Central Australian Aborigines of the Warlbiri Tribe, and its validity confirmed (except for confusion between sound expression of love and reverence). The function of essentic form is illustrated in music: (1) In the formation of melodies. The theory predicts how the essentic form can generate a finite set of melodies expressing similar quality: specifically how duration and melodic interval of components are mutually dependent within this set. (2) How particular amplitude contours in music relate to essentic form. (3) As a novel means of music analysis. (4) As a guiding influence in composition, improvisation and performance. A central theme underlying the investigation is a continuing attempt to discover through successive approximation the clearest dynamic expression of specific qualities, a goal shared with artistic aspiration.

ACKNOWLEDGMENT

The authors express their gratitude to Janice Walker for her extensive assistance and field work in the study involving Aboriginal Australians. Thanks are also due to Mark Dobkin and David Terrazas for assistance in the motor and visual perception experiments, to Mark Dobkin for discussions and assistance with preliminary trials involving the sound transform experiments, to Brian McMahon for assistance with analysis of the data and to Dorothy Capelletto for much assistance with the manuscript. This work was aided in part by a grant from the Commonwealth Education Research and Development Committee of Australia.

REFERENCES

Brown, B.L., and Lambert, W.E., 1976, A cross-cultural study of social status makers in speech, Can.J.Behav.Sci./Rev.Can.Sci.Comp., 8(1):
Brown, B.L., Strong, W.J., and Rencher, A.C., 1974, Fiftyfour voices from two: the effects of simultaneous manipulations of rate, mean fundamental frequency, and variance of fundamental frequency on rating of personality from speech, J.Acoust.Soc.Am., 55(2):

Clynes, M., 1968, Essentic form-aspects of control, function and measurement, Proceedings of 29th Annual Conference of Engineering in Medicine and Biology, Houston, Texas.

Clynes, M., 1969a, Towards a theory of Man: Precision of essentic form in living communication, in: "Information Processing in the Nervous System," K.N. Leibovic, and J.C.Eccles, eds., Springer, New York.

Clynes, M., 1969b, Cybernetic implications of rein control in perceptual and conceptual organization, in: "Rein Control, Or Unidirectional Rate Sensitivity, A Fundamental Dynamic and Organizing Function in Biology, "M.Clynes, ed., Annals N.Y.Acad.Sci., 156(2):629-671

Clynes, M., 1970, Toward a view of Man, in: "Biomedical Engineering Systems, "M.Clynes, and J.H.Milsum, eds., McGraw-Hill Book Co., New York.

Clynes, M., 1973, Sentography: Dynamic forms of communication of emotion and qualities, Computers in Biol.and Med., 3: 119-130.

Clynes, M., 1975, Communications and generation of emotion through essentic form, in: "Emotions - Their Parameters and Measurement," L.Levi, ed., Raven Press, New York.

Clynes, M., 1977, "Sentics: The Touch of Emotions," Doubleday/Anchor, New York.

Clynes, M., 1980, The communication of emotion: Theory of sentics, in: "Theories of Emotion," R.Plutchik, and H.Kellerman, eds., Academic Press, New York.

Cooke, D., 1959, "The Language of Music," Oxford University Press, London and New York.

Dillon, H.A., 1979, "The Perception of Musical Transients," Doct.thesis, University of New South Wales, Sydney.

Eibl-Eibesfeldt, I., 1973, The expressive behavior of the deaf-and-blind born, in: "Social Communication and Movement," M.von Cranach, and I.Vine, eds., Academic Press, New York.

Eibl-Eibesfeldt, I., 1980, Strategies of social interaction, in "Theories of Emotion," R.Plutchik, and H.Kellerman, eds., Academic Press, New York.

Ekman, P., and Friesen, W.V., 1976, Measuring facial movement, Environ. Psychol./Non-Verb.Behav., 1(1):

Ekman, P., Friesen, W.V., and Scherer, K.R., 1976, Body movement and voice pitch in deceptive interaction, Semiotica, 16:23-27.

Fonágy, I., and Magdics, K., 1963, Emotional patterns in intonation and music, Phonetik, 16:293-326.

Fonágy, I., 1976, la mimique buccale, Phonetica, 33:31-44.

Gabrielsson, A., 1979, Experimental research on rhythm, Human.Assoc.Rev., 30:69-92.

Kotlyar, G.M., and Morozov, V.P., 1976, Acoustical correlates of the emotional content of vocalized speech, Sov.Phys.Acoust., 22:208-211.

Langer, S.K., 1953, "Feeling and Form: A Theory of Art Developed from Philosophy in a New Key," Routledge & Kegan Paul, London.

Langer, S.K., 1973, "Mind: An Essay on Human Feeling, " Vol.2, Johns Hopkins University Press, Baltimore.

Mozart, L., 1756, Violinschule, "A Treatise on the Fundamental Principles of Violin Playing," trans. E.Knocker, 1948, Oxford University Press, London.

Osgood, C.E., May, W.H., and Miron, M.S, 1975, "Cross-Cultural Universals of Affective Meaning," University of Illinois Press, Urbana.

Ostwald, P.F., and Peltzman, P., 1974, The cry of the human infant, Sci.Am. (March)

Piechowski, M.M., 1981. The logical and the empirical form of feeling, J. of Aesthetic Education. Vol.15, No 1, pp 31-53.

PLutchik, R., and Kellerman, H., eds., 1980, "Theories of Emotion," Academic Press, New York and London.

Schenker, H., 1935, "Der Freie Satz," Universal Edition, Vienna.

Scherer, K.R., 1979, Non-linguistic vocal indicators of emotion and psychopathology, in "Emotions in Personality and Psychopathology". C.E.Izard, ed., Plenum Press, New York.

Schnabel, A., 1942, "Music and the Line of Most Resistance," Princeton University Press, Princeton, N.J.

Schweitzer, A., 1905, "J.S. Bach, le poète," Breitkopf & Hartel, Leipzig.

Williams, C.E., and Stevens, K.N., 1972, Emotions and speech: Some acoustic correlates, J.Acoust.Soc.Am., 52:1238-1250.

Chapter V

A GRAMMATICAL PARALLEL BETWEEN MUSIC AND LANGUAGE

Ray Jackendoff[1] and Fred Lerdahl[2]

[1]*Brandeis University*
 Waltham, Massachusetts, USA
[2]*Department of Music*
 Columbia University
 New York, N.Y., USA

1. INTRODUCTION TO GENERATIVE MUSIC THEORY

For a number of years we have been developing a formal theory of tonal music, based on the goals and methodology of generative linguistics. Without any intention on our part, one aspect of our theory has proved to be closely analogous to some recent developments in phonological theory. In this paper we will describe the parallelism.

The goal of a generative music theory is to provide an account of the musical intuitions of a listener experienced in a particular tonal musical idiom. By 'musical intuitions' we mean the unconscious principles by which the listener experienced in the idiom organizes what he hears, beyond simple registering of such surface features as pitch, attack, duration, volume and timbre. It should be made clear that we take musical intuitions as in large part distinct from anything the listener has been taught formally (though formal training may enhance musical intuition). The theory is thus explicitly psychological, in that it is concerned not with the organization of music in and of itself, but with the organization that the listener is capable of hearing.

Two sorts of questions must be addressed by the theory. First, what sorts of musical organization do listeners hear? An attempt to answer this question takes the form of what might be called an ANALYTIC SYSTEM (for instance, numbering chords as in traditional harmony, assigning poetic feet to musical rhythms as Cooper and Meyer, 1960, or giving a layered 'Schenkerian' analysis). In common with other music-theoretic traditions, we want to develop an analytic system which is capable of expressing what the listener hears.

But our theory must address a second question which is not explicitly a part of other traditions: if an analysis models what organization the listener hears, what is it that the listener knows that has enabled him to arrive at this organization? To answer this question, we have tried to develop an explicit formal MUSICAL GRAMMAR that models the listener's connection between the presented musical surface and the organization or organizations he attributes to the music. The grammar takes the form of a SYSTEM OF RULES which assigns analyses to pieces. By contrast, previous approaches have left it to the analyst's intuition to decide how to fit an analysis to a particular piece.

Thus a theory of musical intuition has at least two parts, an analytic system and a formal grammar. However, still another question must be asked. To what extent is the experienced listener's knowledge of a musical idiom learned, and to what extent is it part of an innate musical capacity or general cognitive capacity? A formal theory of musical idioms, viewed individually and as a body, will make possible substantive hypotheses about those aspects of musical understanding that are innate.

Readers at all acquainted with generative linguistics (for general expositions, see Chomsky, 1965, 1972, 1975) will recognize the similarity of our research goals to those for the study of language. Linguistic theory is an attempt to describe the linguistic intuitions of a native speaker of a human language. GENERATIVE linguistics seeks this description in terms of a formal grammar which models the speaker's knowledge of his language. Because many people have thought of using generative linguistics as a model for music theory, it is worth pointing out what we take to be the significant parallel: the combination of psychological concerns and the formal nature of the theory. Formalism alone is to us uninteresting, except in so far as it serves to express psychologically interesting generalizations and to make empirical issues more precise.

Previous attempts to apply linguistic methodology to music have proven relatively uninteresting because they attempt a more or less literal translation of linguistic theory into musical terms, for instance looking for musical parts of speech, or deep structures, or transformations, or semantics. (The most prominent example of such work is Bernstein, 1976. While we disagree with most of the specifics of Bernstein's work, we concur in our overall goals. See Jackendoff, 1977, for further discussion of Berstein.) We believe that a generative music theory, beyond the general principles stated above, must be sought in purely musical terms, uninfected by the substance of linguistic theory. If substantive parallels between the two theories emerge (as they in fact have in a number of areas), they are to be regarded as simply an unexpected bonus: we are concerned above all with developing a theory of MUSIC.

Another mistake made in some previous attempts to apply generative liguistics to music is to regard a linguistic grammar as a device to manufacture grammatical sentences. Under this interpretation, a musical grammar should be an algorithm that composes pieces of music. (An example of this approach is Sundberg and Lindblom, 1976.) In stating his criticisms and apprehensions of a music theory based on generative linguistics, Babbitt (1972) has such a conception in mind. However, it was pointed out by Chomsky and Miller (1963), and it has been an unquestioned assumption of actual research in linguistics, that what is really of interest in a generative grammar is the structure it assigns to sentences, not which strings of words are or are not grammatical sentences. Our theory of music is therefore based on structural considerations; it reflects the importance of structure by concerning itself not with the composition of pieces but with assigning structures to already existing pieces.

This view of grammar leads to a crucial difference between the research paradigms of linguistics and music theory, revealing a way in which music is not very much like language at all. In a linguistic grammar, perhaps the most important distinction is grammaticality - whether or not a given string of words is a sentence of the language in question. A subsidiary distinction is ambiguity: whether a given string is assigned two or more structures with different meanings. In music, on the other hand, grammaticality per se plays a far less important role, since almost any passage of music is potentially vastly ambiguous - that is, it is much easier to construe music in a multiplicity of ways. The reason for this is that music is not tied down to specific meanings and functions as language is. In a sense, music is pure structure, to be 'played with' within certain bounds. Thus the interesting musical issues usually concern what is the most coherent or 'preferred' way to hear a passage. Musical grammar must be able to express these preferences among interpretations, a function that is largely absent from generative linguistic theory.

Our music theory specifically addresses those aspects of musical structure that are hierarchical in nature. It is therefore not directly concerned with such undoubtedly important matters as thematic development, although these often play a role in the analysis. We have identified four distinct hierarchical structures which are simultaneously imposed on a passage of music to form its structural description (or analysis): grouping structure, metrical structure, time-span reduction, and prolongational reduction. Briefly, grouping structure describes the segmentation of the music into motives, phrases and sections. Metrical structure describes the regular, hierarchical pattern of beats which the listener attributes to the music. The two reductions ascribe degrees of relative importance to all the pitch-events (notes or chords) of the passage, but with respect to different criteria. In time-span reduction, importance is measured with respect to the other pitch-events in the same time-span, where a time-span is a rhythmic unit constructed out of an interaction of grouping and metrical structure. Prolongational reduction also develops a hierarchy of pitch stability, but in rather different terms. It emphasizes the connections among pitch-events, establishing their continuity and pro- gression, their movement toward tension or relaxation. It is the component of our theory most closely corresponding to a Schenkerian analysis.

The structure of greatest interest for the present paper is the time-span reduction. It turns out that the formalism we have employed to express the time-span reduction is a notational variant of a notation in linguistics for a hierarchical phonological structure called PROSODIC STRUCTURE. The next section will demonstrate this relationship. We will then ask whether the relationship is an accident, or if it rests on a principled basis. In an effort to answer this question, we will explore in turn the theory of time-span reduction and the theory of prosodic structure.

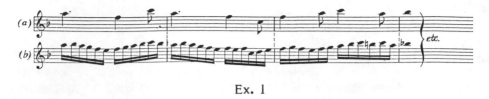

Ex. 1

2.   TIME-SPAN REDUCTION AND PROSODIC STRUCTURE

2.1   Time-span Reduction

It is an obvious intuition about music that some musical passages can be heard as ornamented versions, or ELABORATIONS, of others. For instance, despite the surface differences in pitches and durations between (a) and (b) in Ex. 1, both passages from the Finale of Beethoven's "Pastoral" Symphony, the listener has no difficulty in recognizing (b) as an elaboration of (a), the main theme. The inverse of elaboration also occurs in music, for example when a popular song is played in 'stop-time' to accompany a tap dancer. Despite the fact that the 'stop-time' version has fewer notes in it, and the notes are in different rhythmic relationships, the listener readily accepts it as a version of the song, one in which relatively ornamental events have been omitted, leaving a 'skeleton' or reduction of more essential parts.

More complex is the situation where two or more passages are both heard as elaborations of an abstract structure that is never overtly stated. Bach's "Goldberg Variations" are a particularly magnificent example of this kind of organization. How is the listener able to recognize, beneath the seemingly infinite variety of the musical surface, that the Aria and 30 variations are all variations of one another? Why do they not sound like 31 separate pieces? The answer is that the listener relates them all, more or less unconsciously, to an abstract "skeleton" consisting of important events common to them all.

Such relationships are needed not just for the analysis of pre-existing music. In any musical tradition that involves improvisation on a given subject (for example, jazz and raga), the performer must actively employ knowledge of principles of ornamentation and variation in order to produce a coherent improvisation.

It is worth mentioning here that psychologists have for a long time recognized transposition of a musical passage as a way of changing a musical surface that preserves recognizability; they took this as important evidence for a mental representation that involves not just a list of pitches, but an abstract representation in which relations among pitches are more important that the actual pitches themselves. However, for whatever reasons, little seems to have been done within psychology to extend these observations to any great extent (though a certain degree of generalization Dowling, 1978). The examples just presented are exactly the sort that should be of interest in this regard, for ornamentation, variation and simplification provide evidence for musical cognition of relationships not just between adjacent pitch-events, but at potentially large distances between structurally important events. Thus the study of musical reductions and the processes producing them from musical surfaces is of great value in extending to a richer class of cases what has long been acknowledged as a psychologically important phenomenon.

Music theorists have of course been aware of principles of ornamentation for hundreds of years. However, it was the insight of the

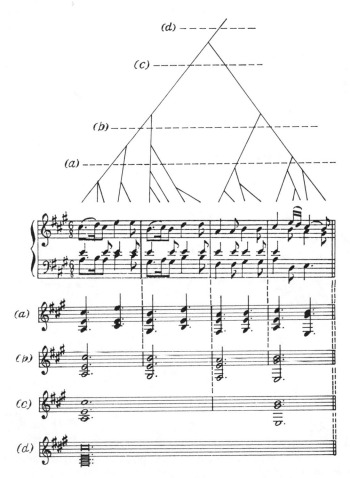

Ex. 2

early 20th century theorist Heinrich Schenker that the organization of an entire piece of music can be conceived of in terms of such principles, and that such organization provides explanations of many of the deeper and more abstract properties of tonal music. Schenker's insight can be restated in our terms as the REDUCTION HYPOTHESIS:

> The pitch-events of a piece are heard in a hierarchy of relative importance; structurally less important (relatively ornamental) events are heard not simply as random insertions, but in relationship to surrounding events of greater importance.

A representation of the relative structural importance of the events in a piece has come to be known as a REDUCTION of the piece, for reasons that will be obvious from an illustration. Ex. 2 represents the time-span reduction of the first four measures of Mozart's Sonata K. 331.* Above the musical text is a tree diagram that constitutes our formal representation for the time-span reduction of the passage. Below the passage is an informal musical interpretation of the tree. Each successive level downwards in the musical illustration results from a deletion of the relatively least important events remaining at the next higher level. The best way to understand Ex. 2 is first to attempt to hear the successive musical levels in rhythm. If the analysis is correct, each level should sound like an intuitively appropriate simplification of the previous level. Thus each level represents a step in REDUCING a piece from its musical surface to a skeleton of relatively important events. At the last level, only the initial event of the passage remains.

Turn now to the tree diagram. Each pitch-event in the musical surface is at the bottom of a branch of the tree. Each branch, with the exception of

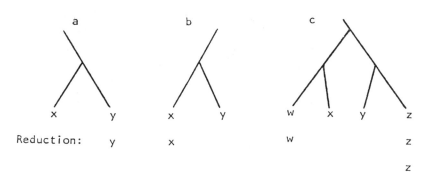

Ex. 3

---

*   As will be pointed out shortly, this is not the only possible kind of reduction. Other analyses may differ both in notation and in selection of important events. They all more or less resemble Ex.2 in general characteristics however.

the branch corresponding to the first event of the piece, terminates at its upper end on another branch. Typical situations are illustrated in Ex. 3. When a branch connected to event x terminates on a branch connected to event y, this signifies that x is less structurally important than y, and that x is heard as an ornament to or elaboration of y. This is the case shown in Ex. 3a. In reducing the passage consisting of x and y, then, y is the event retained; its branch continues upward in the tree. We will call y the HEAD of the passage x-y. Ex. 3b, on the other hand, represents a situation in which x is more important than y and hence is the one retained in a reduction. Ex. 3c illustrates an embedding.

One can think of each musical level as representing a horizontal slice across the tree, showing only the events whose branches appear in that slice. The dotted lines across the tree in Ex. 2 show this correspondence. Note, however, that the tree conveys more information than the musical representation, in that the branching explicitly shows to which surrounding more important event each event is related. It is for this reason that we have adopted the tree notation as the formal representation of the time-span reduction, despite its unfamiliarity.

This brief discussion of time-span reduction is sufficient to motivate an initial comparison with prosodic structure. However, our notion of time-span reduction is not the only notion of reduction in the literature of music theory. (The best known notion of reduction is that of Schenker, 1935); variants of its are commonplace in the theoretical literature.) What all the different theories of reduction share is the belief in a unified hierarchical (or semi-hierarchical) structure for a piece, representing intuitions of relative structural importance. The way these theories differ is in (1) what is taken to be the definition of relative structural importance; (2) what sorts of relationships may obtain between more important and less important events; (3) precisely what musical intuitions are conveyed by the reduction as a result of (1) and (2). Indeed, our theory claims that musical intuitions involve two distinct (though related) reductions differing in just these respects. On our second look at time-span reduction, in section 3, we will treat some of these matters in more detail.

2.2 Prosodic Structure

Traditionally, the theory of phonology has assumed that the sound pattern of language is determined simply in terms of the linear string of phonological segments (or phonemes). However, under this assumption, developed in greatest detail in Chomsky and Halle (1968), many phenomena of stress placement, stress subordination, vowel harmony (in languages such as Turkish), and syllable structure proved resistant to perspicuous treatment. A recent line of research in phonology, first proposed in Liberman (1975) and Liberman and Prince (1977), has developed a theory of PROSODIC TREE STRUCTURES (sometimes also called METRICAL STRUCTURES) that overcomes these difficulties. This theory has stimulated a great deal of work developing and refining the initial formulation (see for example Kiparsky, 1977, 1979; Selkirk, 1978, 1980; Vergnaud and Halle, 1979; and the papers in Safir, 1979) although there are several variants of the theory already in the literature, enough basic agreement exists that we can present a composite version that both does justice to the literature and brings out those characteristics most like time-span reduction.

The rules determining position of word stress in various languages often make use of distinctions among syllable types. This suggests that stress rules should apply not to the simple phonological string, nor to the morphological structure (as in Chomsky and Halle, 1968), but to the syllabic structure. Moreoever, the existence of numerous languages that stress words on every second (or third) syllable suggests that in these languages syllables are themselves organized into larger units, which have been termed FEET. The complete prosodic organization of the word results from aggregating the feet together.

Liberman and Prince (1977) develop a tree notation that expresses the aggregation of syllables into feet and of feet into words. In their notation, each node of the tree dominates either a surface syllable or two other branches, one strong (s) and one weak (w). For example, Ex. 4 illustrates their tree structures for the English words reconciliation (p. 268) and contractual (p. 288).

The purpose of the s and w markings is to express relative degrees of stress. In Chomsky and Halle (1968), as in previous traditions, stress was marked numerically on vowels; (1 stress) was greater than (2 stress), which in turn was greater than (3 stress), and so forth. In addition, all numbered degrees were treated as greater in stress than (unstressed). To employ this formalism in rules, elaborate conventions had to be developed that had little to do with the linguistic insight they were intended to express. In the tree notation, by contrast, main stress falls on the syllable dominated only by ss in the tree (the 'designated terminal element'); subsidiary stresses fall on syllables immediately dominated by s; and unstressed syllables are all immediately dominated by w. In reconciliation, for instance, the main

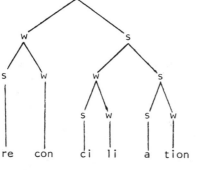
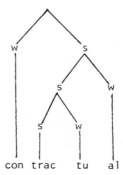

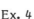
Ex. 4

stress falls on the penultimate syllable, subsidiary stresses fall on re- and
-cil-, and the remaining syllables are unstressed; in contractual, only the
single syllable -trac- is stressed. Thus the tree notation represents relative
stress as explicity relational, i.e. in terms of hierarchical oppositions of ss
and ws. For many reasons this is clearly superior to the theory that assigns
stress in terms of numerical values; and for once a major change in linguistic
theory has not met with vociferous opposition.

2.3 Initial Comparison of the Two Structures

Abstracting away from the musical and linguistic material at the
bottom of the trees, let us examine the trees themselves. In both sorts of
trees, each branch divides into branches that are classified according to a
binary opposition. In the time-span reduction tree, the opposition is head vs.
elaboration; in the prosodic tree, the opposition is strong vs. weak.* This
similarity leads to the observation that the two tree notations are
essentially notational variants. Taking the time-span reduction notion of
HEAD as parallel to the prosodic notion of STRONG, we can establish the
equivalence of structures shown in Ex. 5.

With this equivalence, we can convert a prosodic tree into time-span
reduction notation by systematically substituting time-space configurations
for the corresponding prosodic ones at each node in the tree, i.e. a
right-branching for an s-w configuration and a left-branching for a w-s. Ex.
6 is the time-span notation corresponding to the analyses of reconciliation
and contractual given in Ex. 4. It can readily be seen that Liberman and
Prince's notion of DESIGNATED TERMINAL ELEMENT, that unit
dominated only by ss in a tree, translates into time-span notation as the
HEAD, that unit from which all others branch. Hence the primary stress in
Ex. 6 is indicated by the longest branch in the tree.

It is at least an interesting coincidence that two theories, developed
independently to deal with totally dissimilar phenomena, should have arrived
at equivalent notations to express their analyses. The obvious question to

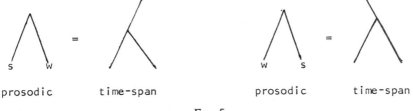

prosodic	time-span	prosodic	time-span

Ex. 5

---

*   One difference, however, is that the prosodic trees permit only one
     weak branch per node, while the musical trees permit more than one
     elaboration per node upon occasion. We return to this difference in
     section 5.

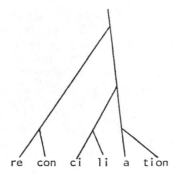 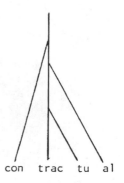

re con cí li a tion   con trac tu al

Ex. 6

ask is whether this equivalence might be more than an accident - whether it reveals some sort of similarity between the intuitions the two theories intend to account for.

To this end, section 3 discusses the principles that determine how a time-span reduction is assigned to a passage of music. Section 4 is a parallel presentation of prosodic theory, bringing out the formal similarities to time-span reduction theory. Section 5 attempts to iron out some discrepancies between the theories, further extending the parallelism.

III.   THE GRAMMAR OF TIME-SPAN REDUCTION

The essential musical intuition expressed by the time-span reduction of a passage is the relative structural importance of the events in the passage with respect to the rhythmic units of the passage. (By contrast, the other reduction in our theory, the prolongational reduction, represents the relative structural importance of events in their role of expressing tension and release - an entirely different sort of intuition.) In order to construct a time-span reduction, one needs three kinds of information: (1) principles for segmenting the passage into rhythmic units, (2) principles that establish the possible relations that may obtain among the events within a rhythmic unit, and (3) principles that establish which of the possible relations actually obtain in the passage in question.

We take up each of these in turn.

3.1   Principles of Segmentation

The notion of 'rhythmic unit' relevant to the time-span reduction is dependent on two of the other hierarchical structures apprehended in music: grouping structure and metrical structure. GROUPING STRUCTURE represents the segmentation of the music into motives, phrases, sections and so forth; we represent it by means of slurs below the musical notation. METRICAL   STRUCTURE   represents   the   hierarchical   arrangement   of beats-points in time where one taps one's feet or claps one's hands in time with the music, separated by regular intervals. We represent metrical structure by means of an arrangement of dots below the music. A dot below a note indicates that a beat is sensed at the attack point of that note; the more dots below a note, the stronger a beat is felt at the attack point of that note. Read horizontally, each row of dots represents a 'level' of metrical structure, i.e. a series of regular intervals of time at which one may hear beats of a given strength.

Ex. 7 illustrates the grouping and metrical structures for two passages of music. 7a is the opening of the Mozart Sonata K. 331 again; 7b is the opening melody of the Mozart G minor Symphony, K. 550.

The intent of the grouping structures should be clear. For example, in Ex. 7a, the first measure is a group, the second measure is a group, the two together form a group, the third and fourth measures together form a group, and the entire passage is a group.

The metrical structures require somewhat more explanation. Each horizontal row of dots indicate a level of metrical regularity. So, in Ex. 7a, the uppermost row designates beats separated by the time interval of an eighth note; the second row designates beats separated by a dotted quarter note (three eighths); the third row designates beats separately by a dotted half note (six eighths or one measure). Each of these is sensed as a domain of metrical regularity. In Ex 7b, the largest level corresponds to a metrical regularity every two measures.

When speaking of a particular metrical level L, it is useful to distinguish between STRONG and WEAK beats of L. In this notation, we can say that a beat of L is strong if it is also a beat of a larger metrical

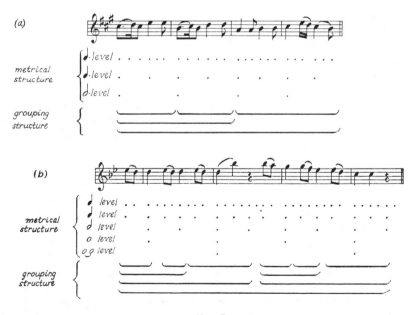

Ex. 7

level, and weak if it is not. So, for example, the first beat of the eighth-note level in Ex. 7a is strong and the second weak; on the other hand, the first beat of the quarter-note level in Ex. 7b is weak and the second strong.

We should make clear the relationship between our formal metrical structure and the metrical indications present in ordinary musical notation, such as time signatures and bar lines. Note that the musical surface, i.e.the music as it strikes the listener's ear, contains no time signatures or bar lines. The pattern of beats must be INFERRED by the listener from the musical surface (and one may often be initially uncertain of the metrical structure of an unfamiliar piece). The role of time signatures and bar lines, then, is as a partial indication of the composer's intended metrical structure; they aid the performer in projecting those distinctions of articulation and stress that help the listener infer the structure. Note also that time signatures and bar lines are of no help in determining intended metrical structure at levels larger than the measure, such as the largest level in Ex. 7b.

Exs. 7a and 7b illustrate two possible ways in which the grouping structure and metrical structure may be related. In 7a, the strongest beat of each group is at the beginning; we will describe such a situation by saying that the grouping and metrical structures are IN PHASE. In 7b, on the other hand, the strongest beat of each group falls somewhere in the middle of the group; we will say that the grouping and meter are OUT OF PHASE. The traditional notion of UPBEAT or ANACRUSIS can be characterized as those beats in a group which precede the strongest beat (the DOWNBEAT). So, for example, Ex. 7a contains no upbeats; but Ex. 7b does, on two levels.

With this understanding of the interaction of grouping and metrical structure, we are now ready to discuss the way the two together produce a segmentation of a passage into rhythmic units, or TIME-SPANS, over which the time-span reduction is defined. At the larger levels, the time-spans are identical to the groups. At the smallest levels, the time-spans can be related to the metrical structure: each beat B defines a time-span TB which consists of the interval of time from B up to but not including the next beat of the same level as B. When the grouping and metrical structures are in phase, these two definitions mesh perfectly. For example, Ex. 8 shows the application of these definitions to Ex. 7a. The grouping remains as before, but directly below each beat of the metrical structure a square bracket has been added that designates the associated time-span. The square brackets, or SUBGROUPS, plus the groups constitute the time-span segmentation of the passage.

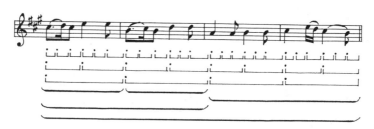

Ex. 8

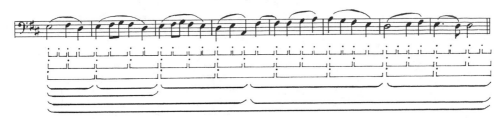

Ex. 9

However when the grouping and metrical structures are out of phase, this simple segmentation will not do. Ex. 9, part of the Finale theme of Beethoven's Ninth Symphony, is a simple illustration of the problem. In this example, the f# on the fourth beat of the fourth measure is interpreted in incompatible ways. According to the subgroup bracketing, it belongs with the rest of the fourth measure, but according to the grouping structure, it belongs with the material in the fifth measure, as an anticipation of the next phrase.

For a number of musical reasons, this contradiction must be resolved in favor of associating this note with material in the group to which it belongs and not with the preceding material. The intuition behind this choice is that upbeats are heard as forming rhythmic units with their downbeats. The correct structure for the Beethoven passage is thus Ex. 10. Note how the subgroups of the half-note level and larger are truncated by the group boundary in the fourth measure, and how an extra AUGMENTED SUBGROUP is added to include the upbeat to the fifth measure.

Ex. 11 illustrates a more complex case, the Mozart G minor Symphony theme given in Ex. 7b.

As a result of this treatment, a piece is exhaustively segmented into time-spans which fall into a strictly hierarchical relationship. Time-spans do not overlap: their definition prevents situations like Ex. 9 from arising. Furthermore, the hierarchy comprises two layers. The inner layer consists of several levels of subgroups, which are defined primarily in metrical terms, with grouping boundaries playing an important secondary role. The outer layer consists of groups; metrical structure plays no role in their definition. As will be seen in section 3.3, the distinction between subgroups and groups bears on the principles determining relative prominence of events in the time-span reduction.

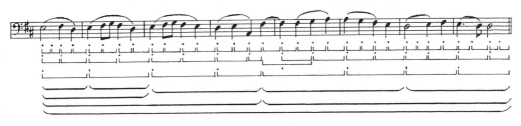

Ex. 10

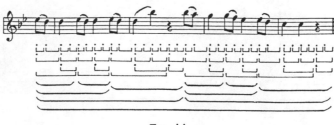

Ex. 11

Given the principles of segmentation, the next step in developing the time-span reduction is to show how the segmentation determines a class of possible tree structures for the passage.

3.2 Principles of Well-formedness for Trees

Section 2.1 presented what we called the Reduction Hypothesis. We can state the Reduction Hypothesis more precisely as a claim that

(1) the relationship of subordination is transitive - if pitch-event x is an elaboration of pitch-event y, and y is an elaboration of z, then x is an elaboration of z;

(2) that every event in a piece is ultimately subordinate to a single event.

Each event in a piece belongs to a number of time-spans, nested one in another from the smallest beat level to the largest group level. If a particular event e is the head of some large time-span, it must also be the head of all the smaller time-spans it belongs to. In turn, this has an important consequence for the way time-span reductions are constructed: the head of a time-span T can be selected from among the heads of the time-spans that T immediately contains, i.e. that are exactly one level smaller than T. This was the principle of reduction illustrated in Ex. 2.

In short, the principles of segmentation into time-spans plus the

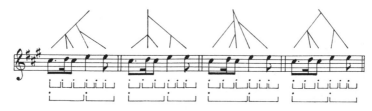

Ex. 12

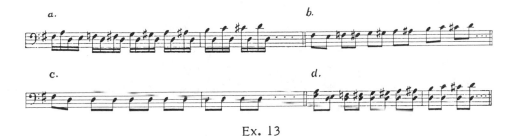

Ex. 13

definition of head in terms of time-span together guarantee that every pitch-event in a piece is included in the time-span reduction, and that the reduction can be constructed in an orderly way, starting by finding heads of all the smallest time-spans and working outward in the hierarchy until a head is selected for the entire piece. Hence these principles create a class of unified hierarchical structures for the entire piece.

However, these principles alone do not create a UNIQUE reduction for every passage. For example, the first measure of the Mozart Sonata has a unique segmentation into time-spans, but any of the trees in Ex. 12 are consistent with this segmentation. What is needed to complete the construction of a time-span reduction is a set of principles of relative prominence, to choose among these possibilities. Before describing the principles of relative prominence, though, we must mention one additional point about the relationship of head to elaboration in the time-span reduction.

In all the time-span reductions illustrated so far, the head of each time-span is simply identical to one of the events within the time-span. However, there are musical situations where this procedure yields intuitively incorrect results. Consider Ex. 13a, from the Bach Suite No. 1 for unaccompanied cello. What one hears in this passage is a counterpoint between a rising line and a sustained d. If at the first level of reduction we

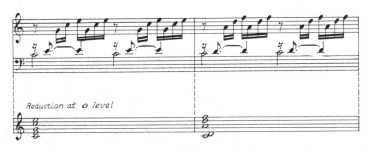

Ex. 14

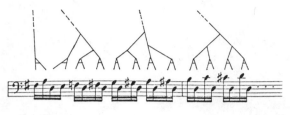

Ex. 15

are obliged to choose either the rising notes (13b) or the ds (13c), we lose the musical sense of the passage. The intuitively correct solution is to fuse the two at the eighth-note level, as in 13d. Similarly, in the C major prelude from Bach's Well-Tempered Clavier, the correct time-span reduction does not consist of single notes, but of the chords which are arpeggiated in the musical surface, as in Ex. 14.

It follows from these examples that the trees for time-span reduction must admit two different kinds of relationships between the events in a time-span T and the head of T. In the first, which we call ORDINARY REDUCTION, the head of T is identical to just one of the events in the time-span; this is the relationship illustrated in all examples prior to Ex. 13. In the second case, the head of T is formed from the FUSION or super-imposition of the heads of the time-spans immediately contained in T. We will indicate fusion in a tree by a small bar between the branches and by making neither of the branches straight. Ex. 15 illustrates the low portions of the tree structure assigned to Ex. 13 by this treatment.

(In addition to ordinary reduction and fusion, time-span reduction trees must express two other ways of forming the head of T from events in it. The first, called transformation, supplies for reduction an event not present at the actual musical surface, but understood to be there in function. The second, called cadential retention, permits the retention of both members of a two-membered cadence where otherwise one of the members would have been reduced out; in effect, it treats the two-membered cadence as a syntactic unit. While we cannot go further into detail here, we do want the reader to understand that the normal head-elaboration relationship is not the only possible way of constructing a reduction, though it is by far the most common. The existence of these other sorts of relationships reduces the strict parallel with phonology.)

3.3 Principles of Relative Prominence

The principles for choosing the head of a time-span cannot be stated in the categorical terms characteristic of rule systems in linguistics, i.e. there is no set of necessary and sufficient conditions for an event to be head of a time-span. Rather, these principles operate along lines first (to our knowledge) made explicit by Wertheimer (1923) and characteristic of a wide variety of aspects of both visual and musical perception. These rules are called PREFERENCE RULES because they all take the form "Prefer an analysis with property x". There are about nine preference rules involved in selecting the head of a time-span.

Preference rules have the following characteristics:

(1) any one alone, in the absence of other evidence, is a sufficient condition for choosing an analysis;

(2) when two or more preference rules apply, they may either reinforce each other or conflict;

(3) when preference rules reinforce each other, they strengthen the salience of analyses they pick out;

(4) when preference rules conflict, they weaken the salience of analyses each one individually picks out;

(5) if one preference rule (or combination of preference rules) is sufficiently stronger than another, it can override the other's preferences in situations of conflict.

With the general properties of preference rules in mind, we can mention the more important preference rules specific to choosing time-span reductions. Two major rules are these:

Preference Rule 1: Of the possible choices for head of a time-span T, prefer a choice that is in relatively strong metrical position.

Preference Rule 2: Of the possible choices for head of a time-span T, prefer a choice that is relatively harmonically consonant.

To see how these rules operate, consider Ex. 16, the time-span reduction of the Mozart sonata again, this time with the time-span segmentation marked in. (The musical notation of the reduction also includes a level omitted from Ex. 2.)

In the time-span marked [a] in Ex. 16, there is a choice among three pitch-events, the first and third of which are identical and more harmonically stable than the second. However the first is also on the strongest beat of the measure, while the second and third are in weaker positions. Hence Preference Rule 1 chooses the first event as head of time-span [a]. Similar considerations obtain in each of the half-measure time-spans in the first three measures.

In the time-span marked [b] (the entire first measure), the head must be chosen from the heads of the two halves. The head of the first half (time-span [a]) is in stronger metrical position than the head of the second half; it is also harmonically more stable, since it is a root position chord and the head of the second half is a first inversion. Hence both preference rules choose the first chord of the measure as the head. The second measure behaves in similar fashion.

So far the preference rules have encountered no conflicts. However, next consider time-spans [c] and [d], both in the fourth measure. In each of

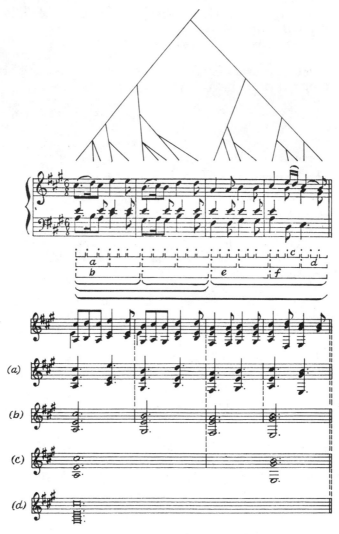

Ex. 16

these, the first event is in stronger metrical position, but the second event is harmonically more stable. The intuitively correct analysis chooses the second event as the head; in other words, Preference Rule 2 has overridden Preference Rule 1 in these cases. However, the conflict between the rules is not without effect; both of these time-spans are examples of APPOGGIATURA, a well-known expressive device in which a dissonance on

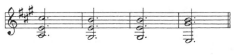

Ex. 17

a strong beat resolves to a consonance on a weak beat. We claim that the peculiar expressive force of the appoggiatura is due at least in part to the tension engendered by the conflict between preference rules.

Next examine time-span [e], the entire third measure. Here the head of the first half is a dissonant f♯-e-a chord, and the head of the second half is a relatively consonant first inversion V (E major) chord. Consistency in treatment would suggest that the relatively consonant chord should be selected in spite of its relatively weak metrical position - entirely parallel to time-spans [c] and [d]. However the intuitively correct analysis seems to choose the first chord. To hear this, substitute g♯-e-b for f♯-e-a in line (b) of the musical notation for the reduction, as in Ex. 17. This should definitely sound less like the original piece than the version in Ex. 16. Does this mean that the preference rules act inconsistently and arbitrarily?

No: rather it means that there is another preference rule applying in this situation whose effect was not detected in the other cases. The rule is roughly of the following form (actually it can be decomposed into two or three independent principles):

> Preference Rule 3: Of the possible choices for head of a time-span T, prefer the one that makes the best melodic and harmonic connections with adjacent time-spans.

Notice how in line (b) of Ex. 16, the melody and bass line move stepwise from each measure to the next, whereas in Ex. 17 the melody gets stuck on b by the second measure and the bass has to skip down from the third measure to the fourth. Without going into details of voice-leading, it appears that these factors contribute to line (b) sounding superior to Ex. 17. Thus we can claim that in time-span [e], Preference Rule 3 favors the first event in the measure as head; combined with Preference Rule 1, its weight can override Preference Rule 2, which favors the second half of the measure. In other words, Rule 2 alone wins out over Rule 1 in time-spans [c] and [d], but it loses to the combination of Rules 1 and 3 in time-span [e].

Notice, by the way, that Preference Rule 3 makes use of information outside the time-span being analyzed in order to make a choice. Such nonlocal rules are common among the rules of our music theory, and they account for much of the richness of musical perception. More generally, such rules account for Gestalt effects in perception, where an analysis cannot be built up from amalgamation of its separate parts: they make the analyses of the parts interdependent on one another.

Finally consider time-span [f], consisting of the entire fourth measure. Here the head of the first half is a tonic chord on a strong beat, and the head of the second half is a (less consonant) dominant chord on a weak beat.

All discussion so far would indicate that the former is strongly favored, since both Preference Rules 1 and 2 pick it out as head. Nonetheless, intuition favors choosing the dominant chord as head.

Again the reason for this apparent inconsistency is that there is an as yet unmentioned preference rule at work. An extremely important principle of musical organization is the use of CADENCES - specified musical formulas - at the ends of larger-level groups, providing clear points of articulation in the music. Because of their role in making structure clear, cadences assume great structural importance in time-span reduction. We can state this importance as a further rule:

> Preference Rule 4: In choosing the head of a time-span T, STRONGLY prefer a cadential event that articulates the end of a group.

It so happens that the dominant chord in time-span [f] constitutes a cadence for the entire four-measure group in Ex. 16; this is the only cadence in the passage. Hence Preference Rule 4 applies to it. The use of "strongly" in this rule is intended to signify that the rule overrides even the powerful combination of Preference Rules 1 and 2, resulting in the choice of the cadence as head of time-span [f].

Note that Preference Rule 4 again depends on information outside the time-span under analysis. If time-span [f] were in a different position in the phrase, say the third measure, the dominant chord would not constitute a cadence and so the rule would not apply. As a result the local preferences of Rules 1 and 2 would prevail, choosing the tonic chord as head.

While this has by no means been an exhaustive discussion of the time-span reduction preference rules, we hope to have given the reader a general idea of how they interact to provide a favored choice of head for each time-span of the piece. It is important to notice how different preference rules come into play at different points. In particular, Preference Rule 1 refers to metrical position, a distinction that arises only at relatively small levels of analysis - essentially subgroups and small groups. At larger levels, such as sections of a piece, there are no salient distinctions of metrical strength, and Preference Rule 1 ceases to play a role. On the other hand, Preference Rule 4 refers to a distinction important to just such larger groups, the distinction between cadences and noncadences. Furthermore, in the middle-sized time-spans where the two interact, such as time-span [f] above, the demands of the larger context prevail.

To sum up the grammar of time-span reductions, then, there are three components. First, a set of segmentation rules produces an exhaustive segmentation of the musical surface into a layered hierarchy of time-spans, with subgroups at smaller levels and groups on larger levels. Second, the segmentation of the surface determines a set of possible time-span reduction trees, such that every time-span has a head selected out of the heads of the time-spans it immediately contains. Third, the choice of head for each time-span is determined by a set of preference rules that are sensitive to metrical, harmonic, voice-leading and cadential properties of the time-span.

The reader may be curious about the extent to which these principles are characteristic of only classical Western tonal music or of tonal music in general. Our guess is that the main grammatical differences between idioms lie only in the specification of what counts as relative consonance or dissonance, what counts as good voice-leading and what formulas function as cadences. In other words, the formal organization of the grammar is universal, and the rules themselves are largely universal - all that varies is the specific pitch relations mentioned in the rules. This is not to say, of course, that there are not other differences elsewhere in musical grammar.

The next section will show how the grammar of prosodic structure is organized along precisely parallel principles.

4. THE GRAMMAR OF PROSODIC STRUCTURE

The version of hierarchical phonology most similar to the grammar of time-span reduction is that developed by Selkirk (1978, 1980). More than other approaches, Selkirk makes clear the distinction between rules of segmentation, rules that build tree structures on the basis of the segmentation, and rules that determine relative prominence of sister branches in the trees (though these distinctions are implicit in all the other approaches as well). Thus in order to bring out the parallelism between music and language, we will present a form of Selkirk's theory, slightly modified from her presentation but preserving its essential insights.

4.1 Principles of Segmentation

Although the pioneering study by Liberman and Prince (1977) makes use of the notions of syllable and foot, their formal role in the theory is left somewhat unclear. Selkirk, however, argues that syllables and feet must be explicitly marked as such, as PROSODIC CATEGORIES, and that these categories play a role in the formal statement of various phonological processes. In addition, Selkirk argues for the existence of other, larger, prosodic categories of WORD, PHONOLOGICAL PHRASE, INTONATIONAL PHRASE and UTTERANCE. The result is a segmentation of the phonological string into a complex hierarchy that corresponds only in part to syntactic structure. For example, Ex. 18 is the segmentation of the sentence In Pakistan, Tuesday is a holiday. The levels to the left identify the prosodic categories.

Notice an important way in which this structure is unlike syntactic structure and like time-span segmentation. Whereas in syntactic structure a category may recur inside one of its constituents (for instance NP inside PP inside NP), this is impossible in the phonological segmentation. Words, for example, may contain feet but may not be contained in them. Thus phonological segmentation is a layered hierarchy in the same sense as time-span segmentation, where groups may contain subgroups but may not be contained in them.

The principles for segmentation into feet vary among languages. Selkirk argues that French essentially has primarily monosyllabic feet. Vergnaud and Halle (1979), examining the literature on a wide variety of

In Pa ki stan Tues day is a ho li day

syllable level	
foot level	
word level	
phon. phr. level	
int. phr. level	
utterance level	

Ex. 18

languages, find three other sorts of foot-formation rules: those establishing bisyllabic feet, those establishing trisyllabic feet and those establishing feet of unlimited length (bounded by word boundaries or syllables of a specified type). English appears to have monosyllabic, bisyllabic and trisyllabic feet, depending on the content of the syllables gathered up into a foot. The relevant factors are the tenseness of the syllable's vowel and the nature of the consonants if any, at the end of the syllable. So far as is known, syllable types are not distinguished for prosodic purposes in ANY language by the nature of their initial consonant(s). Here are some examples.

19a is a monosyllabic foot; 19b is a bisyllabic foot; 19c is a trisyllabic foot, which like all trisyllabic feet in English, begins with a bisyllabic foot. 19d, by contract with 19b, is a bisyllabic word consisting of two monosyllabic feet; the difference between this and 19b accounts for the fact that its second syllable bears secondary stress and that of 19b does not.

An interesting aspect of English foot formation is the behavior of unstressed syllables at the beginning of a word. In one proposed treatment of them, the structure of words like attire, vanilla and America is as in Ex.

a. flounce b. modest c. Pamela d. gymnast

syllable level	
foot level	
word level	

Ex. 19

	attire	vanilla	America
syllable level	⎵ ⎵⎴	⎵ ⎵ ⎵	⎵ ⎵ ⎵ ⎵
foot level	⎿ ⎴⎴	⎿ ⎴⎴	⎿ ⎴⎴
word level	⎿_____⎤	⎿_____⎤	⎿_____⎤

Ex. 20

20 (though the mechanism for deriving this structure has been open to dispute - see Selkirk 1980). In Ex. 20 we see an unstressed initial syllable preceding a monosyllabic, a bisyllabic and a trisyllabic foot. The initial syllable is not simply an odd·syllable added at the beginning of the word, but is adjoined to the rest as the beginning of an extra foot level. In the present connection this solution is particularly significant because of its parallel with the treatment of upbeats in time-span segmentation (see Exs. 10, 11). In each case, a weak segment separated by a major boundary (group boundary in music, word boundary in language) from the preceding strong segment is instead adjoined to the following segment. Hence beyond the formal parallel of a layered hierarchy in both grammars, the segmentation rules display an interesting substantive parallel as well.

Turning to the next layer of the hierarchy, the segmentation into words is obvious. We only have to note that compounds such as <u>blackboard</u> and <u>labor union</u> have two word levels: However, it remains to show how the feet of a multifoot word are structured. Selkirk, following Liberman and Prince, gathers the two right-most feet into a segment, then gathers that with the next to the left, and so on until the left-hand boundary of the word is reached. For example, <u>reconciliation</u>, with three feet, receives the structure in Ex. 22.

Looking at a large variety of languages, Vergnaud and Halle (1979) conclude that the rule for structuring the feet of an English word is typical. The only major difference that appears is that in some languages the gathering of feet begins at the left and works right-ward, in the mirror image of the English rule. Halle has suggested (personal communication) that one should expect similar mirror-image phenomena in time-span segmentaton in music. Recall that the normal gathering of subgroups into

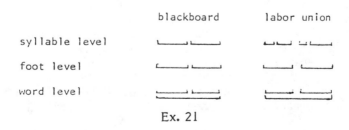

	blackboard	labor union
syllable level	⎿___⎤⎿__⎤	⎵⎵ ⎵⎿__⎤
foot level	⎿_____⎤⎿__⎤	⎿__⎤ ⎿__⎤
word level	⎿_____⎴⎴	⎿__⎤ ⎿__⎤

Ex. 21

reconciliation

syllable level

foot level

word level

Ex. 22

larger subgroups has the strong beat on the left, in the exposition of section 3. However, as Halle predicted, there turns out to be a musical idiom in which the strong beat is on the RIGHT-hand end of subgroups: the gamelan music described by Becker and Becker (1979). Hence the cross-liguistic possibilities for foot formation parallel the cross-idiom possibilites for subgroup formation.

The larger levels of the prosodic structure - phonological phrase, intonational phrase, and utterance - have been less extensively studied than syllables, feet and words. However, Selkirk's preliminary work indicates that the rules determining segmentation at these levels are not very different from the rules discussed so far, except that they make use of syntactic as well as phonological properties to establish boundaries.

To sum up, we find that prosodic structure, like time-span reduction, is based on a segmentation of the surface string into a layered hierarchy. It appears that each layer (subgroups and groups in music; syllables, feet, words, etc. in language) in itself provides at least one level that completely analyzes the string, and of course there may be more than one such level. We next turn to the principles that define the possible trees associated with a phonological segmentation.

4.2 Principles of Well-formedness for Trees

The principles of segmentation have been developed in such a way that each segment at each level immediately contains either one or two segments of the next smaller level (this should be evident from examination of the structures in Exs. 18-22). Each of the smallest segments (syllables in the version of the theory presented here) is attached to the bottom of a branch. If a segment s_1 is the only segment immediately contained in the segment of the next larger level, nothing happens in the tree. If segments s_1 and s_2 are both immediately contained in the same segment s_3 of the next larger level, the branches corresponding to s_1 and s_2 are joined into a branch corresponding to s_3; one of the two constituent branches is labelled s (strong) or w (weak). If this process is carried out recursively, all the way to the largest levels of segmentation, the result is a well-formed tree of the sort illustrated in section 2.2, expressing relative prominence of all the segments of the phonological string.

So far we have constructed a set of POSSIBLE prosodic trees corresponding to a particular segmentation. What is needed in addition is a

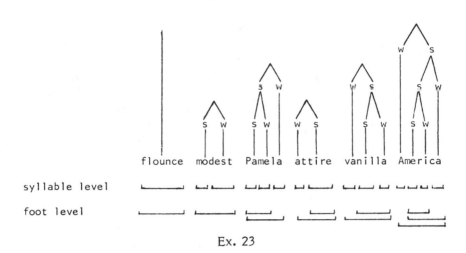

Ex. 23

set of rules of prominence to ascertain, for each branching in the tree, which branch is s and which w.

4.3 Rules of Relative Prominence

Each of the layers in the prosodic hierarchy has a characteristic rule or set of rules for determining relations of prominence. Starting from the innermost layer, the aggregation of syllables into feet, the rule for English is as follows:

Prominence Rule 1:   a. In a foot that immediately contains two syllables, the first syllable is strong.

                     b. In a foot that immediately contains a foot and a syllable, the foot is strong.

This rule results in the following trees for flounce, modest, Pamela, attire, vanilla and America (segmentation from Exs. 19, 20). Recall that main stress goes on the syllable dominated only by ss.

Vergnaud and Halle (1979) show that there are languages in which the counterpart of Rule 1a has the reverse effect, marking the second syllable strong.

The next layer in the hierarchy is the aggregation of feet into words. Liberman and Prince (1977) give the following rule for English:

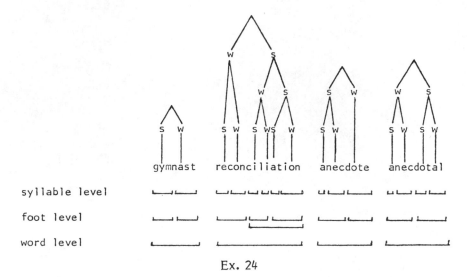

syllable level

foot level

word level

Ex. 24

Prominence Rule 2 (Lexical Category Prominence Rule): In a segment immediately containing two feet, the second is strong if and only if it branches.*

This rule results in the following trees for gymnast, reconciliation, anecdote and anecdotal. Notice in particular the contrast between the last two of

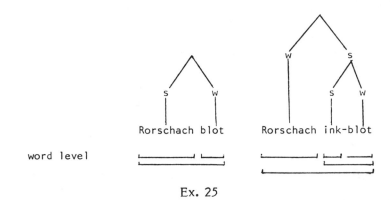

word level

Ex. 25

_____

*   Prominence Rule 2 is subject to a number of classes of exceptions, discussed at length by Liberman and Prince.

these, where the extra syllable -al causes the second foot of anecdotal to branch, in turn altering the tree and shifting stress to -do-.

A similar rule governs the aggregation of words into larger words:

Prominence Rule 3 (Compound Stress Rule): In a word immediately containing two words, the second is strong if and only if it branches into two words.

This rule accounts for the contrast between main stress on Rorschach in Rorschach blot and on ink in Rorschach ink-blot: in the latter only, the second word on the next-to-largest level of segmentation branches into two words. (Ex. 25 shows segmentation and tree structure only from word level up.) Notice that the rule specifies branching into two WORDS rather than just branching as in the previous rule. The reason for this is that the rule is not sensitive to the number of syllables or feet in the constituent words. For example, in both labor day and labor union, main stress falls on labor even though the union branches into two syllables.

Finally the aggregation of words into phonological phrases is governed by this rule from Liberman and Prince (1977):

Prominence Rule 4 (Nuclear Stress Rule): In a phonological phrase that immediately contains two phonological phrases or words, the second is strong.

This rule accounts for the stress patterns or phrases like three red hats and John ate Bill's peach (represented here only from word level up).

At the level of phonological phrase there also appears a prominence

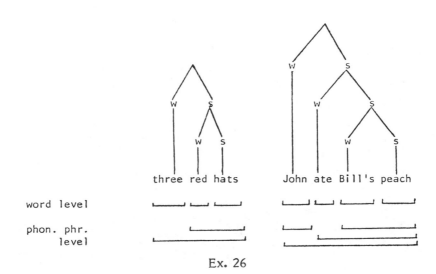

| word level |
| phon. phr. level |

Ex. 26

rule that bears a more patent resemblance to rules of musical structure than the four preceding rules. This is Liberman and Prince's rule of Iambic Reversal, also commonly called the Rhythm Rule. The effect of this rule is to shift stress leftward in certain situations. For example, the words thirteen and Tennessee have strongest stress on the last syllable when spoken in isolation; but in the phrases thirteen men and Tennessee air their strongest stresses are on the initial syllable. Liberman and Prince's explication of the rule is in terms of a metrical structure not unlike the musical metrical structure described briefly in section 3.1.

The general idea behind the Rhythm Rule is that the stresses of a linguistic phrase form a hierarchical metrical pattern, with relatively heavy stresses corresponding to relatively strong beats, and relatively weak stresses corresponding to relatively weak beats. The ideal metrical structure is one in which relatively strong and relatively weak beats alternate; in particular, two relatively strong beats are preferably not

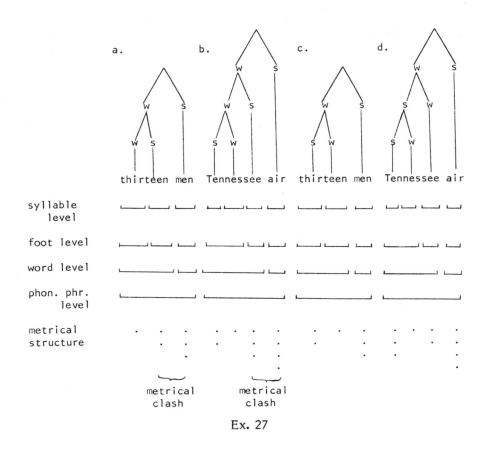

Ex. 27

adjacent to one another. It is just such a situation that arises in the juxtaposition of <u>thirteen</u> with <u>men</u> and <u>Tennessee</u> with <u>air</u>: the strongest stress is on the second word, and the next strongest is on the final syllable of the first word. The Rhythm Rule alters this undersirable situation by reversing the largest w and s of the first word, thereby separating the second-strongest stress from the strongest by a relatively weak stress. For example, instead of Ex. 27a and b, the tree structures one would expect given the stress patterns of the individual words, the Rhythm Rule yields the structures in Exs. 27c and d. Beneath the segmentation is the metrical structure assigned to the tree; the number of dots below a syllable is proportional to its relative prominence in the tree.

The Rhythm Rule can therefore be thought of as a rule that makes prosodic structure conform more closely to an ideal metrical pattern. Despite the differences in formulation, the kinship of this rule to musical Preference Rule 1 ("Of the possible choices for head of a time-span, prefer a choice that is in relatively strong metrical position") is clear. The major difference between the two is that in the musical rule, the metrical structure is fixed in advance and the time-span structure is chosen so as to conform to it; whereas in the phonological rule, the metrical structure is established in terms of the tree, and the tree is chosen so as to optimize the resulting metrical pattern. This difference is probably a consequence of the fact that musical events are organized around a fixed and regular metrical structure which must be maintained throughout. In language, by contrast, the rhythm is flexible and is not required to conform to any particular pattern. Note that either of these practices may be altered: in recitative, the fixed meter of most music is abandoned and more flexible speech-like rhythms appear; in poetry, a fixed meter is imposed to which the linguistic stresses must correspond (see Halle and Keyser, 1971; Kiparsky, 1977 for discussion). Thus we can conclude that the relation of relative prominence to metrical structure is substantially the same in music and language; the difference between musical Preference Rule 1 and the prosodic Rhythm Rule is a function largely of the different metrical practices of the two media.

5.   SOME DISCREPANCIES

The last two sections have shown that time-span reduction and prosodic structure are not only represented by equivalent tree notation; they are the products of grammars that carry out formally parallel operations on musical and phonological strings. In each case, the string is segmented into a layered hierarchy, in which each layer provides at least one exhaustive segmentation. A set of possible tree structures is defined in precisely parallel fashion over the segmentations; and preference rules or prominence rules determine which of the possible trees is the correct one. Furthermore, two substantive parallels have appeared: the treatment of augmented time-spans and augmented feet, with group boundaries and word boundaries playing equivalent roles; and the relationship of metrical structure to choices made by the prominence rules.

Of course the nature of the strings being segmented and most of the substance of the rules in the two theories are quite different. This only serves to make the formal parallels all the more striking, particularly since the two theories were developed independently and were designed to account for radically different sorts of intuitions. Before drawing further conclusions, however, we should turn to some formal respects in which the two theories differ, and discuss how they might be resolved.

In time-span theory, most of the branching we have discussed has been binary; i.e. each time-span above the smallest level contains to time-spans of the next smaller level. However, in a triple meter (such as the 6/8 of Mozart K. 331), ternary branching appears at a certain subgroup level. Moreover, it is not inconceivable for a group to contain three or more small groups; for example, in strophic songs and variation forms, the largest segmentation of the piece is usually into as many groups as there are verses or variations. On the other hand, prosodic theory has been formulated in terms of strictly binary branching. Where a foot, for example, contains more than two syllables, the segmentation and resulting tree are constructed using recursive binary branching, as in Ex. 28a, rather than multiple branching as in 28b. Is this a real difference between language and music, or is it just a consequence of the way the two theories happen to be stated?

Here it is not clear to us which theory should give way, or even if either should. On one hand, there seems to be only one use in prosodic theory for recursive binary-branching trees that cannot be equally coded into multiple-branching trees: the assignment of relative degree of subsidiary stress (Liberman and Prince, 1977, p. 259) - certainly an important function.

On the other hand, there is some potential justification for believing in strict binary branching in time-span trees. At subgroup levels, where ternary branching occurs in connection with ternary meter, there is very often motivation for an additional segmentation into 2 + 1 (♩♩) or 1 + 2 (♩♩); the typical "oom-pah-pah" accompaniment can be thought of as a special case of the latter.* At larger levels, intuition seems to support grouping multiple-branching forms such as variations by twos, in the absence of evidence to the contrary. Thus there might be some advantage to imposing strict binary branching on time-span reductions. Whatever the outcome, the discrepancy between prosodic and time-span theory does not seem irreconcilable, or particularly serious.

A much more important difference is in the interpretation of time-span and prosodic trees. As observed in section 4.2, a branch at any level of a time-span tree stands for a single pitch-event, which is elaborated by all the events whose branches are subsidiary to it. In a prosodic tree, however, a branch is taken to stand for an entire prosodic constituent containing strong and weak parts. If the trees are interpreted so differently, can the theories really be parallel?

The contrast between the two interpretations is not unlike that between

---

*   Kiparsky (1977) shows that so-called triple meters in poetry (dactylic and anapestic) must be treated as duple meters with a divided weak position. The consequences of this for music are however unclear.

two interpretations of metrical accent in music itself. One view, that of Cooper and Meyer (1960), is that metrical weight is (in our terms) a property of time-spans - that metrical weight has duration. In Lerdahl and Jackendoff (in press), we argue against such a view and for one in which metrical weight is a property of beats - points in time - rather than time-spans. The argument is essentially that subsidiary elements of 'strong' time-spans (i.e. time-spans beginning on a relatively strong beat) are in fact no stronger than subsidiary weak elements of 'weak' time -spans. For example, in a 4/4 measure, the second beat does not receive more weight than the fourth by virtue of being in the 'strong' time-span 1-2 as opposed to the 'weak' time-span 3-4. The same argument applies to time-span reduction: low-level elaborations of relatively important events are themselves no more important than equally low-level elaborations of less important events. In other words, strength relative to other time-spans inheres only in the head and not in the time-span as a whole. Thus it would be incorrect to change the interpretation of time-span trees to conform to phonological theory.

On the other hand, it does make some sense to reinterpret prosodic structure in time-span reduction terms. When main stress is applied to a phrase on the basis of a prosodic tree, it is not spread over an entire strong constituent, but is applied to the designated terminal element (the head) alone. Unstressed syllables are of equivalent strength whether they are in a relatively strong or relatively weak constituent. Hence certain aspects of our argument against Cooper and Meyer's interpretation of metrical weight in music are germane here too, suggesting that the musical interpretation of the hierarchical structures common to time-span and prosodic theory is the correct one.

At first glance the notion that a phonological string has a reduction like a musical string may seem rather odd. For example, the tree for reconciliation (Ex. 6) indicates a level of reduction of the form re--ci--a,

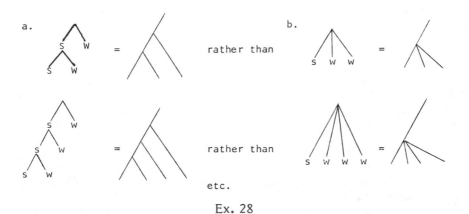

Ex. 28

one of the form re--a, and finally one consisting of the main stressed syllable a alone. This is hardly comprehensible in morphological, syntactic, or semantic terms. However, at the phonological level of linguistic representation we are dealing not only with linguistic information but also with its perceptual and motor organization. It is not at all incomprehensible to think of something like a prosodic reduction being implicated in the way a phonological string is perceived - with relatively strong syllables being identified first, or in the way it is produced - with the stronger syllables being the axes around which other speech movements are marshalled. If this is a plausible view, the parallelism between music and language is still deeper.

6.   GENERAL IMPLICATIONS

However the discrepancies we have just discussed are eventually resolved, the similarity with the theory of prosodic structure seems to us to be a much more significant parallelism between music and language than has ever, to our knowledge, been pointed out. Its persuasiveness arises in large part from the point-by-point correspondence of abstract aspects of the proposed grammars, rather than from superficial analogies between the two media.

To see the force of the argument, notice, by contrast, that similarities between SYNTACTIC and musical structure (for example those proposed by Bernstein, 1976) have not proven to be fruitful avenues of investigation. To be sure, the syntaxes of language and music are both hierarchical; but here the syntactic parallelism stops, since linguistic syntax has grammatical categories (noun, verb, noun phrase, etc.), and musical syntax does not. Furthermore, linguistic trees represent 'is-a' relations: a verb followed by a noun is a verb phrase. By contrast, a pitch event is an elaboration of another pitch event. In short, the relations among entities in linguistic and musical syntax are fundamentally different.

Why then should there be such a parallelism? Given that both theories are attempts to account for human cognitive abilities, the existence of parallelism between them implies a claim that these areas are a respect in which human musical and linguistic capacities overlap. In other words, both capacities make use of some of the same organizing principles to impose structure on their respective inputs, no matter how disparate these inputs are in other respects.

However, if this claim is true, it would be surprising if music and language were the ONLY human abilities so structured. Rather, we should be led to look for something closely analogous to time-span structure in many human abilities under the rubric of 'temporal patterning', from event perception to motor control to the planning of extended strategies of behavior. In particular, we should expect the notion of HEAD/ELABORATION to figure prominently in psychological theories of temporal organization.

As suggestive evidence that this may be the case, Lasher (1978) analyzes sequences of ballet steps, finding that they are invariably interpreted as a sequence of major movements, each preceded by preparatory movements. Such a description is easily seen to be a variant of time-span reduction principles, with the major movements serving as heads of larger segments, and the preparatory movements as their elaborations. (Notice how this description is more highly structured than one articulated only in terms of 'chunking', since it accords to one element of each 'chunk' the privileged status of head.)

Whether or not further kinds of organization are eventually amenable to more rigorous treatment along our lines, our main point should be clear: the similarity between prosodic and musical structure ought to be used as a point of triangulation for approaching an account of other temporally structured cognitive capacities.

SUMMARY

The authors have developed a generative music theory which characterizes, by a set of formal rules, the musical intuitions of a listener experienced in a tonal idiom. One part of the theory, called time-span reduction, assigns to pitches a hierarchy of structural importance with respect to their position in rhythmic structure. Independently, recent research in linguistic theory has resulted in a new formulation of syllabic and word stress, called prosodic tree structures. This paper draws an extensive parallelism between prosodic tree structures and time-span reduction.

Because music and language are generally dissimilar phenomena, this particular similarity is exceptionally striking. After outlining the basic conceptions of time-span reduction and prosodic tree structures, the body of the paper demonstrates a point-by-point correspondence in the form of their grammars, and suggests a few substantive correspondences as well. The paper closes with a discussion of some formal discrepancies and with remarks on the psychological implications of this parallel between music and language.

ACKNOWLEDGMENT

We are grateful to the National Endowment for the Humanities for a fellowship to Jackendoff in 1978, during which much of the research reported here took place. Our notion of time-span reduction owes a great deal to David Lewin's unpublished analysis of the Schubert song "Morgengruss". For advice and comments on our treatment of prosodic structure, we must particularly thank Morris Halle, Samuel Jay Keyser, Alan Prince, and Lisa Selkirk.

The subject of this article is treated more fully in Lerdahl and Jackendoff (in press). A preliminary presentation of the theory appears in Lerdahl and Jackendoff (1977).

REFERENCES

Babbitt, M., 1972, Contemporary music composition and music theory as contemporary intellectual history, in: "Perspectives in Musicology," B. S. Brook, et al., eds., Norton, New York.

Becker, J., and Becker, A., 1979, A grammar of the musical genre SREPEGAN, J. Mus. Theory, 23(1): 1-44.

Bernstein, L., 1976, "The Unanswered Question : Six Talks at Harvard," Harvard University Press, Cambridge, Ma.

Chomsky, N., 1965, "Aspects of the Theory of Syntax," MIT Press, Cambridge, Ma.

Chomsky, N., 1972, "Language and Mind," Harcourt Brace, New York.

Chomsky, N., 1975, "Reflections on Language," Pantheon, New York.

Chomsky, N., and Halle, M., 1968, "The Sound Pattern of English," Harper & Row, New York.

Chomsky, N., and Miller, G., 1963, Introduction to the formal analysis of natural languages, in: "Handbook of Mathematical Psychology," Vol. II., Luce, Bush, and Galanter, eds., Wiley, New York.

Cooper, G., and Meyer, L., 1960, "The Rhythmic Structure of Music," University of Chicago Press, Chicago.

Dowling, W.J., 1978, Scale and contour: two components of a theory of memory for melodies, Psych. Rev., 85(4):341-354.

Halle, M., and Keyser, S.J., 1971, "English Stress," Harper & Row, New York.

Jackendoff, R., 1977, Review of Bernstein, "The Unanswered Question: Six Talks at Harvard," Language, 53(4):883-894.

Jackendoff, R., and Lerdahl, F., in press, Generative music theory and its relation to psychology.

Kahn, D., 1976, "Syllable-based generalizations in English Phonology," Ph.D diss., MIT, dist. by the Ind. Univ. Linguistics Club.

Kiparsky, P., 1977, The rhythmic structure of English verse, Ling. Inquiry, 8(2):189-248.

Kiparsky, P., 1979, Metrical structure assignment is cyclic, Ling. Inquiry, 10(3):421-442.

Lasher, M., 1978, "A Study in the Cognitive Representation of Human Motion," Unpubl. Ph.D. diss., Columbia University, New York.

Lerdahl, F., and Jackendoff, R., 1977, Toward a formal theory of tonal music, J. Mus. Theory, 21(1):111-171.

Lerdahl, F., and Jackendoff, R., 1981, On the theory of grouping and meter, Music. Quart., LXVII.4.

Lerdahl, F., and Jackendoff, R., in press, "A Generative Theory of Tonal Music," MIT Press, Cambridge Ma.

Liberman, M., 1975, "The Intonational System of English," Ph.D. diss.,MIT, dist. by the Ind. Univ. Linguistics Club.

Liberman, M., and Prince, A., 1977, On stress and linguistic rhythm, Ling. Inquiry 8(2):249-336.

Safir, K., ed., 1979, "MIT Working Papers in Linguistics," Vol. 1. MIT Dept. of Linguistics and Philosophy, Cambridge.

Schenker, H., 1935, "Der freie Satz," Universal Edition, Vienna.

Selkirk, E., 1978, "On Prosodic Structure and its Relation to Syntactic Structure," Unpubl. mimeo, Univ. of Masachusetts Dept. of Linguistics, Amherst, Ma.

Selkirk, E., 1980, The role of prosodic categories in English word stress, Ling. Inquiry 11(3).

Sundberg, J., and Lindblom, B., 1976, Generative theories in language and music description, Cognition, 4:99-122.

Vergnaud, J.R., and Halle, M., 1979, "Metrical Structures in Phonology - a Fragment of a Draft," Unpub. mimeo, MIT.

Werner, O., and Topper, M.D., 1976, On the theoretical unity of ethnoscience, lexicography and ethnoscience ethnographies, in: "Georgetown University Round Table of Languages and Linguistics 1976," C. Rameh, ed., Georgetown University Press, Washington, D.C.

Wertheimer, M., 1923, Laws of organization in perceptual forms, in: "A Source Book of Gestalt Psychology 1938", W.D. Ellis, ed., Routledge & Kegan Paul, London.

ORGANIZATIONAL PROCESSES IN MUSIC

Diana Deutsch

Center for Human Information Processing
University of California at San Diego
La Jolla, California, USA

In this paper we shall examine musical organization from several points of view. First we shall consider how the listener sorts the components of a musical configuration into separate groupings. Next we shall discuss some issues involving the formation of musical abstractions so as to lead to perceptual equivalences and similarities. And finally, hierarchical organization in music will be considered.

Basically there are two issues involved in examining grouping mechanisms. First we may enquire into the nature of the stimulus attributes with respect to which grouping principles operate. When presented with a musical configuration, our auditory system may form groupings according to some rule based on the frequencies of its components, on their amplitudes, on the spatial locations from which they emanate, or on the basis of some complex attribute such as timbre. All these attributes can indeed function as bases for grouping, depending on the type of configuration presented.

Second, assuming that organization takes place on the basis of some dimension, what are the rules governing grouping along this dimension? The Gestalt psychologists proposed that we form groupings on the basis of various simple principles. One is the principle of Proximity, which states that groupings are formed out of elements that are close together in preference to those that are spaced further apart. In Figure 1a, for example, the closer dots appear to be grouped together in pairs. Another Gestalt principle is that of Similarity, which states that configurations are formed out of like elements. For example, in Figure 1b, we perceive one set of vertical rows formed by the filled circles and another set formed by the unfilled circles. A third principle is that of Good Continuation. As illustrated on Figure 1c, elements that follow each other in a given direction tend to be perceived together: in this case the dots are perceptually grouped so as to form the two lines AB and CD. Fourth, the principle of Common Fate states that elements which move in the same direction are perceptually linked together (Wertheimer, 1923). It seems reasonable to

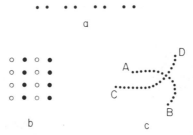

Fig. 1.   Configurations illustrating the Gestalt principles of Proximity, Similarity and Good Continuation.

suppose that grouping in conformity with such principles enables us to interpret our environment most effectively (Bregman, 1978; Gregory, 1970; Hochberg, 1974; Sutherland, 1973). For example, in the case of vision, proximal elements are more likely to be part of the same object than more distal elements. Analogously, similar elements are more likely to belong to the same object than dissimilar ones. In the case of hearing, similar sounds are likely to be coming from the same source and different sounds from different sources. A sequence that changes smoothly in frequency is likely to be coming from a single source. Components of a complex sound spectrum that rise and fall synchronously are also likely to be coming from a single source.

A further point should here be made. When we hear a tone, we attribute to it a fundamental pitch, a loudness, a timbre, and a spatial location. So each tonal percept may be described as a bundle of attribute values. If our percept is veridical, this bundle reflects the location and characteristics of the tone presented. But in situations where more than one tone is simultaneously presented, these bundles of attribute values may fragment and recombine in different ways so as to give rise to illusory percepts. So perceptual grouping in music is not simply a matter of forming linkages between different groups of stimuli; rather it involves an initial process in which these stimuli are fragmented into their different attributes, followed by a later process of synthesis in which the values of these attributes are recombined.

The two-channel listening technique involves presenting two sets of auditory stimuli in parallel, either through earphones or through spatially separated loudspeakers. This technique is particularly useful for studying organizational mechanisms in music, since it enables the experimenter to set different attributes in opposition to each other as bases for grouping. Thus, grouping by spatial location may be opposed to grouping by amplitude or by frequency. At the same time, various principles governing grouping along a given dimension may be opposed to each other; for instance the principle of Proximity may be set out in opposition to the principle of Good Continuation.

In one experiment employing this technique, I presented listeners with the two part pattern shown on Figure 2a. It can be seen that this consisted of a major scale, played simultaneously in both ascending and descending form. The sequence was presented through earphones, such that when a tone from the ascending scale was in the right ear, a tone from the descending scale was in the left ear, and successive tones in each scale alternated from ear to ear. This pattern was presented ten times without pause (Deutsch, 1975a, 1975b). The most common percept is illustrated on Figure 2b. It can be seen that this consisted of two melodies, one formed by the higher tones and the other by the lower tones. The higher tones all appeared to be emanating from one earphone and the lower tones from the other. Thus grouping by frequency proximity was here so strong as to cause the tones in one frequency range to be mislocalized to one side of space, and tones in another frequency range to be mislocalized to the other side.

Recently, Butler (1979a) has extended these findings to a broad range of musical situations. He presented this sequence through spatially-separated loudspeakers in a free sound-field environment. The subjects, who were music students, notated separately the sequence that they heard as coming from the speaker on the right and the sequence that they heard as coming from the speaker on the left. In some conditions piano tones were used as stimuli. In addition, difference in timbre and loudness were sometimes introduced between the sounds presented through the different speakers. Regardless of these variations, almost all responses demonstrated grouping by frequency proximity, so that higher and lower melodic lines were heard, each apparently coming from a different speaker. Further, when differences in timbre were introduced between the stimuli presented through the two speakers, the listeners perceived new tone quality, but as though coming simultaneously from both speakers. Thus not only was there a perceptual rearrangement of the spatial locations of tones, but there was also a perceptual rearrangement of their timbres.

In order to find out where these phenomena generalize to other melodic configurations, Butler presented subjects with further two-part contrapuntal patterns. He found that again, virtually all responses reflected grouping by frequency proximity. In each configuration the two simultaneous sequences were perceptually reorganized so that a melody corresponding to the higher

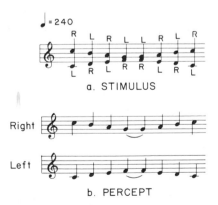

Fig. 2a.   Stimulus pattern producing the scale illusion.
Fig. 2b   The illusion most commonly obtained.

on Figure 4, and each was generated under the four different conditions shown on Figure 5. The error rates in each condition are also shown on Figure 5. In Condition A the melody was presented to both ears simultaneously. As can be seen, identification performance was here very high. In Condition B the component tones of the melody were distributed in quasi-random fashion between the ears, and here identification performance was in contrast very poor. Subjectively one feels compelled in this condition to listen to the pattern coming either from one earphone or from the other, and it is very difficult to integrate the two patterns into a single perceptual stream. Condition C was exactly as Condition B, except that the melody was accompanied by a drone. Whenever a tone from the melody was in the right ear the drone was in the left ear, and whenever a tone from the melody was in the left ear the drone was in the right ear. So both ears always received input simultaneously, even though the components of the melody were still switching from ear to ear exactly as in Condition B. It can be seen that identification of the melody was greatly improved in this condition, and subjectively the difficulty in integrating the two streams essentially disappers. In Condition D a drone again accompanied the melody, but now it was always presented to the same ear as the melody component. This meant that input was again to only one ear at a time, just as in Condition B. And as can be seen, identification performance was again very poor.

This experiment shows that with signals delivered to two spatial locations, temporal relationships between these signals are important determinants of grouping. When the two ears were stimulated simultaneously, grouping by frequency range was easy, so that identification of the melody was readily achieved. However when the inputs to the two ears were clearly separated in time, grouping by spatial location was so powerful as to virtually obliterate the listener's ability to integrate the signals arriving at the two ears into a single perceptual stream.

What happens in the intermediate case, where the signals arriving at the two ears are not strictly simultaneous, but rather overlapping in time? To find out, I investigated the effects of onset-offset asynchronies between the components of the melody and the contralateral drone. This intermediate case found to produce intermediate results. Identification of the melody in the presence of the contralateral drone where the two were

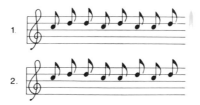

Fig. 4.   Basic patterns used in experiment to study melody identification when the component tones switch between ears. Each pattern was repetitively presented ten times without pause (from Deutsch, 1979).

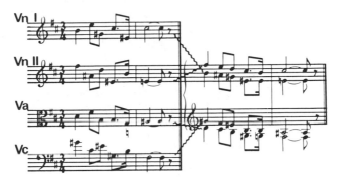

Fig. 3.   Passage from the final movement of Tchaikowsky's Sixth
           Symphony. The combination of the Violin I and Violin II parts
           gives rise to the percept shown on the upper right. The
           combination of the viola and violincello parts gives rise to the
           percept shown on the lower right (from Butler, 1979b).

tones appeared to be coming from one speaker, and a melody corresponding
to the lower tones from the other.

In another paper, Butler (1979b) drew attention to a passage from the
final movement of Tschaikowsky's sixth symphony. As illustrated on Figure
3, the theme and accompaniment are both distributed between the two
violin parts. Yet, the theme is heard as coming from one set of violins and
the accompaniment as from the other. This phenomenon is very striking
even with the instruments arranged in nineteenth century fashion, with the
first violins on one side of the orchestra and the second violins on the other
side.

Such localization illusions may be explained as follows. Given the
complexity of our auditory environment, particularly the presence of echoes
and reverberation, when a sound mixture is presented such that both ears
are stimulated simultaneously, it is not evident from first-order localization
cues alone which components of the total spectrum should be assigned to
which source. Other cues must also provide information concerning the
sources of these different sounds. One such cue is similarity of frequency
spectrum. As described above, similar sounds are likely to be coming from
the same source and different sounds from different sources. So with these
musical examples it becomes plausible to suppose that tones in one
frequency range are coming from one source, and tones in a different
frequency range from another source. The listener therefore reorganizes
the tones perceptually on the basis of this supposition (Deutsch, 1975b). The
general notion of 'unconscious inference' as a basis for perceptual illusions
was proposed in the last century by Helmholtz.

In these experiments the signals arriving at the two ears or from the
two locations were simultaneous. What happens when this isn't so? To examine this issue, I performed an experiment in which subjects were
presented with two simple melodic patterns, and they identified on each
trial which one they had heard (Deutsch, 1979). The two patterns are shown

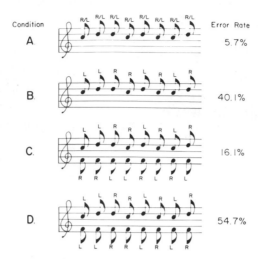

Fig. 5.   Examples of distributions between ears of melody and drone in the different conditions of the experiment, together with error rates in each condition (from Deutsch, 1979).

asynchronous was better than where input was to only one ear at a time, but worse than where the melody and drone were strictly synchronous.

How do we explain these findings? The relationships between waveform envelopes of sound signals are important indicators of whether these signals are coming from the same source or from different sources (following the principle of Common Fate). We should therefore expect that the more clearly the signals arriving at the two ears are separated in time, the greater should be the tendency to treat these signals as emanating from separate sources, and so the greater the tendency to group them by spatial location. If such grouping is powerful enough it should prevent us from forming perceptual linkages between the signals emanating from different sources. Obviously it is necessary, in performing auditory shape analyses, that we not link together the components of different signals, or we would end up with nonsensical percepts (see also Bregman, 1978).

Other experiments on grouping in music have used the technique of presenting a single stream of tones in rapid succession. Much of this work has emphasized the importance of frequency proximity as an organizing factor. For example, when tones in a rapid sequence are drawn from two different frequency ranges the listener perceives, not a single stream of tones but two parallel streams. This perceptual phenomenon forms the basis of the technique of pseudo-polyphony. A sequence of tones which are drawn from two different frequency ranges is played in rapid succession, with the result that the listener hears two melodic lines in parallel.

Now, such rapid sequences of tones have several interesting properties. For example, they are poorly organized in the temporal domain. Temporal relationships are easily perceived between tones in the same frequency range, but are poorly perceived between tones in different frequency ranges. This is manifest in several different ways. For example if one presents a sequence of tones drawn from two different frequency ranges in rapid succession (i.e., at a rate of about 10 per second) perception of the orders of these tones can be very difficult (Bregman and Campbell, 1971). When the presentation rate is slowed down, so that order perception is readily accomplished, there is still a gradual breakdown in temporal resolution with an increase in the frequency disparity between two alternating tones. For instance, a rhythmic irregularity in such a pattern of tones becomes difficult to detect (Van Noorden, 1975).

Another consequence of channeling by frequency proximity was demonstrated by Dowling (1973). He presented two well-known melodies, with their component tones alternating at a rapid rate. He found that when the frequency ranges of these melodies overlapped, recognition was difficult, since their components were perceptually combined into a single stream. But as one of the alternating melodies was gradually transposed, so that their frequency ranges diverged, recognition performance increased.

Another principle by which musical configurations are organized is that of Good Continuation. It has been shown, for instance, that when presented with a rapid sequence of tones, listeners can identify their orders better when they follow a unidirectional frequency change than when they do not (Divenyi and Hirsh, 1974; McNally and Handel, 1977; Nickerson and Freeman, 1974: Warren and Byrnes, 1975).

A further organizing principle is that of Similarity, which is manifest in grouping on the basis of timbre. In classical music, timbre is often used as a marker of sequential configurations (Erickson, 1975). Adjacent phrases are often played by different instruments, to enhance their distinctiveness. Overlaps in frequency range between figure and ground are far more common where different instruments are involved. This reflects the greater perceptual distinctiveness provided by difference in timbre.

Grouping by timbre is reflected in the finding that listeners have extreme difficulty in identifying the orders of rapid sequences of unrelated sounds. This was first demonstrated by Warren, Obsuek, Farmer and Warren (1969). They generated repeating sequences of four unrelated sounds: a high tone, a hiss, a low tone and a buzz. Each sound was 200 msec in duration, and the sounds followed each other without pause. Listeners were found to be quite unable to name the order of the sounds in these repeating sequences. To achieve correct naming, the duration of each sound had to be increased to over half a second.

We next turn to an examination of the types of abstraction that are performed on musical information so as to lead to perceptual equivalences and similarities. The Gestalt psychologists first emphasized that configurations may be perceived as equivalent even when they are composed of entirely different elements, provided that certain relationships between these elements are preserved. A visual shape for example will retain its perceptual identity when it is translated to a different location in the visual field, altered in size, and in some conditions rotated or turned into its mirror image.

Interestingly, one of the first examples given of perceptual equivalence under transformation was a musical one. Von Ehrenfels (1890) pointed out that a melody when transposed retains its essential form, provided that the relations between the individual tones are not changed. In this respect, he claimed, melodies are similar to visual shapes. He was therefore implying an inter-modal analogy where one dimension of visual space is mapped into pitch and the other dimension into time. On this analogy, transposing a melody is like translating a shape to a different location in the visual field.

This leads us to ask whether further equivalences can be demonstrated for musical shapes that are analogous to those for shapes in vision. Schoenberg (1951) argued that transformations similar to rotation and mirror-image reversal in vision result in perceptual equivalences in music also. He proposed on this basis that a row of tones may be recognized as equivalent when it is transformed such that all descending intervals become ascending intervals and vice versa ('inversion'); when it is presented with the order of the tones reversed ('retrogression') or when it is transformed by both these operations ('retrograde-inversion'). Examples of such transformations, together with their visuospatial counterparts are shown on Figure 6.

Whether such transformations do indeed result in perceptual equivalences is a thorny issue. In experiments by Dowling and Fujitani (1971) and White (1960) subjects had considerable difficulty in recognizing certain melodic patterns in retrogression or inversion. However, considerably more experimental work needs to be done before this issue can be properly understood. First, such operations may occur readily, provided that the processing load is not too heavy. Second, it appears from consideration of tonal music that inversion is an operation that may be accomplished readily with respect to highly overlearned pitch alphabets, such as the arpeggiation of a triad, or a diatonic scale; without regard to interval size (Deutsch and Feroe, in preparation).

Another assumption of importance is that of octave equivalence. It is clear from a large amount of general evidence that there is a strong perceptual similarity between tones that are separated by octaves. For this reason it has been suggested that pitch should be regarded as a bidimensional attribute; the first dimension representing overall pitch level, and the second defining the position of a tone within the octave. Psychologists have referred to these two dimensions as 'tone height' and 'tone chroma' (Bachem, 1948; Meyer, 1904; Revesz, 1913; Ruckmick, 1929; Shepard, 1964), and music theorists make an analogous distinction between 'pitch' and 'pitch class' (Babbitt, 1960; Forte, 1973).

This raises the question of whether the principle of octave equivalence should be treated as a perceptual invariant; that is, whether it holds true for all types of musical processing. For example, what happens when we take a melody and place its component tones in different octaves so that pitch class is preserved but the pitches themselves are altered? Does our perceptual system treat such a transformed melody as equivalent to the original?

In one experiment I investigated this question by playing a well-known tune (it was Yankee Doodle) to groups of listeners, and asking them to give its name (Deutsch, 1972). The tune was generated in several different ways. First it was produced without transformation. Then it was generated such that pitch class was preserved (that is, each tone was in its correct position within the octave) but the choice of octave placement varied randomly between three octaves. And finally it was generated as a series of clicks, so that the pitch information was removed entirely, but the rhythm was retained. This was to determine a baseline for identificaton performance with rhythm as the only clue.

These different versions of the tune were presented to separate groups of subjects, who were given no clues as to its identity. As shown on Figure 7, although the untransformed version was recognized by everyone, recognition of the randomized octaves version was no better than where the pitch information was entirely removed. The subjects were then informed of the identity of the tune, and were again played the randomized octaves version, and found that they could now follow it to a large extent. They were therefore able to <u>confirm</u> the identity of the tune, although they had not been able to <u>recognize</u> it when they had been given no prior information. We would therefore expect that, if the listener is provided with certain clues as to what a tune might be, for instance, if he is given its rhythm, its contour, or its name amongst a small list of alternative; and as a result he forms the right hypothesis, he can then confirm this hypothesis using the tonal information provided. Indeed, other studies have shown that when subjects are given ample opportunity for hypothesis testing, recognition performance is much higher, as would be expected on the present line of reasoning (Deutsch, 1978; Dowling and Hollombe, 1977; House, 1977; Idson and Massaro, 1978).

We may in this context consider the use of octave jumps in traditional music. Given the present line of reasoning, such jumps can be made with impunity provided that the musical setting is such as to make the displaced

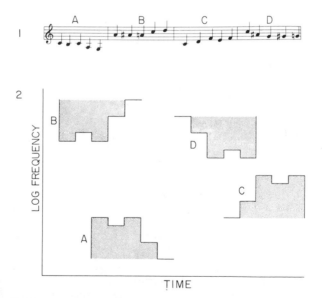

Fig. 6.1   A row of tones presented in prime form (A) inversion (B) retrograde (C) and retrograde-inversion (D).

Fig. 6.2   Visuospatial equivalents.

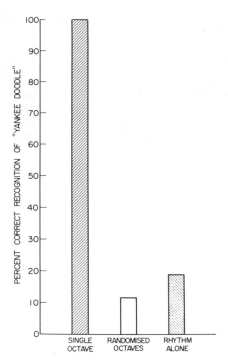

Fig. 7.   Percent correct recognition of the tune "Yankee Doodle" under various presentation conditions. See text for details (from Deutsch, 1972).

note highly probable. We should thus expect that octave jumps would tend to occur mostly in such situations. Indeed this appears to be so. In one such situation a melodic line is presented several times without transformation. A clear set of expectations having thus been established, a jump to a different octave occurs. In another such situation, the harmonic structure is clear and unambiguous, with the result that again the displaced notes are highly probable.

Finally I should like to address the issue of hierarchical structure in music from a psychologist's point of view. Music theorists have long recognized that tonal music is organized in hierarchical fashion (Meyer, 1973; Salzer, 1962; Schenker, 1956, 1973). This raises several questions of interest to psychologists. What processing advantages are to be gained by such organization, and why? Under what conditions are tonal hierarchies more apparent to the listener, and under what conditions are they masked?

First we should note that hierarchical structuring of information is a general cognitive phenomenon. The structure of language is a prime example here, but we also readily form hierarchies of rules, of goals in problem solving, and even visual scenes have been shown to be encoded in hierarchical fashion. So hierarchical structuring in music is a manifestation of a general principle of cognitive organization.

Second we should note that when presented with a serial pattern, regardless of the nature of its elements, recall of such a sequence is enhanced if we can divide this information into subsequences or chunks of three of four items each (Estes, 1972; Wickelgren, 1967). In fact, when given the opportunity to do so, we readily group serial patterns into chunks that are retained as units (Bower, 1972).

A third point to be noted from general studies of cognition is that we encode and retain information much more effectively when it is composed of a relatively small alphabet and further that we can handle several such small alphabets at the same time very well, and much better than a single large alphabet which is composed of the same total number of elements (Mandler, 1967).

A fourth point to note is that if different portions of a sequence of elements can be related to each other by some rule, we need only remember an abstraction and the rule, in order to retrieve a considerable amount of information. For example, in order to remember the sequence A B C D B C D E C D E F we need only remember that a higher level sequence traversing the English alphabet acts on a lower level sequence consisting of four steps up this alphabet. Here again, this type of cognitive manipulation occurs with all kinds of information (Restle, 1970: Restle and Brown, 1970; Simon. 1972: Simon and Kotovsky, 1963; Simon and Sumner, 1968; Vitz and Todd, 1969).

Tonal music appears to have evolved in accordance with such principles of cognitive organization. Musical hierarchies involve limited alphabets which may differ from one structural level to another. For example a higher-level subsequence based on a triad may act on a lower-level subsequence based on a diatonic scale. Further, a segment of music tends to be limited to very few items at any one hierarchical level. even though the segment taken in its entirety may be very long. Also, there are often abstract rules governing relationships between subsequences which allow for considerable economy of memory storage. A hierarchical model for the internal representation of pitch sequences in tonal music has recently been advanced (Deutsch and Feroe, in preparation).

In a recent experiment memory for tonal sequences that were hierarchically structured was compared with memory for those that were not (Deutsch, in press). There was a second factor that was also considered. This concerns the influence of temporal segmentation on the ability to utilize such hierarchies. Temporal proximity may act as a very strong grouping principle, and may mask grouping on other principles (Bower and Springston, 1970; Handel, 1973; Restle, 1972). So it was predicted that temporal grouping in accordance with tonal structure would result in somewhat enhanced performance, and that grouping in conflict with such structure would give rise to performance decrements.

In this experiment, four structured sequences were employed, and these are shown on Figure 8a. It can be seen that each consisted of a higher-level subsequence of four elements that acted on a lower-level subsequence of three elements. From each of these, another sequence was constructed, which consisted of the identical set of tones, but arranged in haphazard fashion. These are shown on Figure 8b. The average interval size formed by adjacent tones in the unstructured sequences was near-identical to the

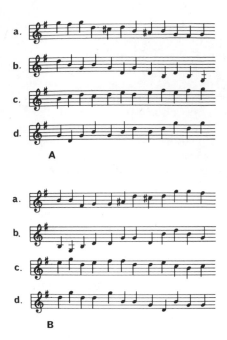

Fig. 8.   Sequences employed to study utilization of structure in recall.
The sequences in A can each be described as a higher-order subsequence of four elements that act on a lower-order subsequence
of three elements. The sequences in B are unstructured (from
Deutsch, in press).

average interval size formed by adjacent tones in the structured sequences.

These eight sequences were each presented in three temporal configurations. In the first, the tones were spaced at equal intervals; in the second
they occurred in four groups of three; and in the third they occurred in three
groups of four.

There were therefore six conditions in the experiment. Figure 9
displays the percentages of tones correctly recalled at each serial position
in these different conditions. It can be seen that large effects of both tonal
structure and temporal segmentation were obtained. For structured
sequences that were segmented in accordance with structure the
performance level was extremely high. For structured sequences with no
temporal segmentation the performance level was again very high, though
slightly lower. But, for structured sequences that were segmented in
conflict with structure, the performance level was considerably reduced.
For unstructured sequences performance levels were considerably lower
than for structured sequences that were either not segmented or that were
segmented in accordance with structure.

Examining the serial position curves further, we may note that typical
bow-shaped curves are apparent, and that in addition discontinuities appear
at boundaries between temporal groups. This type of configuration, which is

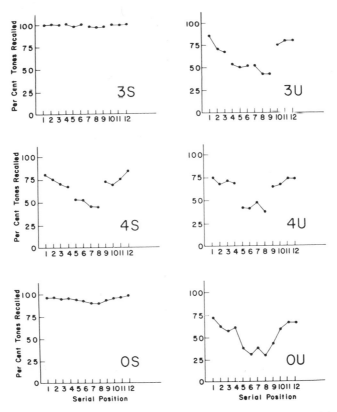

Fig. 9. Serial position curves for the different conditions of the experiment. 3s: structured sequences segmented in temporal groups of three; 4s: structured sequences segmented in temporal groups of four; OS: structured sequences with no temporal segmentation; 3U unstructured sequences segmented in temporal groups of three; 4U: unstructured sequences segmented in temporal groups of four; OU: unstructured sequences with no temporal segmentation.

very similar to that obtained by Bower and Winzenz (1969) with verbal materials, implies that temporal groups tend to be coded as units or chunks, and to be retained or lost independently. A further measure of interitem association is the transition shift probability (or TSP), defined as the joint probability of either a correct response following an error on the previous item, or of an error following a correct response on the previous item. If groups of elements tend to be retained or lost as chunks, then the TSP values should be smaller for transitions within a chunk, and larger for the transition into the first element of a chunk. Figure 10 displays the TSP values for sequences segmented in temporal groups of three and four respectively. The TSP after each pause is shown by shading. It can be seen that the TSPs are larger on the first element of each temporal group than on

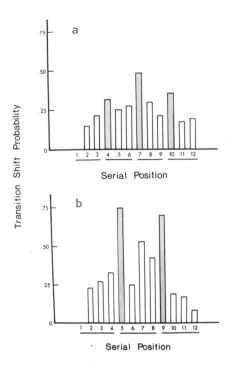

Fig. 10.   Transition shift probabilities for sequences segmented in temporal groups of three (a) and temporal groups of four (b).

the other elements.   This is as expected on the assumption that pauses define subjective chunks that tend to be retained or lost independently; and these results are again very similar to those obtained by others with verbal materials (Bower and Springston, 1970).

This experiment entails several conclusions. First, it demonstrates that listeners perceive hierarchical structures that are present in tonal sequences and can utilize these structures in recall. For the structured sequences employed in this study, the listener need only retain two chunks of three or four items each; however, for the unstructured sequences, no such parsimonious encoding was possible. The unstructured sequences therefore imposed a much heavier memory load, with resultant performance decrements. Second, the experiments demonstrate that temporal segmentation has a profound effect on perceived structure, as has been noted by others with the use of different materials. Temporal segmentation in accordance with structure resulted in somewhat enhanced performance; temporal segmentation in conflict with structure led to severe performance decrements. On our present line of reasoning, when temporal grouping is in conflict with tonal structure, there results a less parsimonious representation, which in turn leads to decrements in recall. Such findings are in accordance with musical practice, in which groupings based on tonal structure tend to coincide with groupings based on temporal structure.

In this review, musical organization has been considered at several levels: from the mechanisms involved in separating out the components of a complex sound spectrum so that multiple streams of tones are perceived, to those underlying the generation of tonal hierarchies. The system involved is clearly very complex, but an understanding of how we organize musical information is beginning to emerge.

SUMMARY

The organization of musical information is examined at several levels. Grouping mechanisms are first considered. When presented with a complex musical configuration, our auditory system forms groupings according to some rule based on the frequencies of its components, on their amplitudes, on the spatial locations from which they emanate, or on the basis of some complex attribute, such as timbre. The decision as to which attribute is used as a basis for grouping depends on the characteristics of the configuration presented. The principles governing grouping along any given dimension are examined. These include various Gestalt principles, such as Proximity, Similarity and Good Continuation. Some issues involving the formation of higher-order abstractions in music are next considered. Finally, hierarchical structure in music is considered, together with the interaction between tonal structure and temporal segmentation.

ACKNOWLEDGMENT

The work of this chapter, based on a review paper given at the Third Workshop on Physical and Neuropsychological Foundations of Music, held at Ossiach, August 1980, was supported by United States Public Health Service Grant MH 21001.

REFERENCES

Babbit, M., 1960, Twelve-tone invariants as compositional determinants, Mus. Quart., 46:246-259.
Bachem. A., 1948, Note on Neu's review of the literature on absolute pitch. Psychol Bull., 45:161-162.
Bower, G.H., 1972, Organizational factors in memory, in: "Organization of Memory," E. Tulving and W. Donaldson, eds., Academic Press, New York.
Bower, G.H., and Springston, F., 1970, Pauses as recoding points in letter series, J. Exp. Psychol., 83:421-430.
Bower, G.H., and Winzenz, D., 1969, Group structure, coding and memory for digit series, J. Exp. Psychol. Monographs, 80.2:1-17.
Bregman. A.S., 1979, The formation of auditory streams, in: "Attention and Performance VII," J. Requin, ed., Erlbaum, Hillsdale.
Bregman. A.S., and Campbell, J., 1971, Primary auditory stream segregation and perception of order in rapid sequence of tones, J. Exp. Psychol., 89:244-249.

Butler, D., 1979(a), A further study of melodic channeling, Perc. and
    Psychophys., 25:264-268.
Butler, D., 1979(b), Melodic channeling in musical environment, Res. Symp.
    Psychol. and Acoust. Music, Kansas.
Deutsch, D., 1972, Octave generalization and tune recognition, Perc and
    Psychophys., 11:411-412.
Deutsch, D., 1975(a), Two-channel listening to musical scales, J. Acoust.
    Soc. Am., 57:156-1160.
Deutsch, D., 1975(a), Musical illusions, Scient. Am., 233:92-104.
Deutsch, D., 1978, Octave generalization and melody identification, Perc.
    and Psychophys., 23:91-92.
Deutsch, D., 1979, Binaural integration of melodic patterns, Perc. and
    Psychophys., 25:399-405.
Deutsch, D., in press. The processing of structured and unstructured tonal
    sequences, Perc. and Psychophys.
Deutsch, D., and Feroe, S., in press, The internal representation of pitch
    sequences in tonal music.
Divenyi, P.L., and Hirsch, I.J., 1974, Identification of temporal order in
    three-tone sequences, J. Acoust. Soc. Am., 56:144-151.
Dowling, W.J., 1973, The perception of interleaved melodies, Cog.
    Psychol., 5:322-337.
Dowling, W.J., and Fujitani, D.S., 1971, Contour, interval and pitch
    recognition in memory for melodies, J. Aoust. Soc. Am., 49:524-531.
Dowling, W.J., and Hollombe, A.W., 1977, The perception of melodies
    distorted by splitting into several octaves. Effects of increasing
    proximity and melodic conotour, Perc. and Psychophy, 21 60-64.
Ehrenfels, C. von., 1890, Über Gestaltqualitaten "Vierteljahrschrift fur
    Wissenschaftliche Philosophie." 14:249-292.
Erickson, R., 1975, "Sound Structure in Music," University of California
    Press, Berkeley.
Estes, W.K., 1972, An associative basis for coding and organization in
    memory, in: "Coding Processes in Human Memory," A.W. Melton and E.
    Martin, eds., Winston, Washington.
Forte, A., 1973, "The Structure of Atonal Music," Yale University Press,
    New Haven.
Gregory, R.L., 1970, "The Intelligent Eye," McGraw-Hill, New York.
Handel, S., 1973, Temporal segmentation of repeating auditory patterns, J.
    Exp. Psychol., 101:46-54.
Hochberg, J., 1974, Organization and the Gestalt tradition, in: "Handbook of
    Perception," Vol. I, E.C. Carterette and M.P. Friedman, eds.,
    Academic Press New York.
House, W.J., 1977, Octave generalization and the indentification distorted
    melodies, Perc. and Psychophys., 21:586-589.
Idson, W.L., and Massaro, D.W., 1978, A bidimensional model of pitch in the
    recognition of melodies, Perc. and Psychophys., 24:551-565.
Mandler, G.. 1967, Organization and memory, in, "The Psychology of
    Learning and Motivation," Vol. 1, K.W. Spence and J.A. Spence, eds.,
    Academic Press, New York.

McNally, K.A., and Handel, S., 1977, Effect of element composition on streaming and the ordering of repeating sequences, J. Exp. Psychol: Human Perc. and Perf., 3:451-460.

Meyer, L.B., 1973, "Explaining Music: Essays and Explanations," University of California Press, Berkeley.

Meyer, M., 1904, On the attributes of the sensations. Psycho. Rev., 11:83-103.

Meyer, M., 1914, Review of G. Revesz, Zur Grundlegung der Tonpsychologie, Psychol. Bull., 11:349-352.

Noorden, L.P.A.S. van, 1975, "Temporal Coherence in the Perception of Tone Sequences," unpubl. doctoral dissertation, Technische Hogeschool Eindhoven.

Restle, F., 1970, Theory of serial pattern learning: Structural trees, Psychol. Rev., 77:481-495.

Restle, F., 1970, Serial patterns: The role of phrasing, J. Exp. Psychol., 92:385-390.

Restle, F., and Brown, E., 1970, Organization of serial pattern learning, in: "The Psychology of Learning and Motivation: Advances in Research and Theory," Vol. 4, G. Bower, ed., Academic Press, New York.

Revesz, G., 1913, "Zur Grundlegung der Tonpsychologie," Feit, Leipzig.

Ruckmick, C.A., 1929, A new classification of tonal qualities, Psychol. Rev., 36:172-180.

Salzer, F., 1962, "Structural Hearing," Dover, New York.

Schenker, H., 1956, "Neue Musikalische Theorien and Phantasien: Der Freie Satz," Universal Edition, Vienna.

Schenker, H., 1973, "Harmony," O. Jones, ed. and annot., E.M. Borgese, transl., MIT Press, Cambridge, Ma.

Schoenberg, A., 1951, "Style and Idea," Williams & Norgate, London.

Shepard, R.N., 1964, Circularity in judgements of relative pitch, J. Acoust. Soc. Am., 36:2345-2353.

Simon, H.A., 1972, Complexity and the representation of patterned sequences of symbols, Psychol. Rev., 79:369-382.

Simon, H.A., and Kotovsky, K., 1963, Human acquistion of concepts for sequential patterns, Psychol. Rev., 70:534-546.

Simon, H.A., and Sumner, R.K., 1968, Pattern in music, in: "Formal Representation of Human Judgment," B. Kleinmuntz, ed., Wiley, New York.

Sutherland, N.S., 1973, Object recognition, in: "Handbook of Perception" Vol. III. E.C. Carterette and M.P. Friedman, eds., Academic Press, New York.

Vitz, P.C., and Todd, T.C., 1969, A coded element model of the perceptual processing of sequential stimuli, Psych. Rev., 76:433-449.

Warren, R.M., and Byrnes, D.L., 1975, Temporal discrimination of recycled tonal sequences: Pattern matching and naming of order by untrained listeners, J. Acoust. Soc. Am., 18:273-280.

Warren, R.M., Obusek, C.J., Farmer, R.M., and Warren, R.P., 1969, Auditory sequence: Confusions of patterns other than speech or music, Science, 164:586-587.

Wertheimer, M., 1923, Untersuchung zur Lehre von der Gestalt II, Psychol. Forschung, 4:301-350.

White, B., 1960, Recognition of distorted melodies, Am. J. Psychol.,
    73:100-107.
Wickelgren, W.A., 1967, Rehearsal grouping and the hierarchical
    organization of serial position cues in short-term memory, Quart. J.
    Exp. Psychol., 19:97-102.

SPEECH, SONG, AND EMOTIONS

Johan Sundberg

Department of Speech Communication and Music Acoustics
Royal Institute of Technology
Stockholm, Sweden

INTRODUCTION

Emotions are of course closely related to the sound of the voice. Mostly, 'we judge from the voice' rather well in what state of emotion a speaker is . One and the same sentence can be pronounced in a vast number of different ways, and the way it is pronounced reveals among other things the speaker's state of emotion. Among phoniatrists, it is a general clinical observation that stress may influence a speaker's use of his voice, sometimes to the extent that a voice problem develops. As regards singing, the main intonation contour, which we may consider as sort of 'macro-intonation', is decided by the composer. Also, we may assume that it is up to the singer to guide, within the framework of this macrointonation, the listeners' associations to the state of emotion which the text intends to reflect. The singer may achieve this effect by means of voice character-istics and 'microintonation'. How do these different emotions manifest themselves in speech and singing?

Different investigators have applied different strategies in attempts to find an answer to the last mentioned question. Most of them have analyzed the sound, but some have examined production aspects, and one author has studied the interrelationships between gestures and sound. Three reviews on the subject might be mentioned: Crystal (1969), Kramer (1963), Scherer (1979). They treat the combination emotion-voice in a broad sense including, for instance, such aspects as personality judgements based on voice and the influence of stress on voice. In the last mentioned review article summaries of Scherer's own extensive investigations in this field can be found. Several contributions to this topic of voice and emotions were indirectly generated by man's interest in space; when astronauts were shot away to be left alone in space for a while, it became important to collect all means to find out their emotional state. In this chapter, however, we will go into the aspects of neither stress, nor personality. Instead we will con-centrate on the question how specific emotions influence the vocal behavior.

I.   EMOTIONAL SPEECH

Where in the sound of the voice do we find the informaton about the emotional state of the speaker? One possible parameter is the frequency pattern of the voice fundamental, i.e. the phonation frequency pattern, because the course of the phonation frequency can be varied within wide limits without encroaching on the information on the linguistic contents of a sentence. The breathing pattern can also be influenced by emotions, and consequently effects on the subglottic pressure can be expected. If this pressure is raised, loudness and also, to some extent, phonation frequency will increase. Moreover, faster breathing should affect the phrasing of speech. Drying of the mouth is a symptom of certain emotions, as are disturbances of the motor functions e.g., tremor ('shake with anger', 'tremble with fear'). These are a few factors which ought to have some effect on the glottal voice source. Thus there are a number of voice aspects which appear worthwhile to examine in a study of the influence of emotions on the voice.

Lieberman and Michaels (1962) consider voice source parameters. In a series of listening tests they deprived emotional speech, produced by male speakers, of a systematically increased number of acoustic parameters. In this manner they reduced the listeners' ability to correctly identify the emotion underlying different utterances from 85% for non-manipulated speech down to 14% for speech retaining the amplitude modulation only. A great step in this decrease (from 85% to 47%) resulted from the elimination of the supraglottal, or articulatory contributions to the speech signal. Similarly, the phonation frequency movements were found important; a drop in the percentage of correct responses from 47% to 25% resulted when these movements were eliminated. They also found that "the several emotional modes...do not utilize all the acoustic parameters to the same extent." For instance, fear seemed to rely more heavily on amplitude information than other emotions.

Sedláček and Sychra (1963) had 23 actors read one sentence in a number of different ways, so as to express eight emotional states: neutral, love, joy, solemnity, comic, ironic, sorrow and fear. Listening tests with different groups of observers revealed that a correct identification of these modes did not depend on the subject's capability to understand the language spoken in the test phrases. Nor did the cultural background of the observers seem relevant; a group of students from Asia, Africa and Latin America gave practically the same answers as a group of Czech students, who were the only subjects familiar with the language spoken in the test sentences. The authors examined phonation frequency, amplitude, and spectrum in those sentences which showed the best scores in the listening tests. The average phonation frequency was found to be raised in joy, lowered in sorrow, and intermediate in neutral mode. Phonation frequency movements seemed important as well. Thus, one single phonation frequency peak followed by a falling movement appeared typical for sad modes while the occurrence of two peaks during the utterance seemed associated with more active modes.

Trojan (e.g. 1952) found formal evidence (mainly in terms of pupil dimensions) supporting the assumption of two distinct phonatory dimensions associated with the expression of emotions. One dimension has the extremes sparing-voice (Schonstimme) and power-voice (Kraftstimme) and it is said to 'correspond' to the poles of the 'autonomic rhythm'. The other dimension is the pharyngeal width, which, according to Trojan, is used to express pleasure and disgust. Referring to these hypotheses Trojan and Winckel (1957) studied the acoustical consequences of these phonatory and articulatory dimensions. Phonation in sparing- and power-voice modes differed with respect to amplitude, as we might expect, while the articulatory adjustments of the pharyngeal width affect the formant frequencies, as shown by the spectra published in their article.

More recently, Williams and Stevens (1972) consider the voice effects of four emotional states: sorrow, anger, fear and neutral. Actors performed a short spoken play in which different states of emotion were displayed. As regards phonation frequency curve, a neutral state of emotion was found to be associated with slow changes without any sharp contrasts (Fig. 1). The phonation frequency of anger was normally higher than that for a neutral state. Further, a few syllables showed high peaks in the phonation

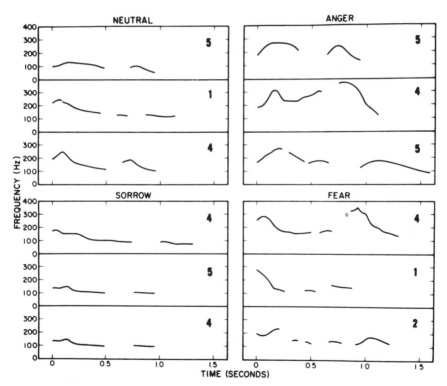

Fig. 1   Phonation frequency curves for the voice of an actor who speaks in the indicated modes several times. Phonation frequency descends slowly in sorrow and exhibits rather wild jumps in the more excited emotional modes. From Williams and Stevens, 1972, J. Acoust. Soc. Am., 52:1238-1250.

frequency contour. Apart from such peaks, the curve is even and continuous. Sorrow presents a completely different pattern. The phonation frequency is low and varies little. It falls slowly almost without interruption until the end of the sentence. Fear was manifested, among other ways, by fast increases and decreases and sharp contrasts.

Statistically the average phonation frequency (Fig. 2) is lowest for sadness, higher in a neutral state and for fear, and highest for anger. The variation is smallest for sorrow and greatest for fear.

The same sentence ("For God's sake!") was pronounced in the shortest time with a neutral state of emotion and in the longest for sorrow. This was due to longer vowel sounds, but mainly because of prolonged consonants. The average number of syllables per second were 4.31 for a neutral state, 4.15 for anger, 3.80 for fear, and 1.91 for sorrow. For sorrow a lack of stability was also observed in the voice source: the individual voice pulses were not similar with respect to the overtone contents. Anger also seems to have higher values for the first formant, probably caused by an exaggerated mouth opening.

A long term average spectrum of speech contains information about the amount of overtones of the voice source. The results (Fig. 3) show that the overtones higher than 1 kHz were most powerful for anger and weakest for sorrow. One can assume that anger is associated with a higher subglottic pressure and maybe a high activity of the adduction muscles. If so, the glottis will close more rapidly in the vibratory cycle and the source spectrum overtones will become stronger. In sorrow, lowered activity of all muscles in general may be the reason for the opposite effect.

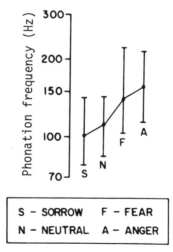

Fig. 2   Median and range of the phonation frequency (points and bars, respectively) for an actor speaking in the emotional situations indicated. Phonation frequency was lowest in sorrow and highest in anger. From Williams and Stevens, 1972, J. Acoust. Soc. Am., 52:1238 1250.

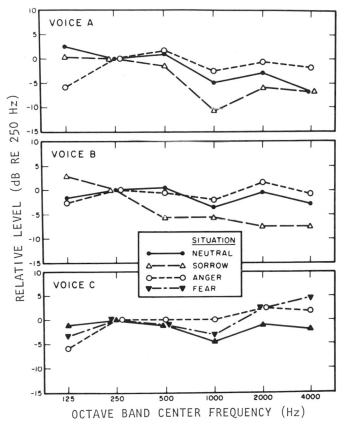

Fig. 3   Averaged spectra of actors speaking in the different modes indicated. Sorrow and neutral show the lowest amplitudes for high overtones. From Williams and Stevens, 1972, J. Acoust. Soc. Am., 52:1238-1250.

A unique piece of evidence in relation to the above has been preserved and may be studied: a recording by a radio journalist who gives an account of the arrival of the airship Hindenburg and the following explosion at Lakehurst, New Jersey, USA on May 6, 1937. A time spectrogram of his voice before and after the explosion shows the following typical differences (Fig. 4): before the catastrophe the phonation frequency shows smooth changes upwards and downwards. After the catastrophe it is higher and varies very slowly but within a larger range. It shows, furthermore, sudden small irregularities, some type of tremor; maybe the newsman is momentarily losing control over his phonation frequency.

In summary, the following 'state-of-emotion-profiles' can be presented for speech, according to Stevens and Williams:

Well here it comes, ladies and gentlemen

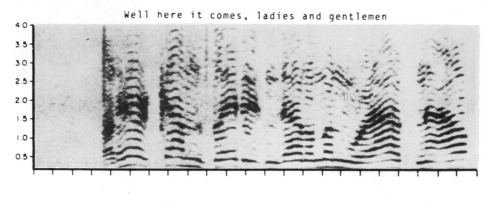

a terrific crash, ladies and gentlemen

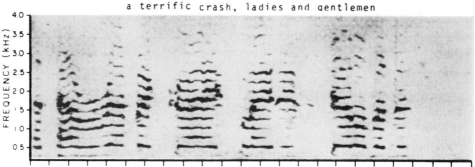

I, I can't talk, ladies and gentlemen

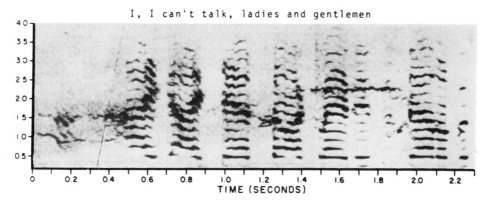

Fig. 4   Time spectrogram of the voice of a radio announcer speaking before (top) and after (middle and bottom) the crash of the Hindenburg. The voice characteristics change drastically when the speaker suddenly witnesses the death of several people. From Williams, Stevens and Hecker, 1969, Aerospace Med., 40:1369-1372.

ANGER: High phonation frequency, almost half an octave above the normal level for neutral speech. The phonation frequency range is greatly expanded. Some syllables are pronounced with high emphasis (increased intensity and sudden increases in phonation frequency) and often a high first formant frequency. The articulation is almost excessively distinct.

FEAR: The phonation frequency is lower compared with anger. Sudden peaks and irregularities are seen in the phonation frequency, The articulation is more precise than in a neutral situation.

SORROW: Little variability in the phonation frequency. The articulation is slow and vowels, consonants, and pauses are long; irregularities can be found in the voice (traces of hoarseness) and the phonation frequency is almost falling monotonously towards the end of the phrase and shows traces of tremor.

NEUTRAL: Neutral speech was generally faster than for the above-mentioned states of emotion. The consonants were often pronounced imprecisely but the vowels show a well-defined pattern with few examples of those irregularities which bear witness to lack of voice control.

II. SINGING WITH EMOTIONAL EXPRESSION

Kotlyar and Morosov (1976) carried out a song-oriented study in which they had eleven professional singers sing a phrase from different songs or arias several times. The singers' task was to create different moods: happiness, sorrow, fear, anger, and neutral. With a proper test procedure they were able to ensure that the singers did in fact succeed with this task. They then measured a number of different acoustic qualities of the song. The result can be seen in Fig. 5. The tempo determined as the average duration of the syllables was fastest for fear and slowest for sorrow. Fear

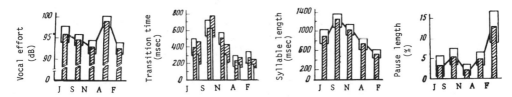

Fig. 5.   The average dependence of some acoustical voice parameters on different emotional modes as produced by professional singers. The modes are indicated as: J = joy, S = sorrow, N = neutral, A = anger, F = fear. In the second graph from the left the hatched column shows the voice onset time and the white column the corresponding value for the decay. Apparently, everything moves slowly in sorrow! The rectangles represent the scatter of the underlying data. From Kotlyar and Morozov, 1976, Sov. Phys. Acoust., 22:208-211.

was also characterized by the longest pauses between syllables. A neutral state of emotion showed the shortest pauses. Anger had the loudest voice amplitude and fear the softest. Sorrow was characterized by the slowest tone onsets, anger and fear the fastest. In this way each mood investigated showed a typical pattern of acoustic characteristics. The authors also tried to find out how much of the whole truth they had been able to identify, by presenting to observers an electronically generated signal whose time dependent characteristics (pitch, loudness, onset etc.) varied in accordance with what they had found was of significance with the studied moods. The signals had no vowels and consonants and consisted only of a sound with variable loudness and pitch. The question asked was whether it was possible for the observers to determine what mood the signal 'represented'. The observers succeeded pretty well with the exception of the case of joy. The signal never really sounded joyful. A possible interpretation of this result is that although the temporal variations they studied are characteristics for the moods, there are also other important signal characteristics, especially in the case of joy. It is not ony by duration of syllables and pauses, by voice amplitude, and by rise and decay time of the tones that one expresses happinesss. Still. those parameters are involved in the pattern of characteristics which are typical of sorrow, fear, anger and a neutral state.

III. EMOTIONAL PHONATION

Fónagy has, alone or in collaboration with others, carried out a series of interesting and stimulating investigations on how the state of emotion affects the way in which speech is produced. Some of them which have a direct relation to how a speaker's mood is unveiled in his speech will be reported upon. Fónagy and Magdics (1963) compared the fundamental frequency of speech with various composers' melodic lines related to 10 different states of emotion: joy, tenderness, longing, coquetry, surprise, fear, plaintiveness, mockery, anger, and sarcasm. Thus the investigation is comparing phonation frequency patterns to what we initially termed macro-intonation.

Fónagy (1962) gives measurements of glottal behavior during emotional speech. Two methods of measurement were used; throat mirror and X-ray tomography. Three speakers articulated the vowel [i] (as in heed) serveral times as if they were in one of seven different states of emotion. Fonagy described the types of voicing in the following way: (1) soft, voiced; (2) soft and unvoiced, as in tender whispering; (3) hard and unvoiced, spiteful whisper; (4) hard and hateful, voiced, pressed phonation, creaky voice; (5) contemptuous growl (purring). Fig. 6 shows typical results in terms of throat mirror pictures. The shaded areas symbolize the ventricular folds, and the white areas the vocal folds. The vocal folds are completely covered by the ventricular folds during tense phonation with glottal fry, and during unvoiced phonation they do not close. The ventricular folds are further apart during tender whispering than during spiteful whisper. As far as the laryngeal ventricle was concerned, it is wide and enlarged during soft, weak, voiced phonations, somewhat smaller during tender whispering and rather small when whispering spitefully. In the last case the larynx tube was so

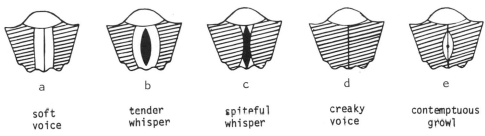

a	b	c	d	e
soft voice	tender whisper	spiteful whisper	creaky voice	contemptuous growl

Fig. 6   Schematized views of the larynx as seen from above by means of a laryngeal mirror during phonation of the vowel in he. The figures pertain to phonation in the emotional modes indicated. The top contour shows epiglottis, the hatched areas the false vocal folds, the white areas the (true) vocal folds, and the black are the glottis. From Fónagy, 1962, Phonetica 8:209-219.

narrow, that if formed a quite narrow passage. During pressed phonation the laryngeal ventricle was squeezed together, somewhat less during contemptuous growl. The vocal folds were thick and looked swollen during contemptuous growling. Fónagy interprets all these emotion-dependent glottal profiles as "pre-conscious expressive gestures".

IV.   EMOTIONAL ARTICULATION

Fónagy (1976) investigated phenomena related to articulation corresponding to the phonatory findings reported above. This investigation concerns the movement patterns of the tongue and the mouth opening during utterances with different emotional background. Distinct effects were established. For instance, a vowel could be produced so far removed from normal, that it partly assumed the characteristics of another vowel. Anger was associated with violent movements between extreme articulatory positions, while tenderness was characterized by slow, more 'tender' movements. In the pronunciation of a menacing expression, the tongue assumed firstly a tense and rather extreme articulatory position in order, as it were, to shoot 'as an arrow' towards the next articulatory position. Disappointment was characterized by a progressive relaxation of the tongue and the soft palate and a decreasing speed of the articulatory movement. Fónagy thinks there is a parallel in this behavior with the emotional paradigm of disappointment: expectation - suspense - disappointment - resignation. In a like way he finds similarities between articulatory movements associated with other states of emotion and the meaning of these states of emotion. Every attitude is expresssed by its own articulation - and as we have seen earlier, also glottal - pattern which reflects the mental contents of the attitude. Fónagy wants to interpret this as a materialization of the state of emotion, a re-interpretation of it into a movement, that is different from a movement which goes with a neutral state. According to Fónagy, a correct interpretation of the state of emotion behind an expression demands, therefore, knowledge of the manner of pronunciation for a neutral state of emotion. Thus, it is the deviations from the (expected) neutral, which carry the information concerning the state of emotion of a speaker.

Another investigation (Fónagy and Bérard, 1972), examines how an actress pronounces a common phrase (Il est huit heures. It is eight o'clock) using as many as 26 different emotional states. Fónagy finds evidence of both glottal and articulatory equivalent of facial gestures. He has also carried out an investigation on how much of the facial expression a listener can infer just from listening to the voice, as one may generally do, for instance, during a telephone conversation (Fónagy, 1967).

V.   EMOTIONAL BODY MOVEMENT AND SOUND

It does not seem too far-fetched to assume, as Fónagy does, the existence of a close correlation between visible and normally invisible body movements. Examples of normally invisible body movements can be found in the laryngeal cartilages, most of which are involved in the regulation of voice pitch. Thus, if it is true that a particular pattern of expressive body movement is typical of a specific emotional mode, then we would expect a corresponding pattern of, for example, vocal pitch in speech produced in that same emotional mode. In other words, it it likely that expressive body movements are translated into acoustic terms in voice production. According to Clynes (1969) phonatory and articulatory gestures are manifestations of a common expressive dynamic form which underlies both the perception and production of expression in different modalities. Clynes (1980) asked subjects to press on a button-like transducer in such a way as to express one of seven emotional modes: anger, hate, grief, love, sex, joy, and reverence. The vertical and horizontal components of the resulting dynamic pressures were recorded. The vertical component was converted into dynamic acoustic parameters, namely the pitch changes and the amplitude envelope of a sinusoidal signal. Clynes then presented these acoustic signals to observers and asked them in a forced-choice test to identify the signal as the expression of an emotional mode. The result showed that this was possible to do with a rather high accuracy. He received about 80% correct responses, which was only slightly lower than when the subjects watched the finger movements (without sound) directly by means of a video tape-recording. It seems that these results can be readily understood if the voice function exemplifies the way body movements may be coded into acoustic signals.

VI.   DISCUSSION

In contrast to most of the studies mentioned earlier which offer an acoustic description. the various papers by Fónagy concern articulatory and phonatory observations, and attempts as does Clynes to put these observations into a general psychological framework. His results support the assumption that there is a relation between the way the voice organs are used and the emotional content of the utterance. The tongue, which shoots 'like an arrow' between extreme articulatory positions in the course of a menacing utterance, can be seen as a symbol of the threat, and its slow movements during tender phonation seem to fit well with the idea of tenderness. A possible reason for this symbolic behavior in phonation and articulation may be a general body language of emotions which exerts its influence also over the behaviour of the voice organs. For instance, it would be typical for sadness and depression that all muscle activity is minimized. A sad person is not really disposed to express himself by means of wild gestures, but tends to minimize movements to a mere hint. Such a low level of muscular activity is also characteristic for the speech tempo. The flat course of the phonation frequency curve, in addition to the generally low average of the phonation frequency suggests a low activity in the crico-thyroid muscles. The low number of overtones of the voice source seems to indicate a low activity in the expiratory muscles, resulting in a low subglottic presssure and hence a low voice intensity. Probably all muscles are as passive as they can be without destroying the communication function of the speech. The opposite is valid in practically all these respects for the angry voice. The level of the phonation frequency is high, high peaks appear in the course of the phonation frequency curve, the voice source is wealthy in overtones, speech tempo is rather fast and, one can assume, the voice intensity is high. This indicates a high but rapidly changing activity in many of the muscles of the speech organs. One can easily imagine the related (visible) violent gestures of an angry person.

Thus, for both sadness and anger one can see a connection between the voice and gestures, and what else could be expected? Those gestures are what we can observe with the eyes: gestures of the speech organ we cannot see; but we can hear their acoustic consequences.

Some further points should be added. There seems to be a relation between the words we use to describe a certain manner of phonation, and that which phonatorically and articularly characterizes this way of phonation. A 'tense' phonation is characterized by high subglottal pressure combined with high adduction activity. One puts high tension on both the expiratory muscles and certain phonation muscles. Presumably, it is this type of conformity which enables us to imagine correctly what a person means when he tries to describe a way of phonation which is characterized by physiological signs that are actually unknown to both speaker and listener. Finally, we have seen above several examples of the influence that the emotional state of a speaker exerts on the ways the voice organ is being used. This seems to explain why the emotional relationship between teacher and pupil has a decisive influence on the result of the voice training. If the atmosphere in the studio is not relaxed, the phonation learnt in that studio is not very likely to be relaxed.

SUMMARY

It is a well known fact that emotions affect the way in which the voice is used; we often judge correctly the emotional mode of a speaker even in cases when we don't understand what the speaker says. This section reviews the research on the influence of emotions on vocal behavior in speech, and also singing, because singing can be regarded as a type of voice use, in which the emotional influence on vocal behavior is systematically exploited. According to results of various investigations, the fundamental frequency, i.e., the voice pitch, and particularly its variability, is very efficient in revealing the emotional state of a speaker, but also the timing of the speech and typical amplitude patterns seem relevant. All voice sound characteristics originate from (i.e., translate into acoustics terms) movements of cartilages and muscles in the voice apparatus. Studies of these movements in emotional speech and how they relate movements of other parts of the body under the influence of emotions are discussed.

ACKNOWLEDGEMENT

This paper is an expanded and translated version of material from the book "Röstlära" (Voice Science) by Johan Sundberg, Proprius Förlag, Stockholm, 1980.

REFERENCES

Clynes, M., 1969, Precision of essentic form in living communication, in: "Information Processing in the Nervous System, K.M. Leibovic, and J.C. Eccles, eds., Springer Verlag, New York.

Clynes, M., 1980, Transforming emotionally expressive touch to similarly expressive sound, Proc. Tenth Int. Acoust. Cong., Sydney.

Crystal, D., 1969, "Prosodic Systems and Intonation in English," Cambridge Univeristy Press, Cambridge, Eng.

Fónagy, I., 1962, Mimik auf glottaler Ebene, Phonetica, 8:209-219.

Fónagy, I., 1967, Hörbare Mimik, Phonetica, 16:25-35.

Fónagy, I., 1976, La mimique buccale, Phonetica, 33:31-44.

Fónagy, I., and Bérard, 1972, "Il est huit heures": contribution a l'analyse sémantique de la vive voix, Phonetica, 26:257-192.

Fónagy, I., and Magdics, K., 1963, Emotional patterns in intonation and music, Z.f. Phonetik, 16:293-326.

Kotlyar, G.M., and Morozov, V.P., 1976, Acoustical correlates of the emotional content of vocalized speech, Sov. Phys. Acoust., 22:208-211.

Kramer, E., 1963. Judgments of personal characteristics and emotions from nonverbal properties of speech, Psych. Bull., 60:408-420.

Lieberman, P., and Michaels, S.B., 1962, Some aspects of fundamental frequency and envelope amplitude as related to the emotional content of speech, J. Acoust. Soc. Am., 34:922-927.

Scherer, K.R., 1979, Non-linguistic vocal indicators of emotion and psychopathology, in: "Emotions in Personality and Psychopathology," C.E. Izard, ed., Plenum Press, New York.

Sedlacek, K., and Sychra, A., 1963, Die Melodie als Faktor des emotionellen Ausdrucks, Fol. Phon. 15:89-98.

Trojan, F., 1952, Experimentelle Untersuchungen über den Zusammenhang zwischen dem Ausdruck der Sprechstimme und dem vegetativen Nervensystem. Fol. Phon. 4:65-92.

Trojan, F., and Winckel, F., 1957, Elecktroakustische Untersuchungen zur Ausdruckstheorie der Sprechstimme, Fol. Phon. 9:168-182.

Williams, C.E., and Stevens, K.N., 1972 Emotions and Speech: Some acoustic correlates, J. Acoust. Soc. Am., 52:1238-1250.

Williams. C.E., Stevens, K.N. and Hecker, 1969, Aerospace Med., 40:1369-1372.

Chapter VIII

PROSODY AND MUSICAL RHYTHM ARE CONTROLLED BY THE SPEECH HEMISPHERE

Hans M. Borchgrevink

Institute of Aviation Medicine
Blindern
Oslo, Norway

INTRODUCTION

Cerebral processing of both speech and music imply analysis and identification of
1   the spectral pattern of complex sound
2.   the temporal sequence pattern of complex sound during a certain time period.

One might hypothesize that speech and musical functions were likely to rely upon common brain mechanisms situated in the same cerebral locations. On the contrary, however, the currently held idea has been for a considerable time that speech perception and production are controlled by the so-called 'dominant' (usually the left) cerebral hemisphere, while musical functions are controlled by the 'non-dominant' (usually the right) hemisphere (e.g. Kimura, 1964).

In 1977 the author demonstrated by the selective anaesthesia of successive hemispheres that musical rhythm as well as the act of singing were processed by the speech hemisphere (Borchgrevink, 1977). This experiment further showed that singing may facilitate speech and vice versa with left (dominant) hemisphere anesthesia, much in the same way as Melodic Information Therapy (M.I.T.) does with aphasia - indicating that the positive effect of M.I.T. (e.g. Sparks and Holland, 1976) might be due to the melody giving access to otherwise barred speech pathways by a 'detour' involving psychological processes in the non-speech hemisphere. The study concluded: "There is a close, but complex, connection between speech function and musical function. Both apparently consist of a multitude of sub-functions, many of which rely upon the same psychological mechanisms. This implies extensive possibilities of interference between the two functions, weakening the concepts of distinct and different cerebral lateralizations for speech function and musical function. Each subfunction may however be distinctively lateralized" (Borchgrevink, 1980a).

The present study was preformed to illuminate further the complex relation between the cerebral processing of speech and musical functions. Preliminary results were reported previously (Borchgrevink, 1979, 1980d).

METHOD

Six intelligent young adults (12-30 years) with unilateral epilepsy were tested during selective intracarotid barbiturate anaesthesia of one hemisphere after the other. The diagnostic purpose of the examination was to find the cerebral lateralization of speech and language function in order to avoid speech pathology induced during planned neurosurgical treatment.

Prior to testing, the patients were individually instructed

1.   to count to a steady tempo,
2.   to sing a certain song with text,
3.   to hum the tune,
4.   to count to the melody repeating 1, 2, 3, 4, 5, 6, 7 as if this was the text of the tune,
5.   to sound a note of the same pitch after it was sung by the investigator,
6.   to sound a note while it was sung by the investigator.

The tune chosen was the first four bars of "Alle Vögel sind schon da", well known to the patients in its Norwegian version and convenient for the purpose of analysis, as it has distinct rhythm, starts and ends on the same note (pitch) - and includes both the rising and falling major triad, as well as the octave.

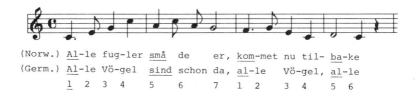

```
(Norw.) Al-le fug-ler små  de     er, kom-met nu til- ba-ke
(Germ.) Al-le Vö-gel  sind schon da, al-le    Vö-gel, al-le
         1  2  3  4    5    6     7  1  2      3   4    5  6
```

In addition, the patients were instructed

7.   to name shown objects,
8.   to recall memorized material (e.g. room number, date),
9.   to do rapid finger movements upon demonstration,
10. to do rapid finger movements on verbal command.

They were generally instructed to continue doing a task repeatedly until a new order was given.

Routine carotis angiography (femoral catheter) was performed on the presumed side of the speech center (based on handedness and other laterality tests). Then the catheter was moved on to the internal carotid on the same side. A reference tape recording (Nagra IV Kudelski tape recorder with Bruel & Kjar 1/2" microphone) was made of the patient's performance on tests 1 to 10, the patient lying in supine position with stretched arms raised 60 degrees. Still tape recording, the patient was asked to start counting, and at digit 7, 75 mg (3 ml) amytal was injected in 2 secs - an amount just sufficient to produce a transient (1-2 mins) contralateral hemiplegia (right body half), and aphasia. In the 3-5 min period before full recovery, the awake and fully conscious patient was asked continuously to count. hum etc. (tests 1 to 10), his responses being tape recorded - as was the running verbal description by the attending neurologist. After full recovery the catheter was moved to the other (right) common carotid artery for carotis angiography, and the procedure was repeated, with the difference that, if aphasia had been produced on the left side, the patient was asked to count to the melody prior to and during the amytal injection. Since singing may facilitate speech (Borchgrevink 1977, 1980a), counting without melody is only performed on the presumed purpose of the diagnostic test - verification of the cerebral lateralization of the speech.

The speech perception deficit, which can be difficult to prove in a non-speaking individual, was registered by asking the anaesthetized, aphasic patient to wave his fingers, first verbally then by visual demonstration (adequate response to visual demonstration and no response to verbal command reflects speech perception pathology).

The following results are based on the comparison between the reference tape recordings made prior to the injection, and the tape recordings made during the injection and recovery periods in the same individual, as judged by musical listeners.

RESULTS

Tape recordings of the effects are given in the phonograph record provided with this work, and were played at the verbal presentation of this paper.

Right Hemisphere Anaesthesia

When counting 1, 2, 3, 4, 5, 6, 7 (in place of the lyrics) to the melody, during right intracarotid amytal injection, four right handed patients abruptly lost control of pitch and tonality - counting monotonously with preserved musical rhythm. Tonal control was gradually regained during recovery. First regained were the gross characteristics of the melodic line ('melodic envelope'), the accuracy of pitch within this gross pattern being the last element to be restored. Consciousness and normal speech comprehension and production were preserved throughout, including the local dialect (prosody, intonation, stress).

Left Hemisphere Anaesthesia

In the four right handers this produced abrupt loss of speech comprehension, speech production and singing ability; normal functions being as suddenly regained - and then were perfectly controlled at once.

One right hander with verified temporal lobe agenesia, as well as one left hander with extensive long standing epileptic activity in the left frontotemporal cortex lost all the above abilities abruptly upon right hemisphere anaesthesia; being unaffected by left hemisphere anaesthesia. The latter patient aged 19 years was unable to pitch a sounded note even in the unanesthetized state, although she had played the piano and received piano lessons since the age of six years.

Shortly after recovery from aphasia, some of the patients demonstrated loss of memory for room number and date, for example. About half an hour post injection these patients would typically fail to recognize familiar objects (keys, matchbox) shown to them shortly after recovery from aphasia and which they had been able to name at that time.

DISCUSSION

All patients were conscious and awake during the injection periods. The injections produced temporary contralateral hemiplegia. Carotis angiography showed no X-ray contrast medium in the contralateral hemisphere. Each patient was tested both before and during selective anaesthesia periods of both the left and the right cerebral hemispheres, and thus the individual served as his own control, in the present paradigm. It is therefore reasonable to assume that the functions absent during selective hemisphere anaesthesia periods were lost because they were controlled by the cortex of the selectively anaesthetized cerebral hemisphere.

Even though the cerebral pathology of the patients may have influenced the results to some extent, the results were so clearly evident that it seems reasonable to conclude, that for the 'normal' righthander the left hemisphere controls speech perception, speech production, prosody (local dialect/stress/intonation), musical rhythm and the act of singing; - whereas the right hemisphere controls pitch and tonality in singing (but not in speech!). Re-examination of the tape recordings of the earlier project (Borchgrevink, 1977, 1980a) confirms these lateralizations of the above elementary functions.

In case of extensive damage to or absence of essential parts of the frontotemporal cortex of the speech hemisphere - which appears to be anatomically and physiologically specialized for speech and language processing from the 7th month of fetal life (Chi et al., 1977; Davis and Wada, 1978) - all functions may be controlled by one hemisphere. The performance of the 19 year old lefthanded patient indicates that the brain in these circumstances gives priority to speech to the extent that speech may suppress musical functions such as pitch control in singing. The other patient with this pattern of lateralization also showed poor musical abilities. This might be due to poor inherited potential for cerebral musical processing, or to lack of adequate stimulation, as in fact there were no musical activities in the life of the patient or of his family. However, he did demonstrate a better performance IQ than his verbal IQ, which may be seen often when speech control has shifted to the non-specialized hemisphere - where it might accordingly have suppressed his musical functions.*

---

*   Lack of preschool musical activities was a common factor in 12

The different cerebral lateralization of pitch/tonality (right hemisphere) and musical rhythm (left hemisphere) explains the greater cerebral
lateralization of chords than of melodies reported in dichotic listening
studies (eg Gordon, 1975), as melody consists of both rhythmic and tonal
elements while chords only contain tonal elements. Accordingly, the
relative predominance of the rhythmic and tonal factors in a melody would
determine the side and degree of lateralization of a given melody -
explaining the discrepancies of earlier dichotic listening reports (eg Kimura,
1964; Gordon, 1975).

It may seem surprising that prosody, the 'musical element of the
language', appears to be controlled by the speech hemisphere. Clearly,
speaking with preserved local dialect necessarily must imply accurate
pitching. However, with right (non-speech) anaesthesia, the patients
typically lost control of musical pitch in singing, but preserved pitching
accuracy in speech. This indicates that physically identical complex sounds
may be controlled by different hemispheres, depending upon whether the
sound is a signal referring to a symbol or concept - or whether the sound is
analysed as non-symbolic 'sound as such'. Patients with right (non-speech)
temporal lobe pathology without aphasia were able to perform the linguistic
(Norwegian) discrimination SIL-SYL (presented verbally by tape) but failed
to discriminate between the same vowels I-Y removed from linguistic
context - and also failed to discriminate between major and minor triads
(Borchgrevink and Reinvang, in prep).

This factor, if not taken into account, may lead to disturbing and
inexplicable discrepancies between the results of apparently identical
studies. It also supports the author's 'model' of the therapeutic effect of
Melodic Information Therapy on speech in aphasia: that the melody added to
speech is the musical element necessary to give access to the speech center
by the musical pathways in the undamaged non-speech hemisphere, restoring
speech function by marking a detour around the destroyed, barred speech
path pathways (Borchgrevick, 1977, 1980a). It also explains why it appears
impossible to remove the melody from the sentences mastered by means of
Melodic Information Therapy without also removing the speech faculty: the
melody is the essential element in finding functional compensatory
pathways. It might accordingly be relevant to improve auditory perception
diagnosis by examining the cerebral lateralization pattern of the patient
(Borchgrevink, 1980b), in order to choose the optimal therapeutic program
for the patient.

Based on the observation that right hemispere trauma has lead to
monotonous speech, prosody has been believed to be controlled by the right,
'musical' hemisphere (eg Tucker et al., 1977), contrary to what was found in
the present study.

The present results show that memory deficits may be recorded in the

---

intelligent, but 'tone-deaf' girls from a Grammar School - indicating
that there might well be a critical age for the acquisition of certain
musical abilities, most likely before the age of 7 years (Borchgrevink, in
prep). If so, the pedagogical consequence would be early, active musical training.

recovery period <u>after</u> the speech faculty is regained, but before full recovery - indicating that memory is even more susceptible to light anaesthesia than speech, both concerning the recall of memorized material and the storage of perceived information. Appearing only in some patients, this also shows that memory storage may be processed by one or by both hemispheres in different individuals, lending support to the relevance of such testing during selective hemisphere anaesthesia, as part of the pre-neurosurgical diagnostic program.

After recovery from anaesthesia it turned out on questioning that the patients apparently did not realize their poor pitching performance during anaesthesia, nor did they register that they were hemiplegic (neglect phenomenon). One patient remarked that he was able to register by vision that his paralysed arm was not raised, as he believed it to be - judged by proprioception.

As musical rhythm and pitch/tonality are seen to be controlled by different cerebral hemispheres, singing and almost any musical performance implies extensive integration and cooperation between the hemispheres. Prosody, the 'musical element of speech', may in early development be initially controlled by the non-speech hemisphere; and then lateralized to the speech hemisphere along with the person's cognitive development in childhood before puberty (Borchevink, 1980c). The well known observation that adults preserve their accent when moving to another place, while small children acquire the accent of the new place where they live, indeed supports this assumption. This may be one of the main differences of first and second language processing, also influencing speech comprehension, as much information is given by prosodic features. Presumably it is the close connection with speech as a symbolic code that makes prosody a speech hemisphere function even though it requires accurate pitching mostly in the same manner as singing does.

SUMMARY

Six intelligent, young adults (12-30) years with unilateral epilepsy were tested with the production of rhythm and melody during selective, intracarotid barbiturate anesthesia of one hemisphere after the other, induced in order to find the cerebral lateralization of speech function, and avoid speech pathology following planned neurosurgical treatment. All injections produced temporary, contralateral hemiplegia. Carotid angiography showed no X-ray contrast medium in the contralateral hemisphere.

When attempting to sing 1, 2, 3, 4, 5, 6, 7 in place of the lyrics of a well-known tune during <u>right</u> intracarotid amytal injection, four right-handed patients lost control of pitch and tonality - counting monotonously with preserved musical rhythm. Tonal control was gradually regained during recovery. Consciousness and normal speech comprehension and production including dialect (stress, prospody, intonation) were preserved throughout, Corresponding <u>left</u> hemisphere anesthesia produced abrupt loss of speech comprehension, production and singing ability, normal functions being as suddenly regained. One right-hander with verified left temporal lobe agenesia, as well as one left-hander with extensive epileptic activity in the left frontotemporal cortex, had speech and musical functions entirely controlled by the <u>right</u> hemisphere, as all above mentioned abilities were abruptly lost upon right hemisphere anesthesia, being unaffected by left hemisphere anesthesia. The latter patient (aged 19) was unable to pitch a sounded note although she had musical training since the age of six years, indicating that speech may suppress tone control when both are controlled by the same (right) hemisphere.*

REFERENCES

Borchgrevink, H.M., 1977, Cerebral lateralization of speech and singing after intracarotid amytal injection, Int. Symp. on Aphasia, Gothenburg.

Borchgrevink, H.M., 1978, Improving auditory perception diagnosis by considering the cerebral lateralization of speech and musical stimuli, 1. Int. Cong for the Study of Child Language, Tokyo.

Borchgrevink, H.M., 1979, Speech, singing, object identification and memory investigated during intracarotid hemisphere anaesthesia, Second Europ. Conf. of the International Neuropsychological Society, Holland. Abs. in INS Bulletin, June 1979, p. 14.

Borchgrevink, H.M., 1980 a, Cerebral lateralization of speech and singing after intracarotid amytal injection, in: "Aphasia: Assessment and Treatment", M. Taylor Sarno & O. Hook, eds., Almquist Wicksell, Stockholm.

Borchgrevink, H.M., 1980 b, Improving auditory perception diagnosis by considering the cerebral lateralization of speech and musical stimuli, in: "Proceedings of the First International Congress for the Study of Child Language", D. Ingram, F.C.C. Peng, and Ph. Dale, eds., University Press of America. Lanham.

Borchgrevink, H.M., 1980 c. Speech perception involves cognition: the influence of concept - reference coherence upon speech perception, submitted to Brain and Language.

Borchgrevink, H.M., 1980 d, Cerebral lateralization of speech, dialect, pitch and rhythm, XVIIIth Int. Cong. of Logopedics and Phoniatrics, Washington D.C. Abs. in Folia Phoniat. (1980), 32(2):168:169.

Borchgrevink, H.M., and Reinvang, I., in prep., The correlation between speech and musical functions in adult aphasics, submitted to Brain and Language.

Chi, J.G., Dooling, E.C.L., and Gilles. F.H., 1977, Left-right asymmetries of the temporal speech areas of the human fetus, Arc. Neurol., 34; 346-348.

Davis, A.E., and Wada, J.A., 1978, Speech dominance and handedness in the normal human, Brain and Lang., 5.1:25-35.

Gordon, H.W., 1975, Hemispheric asymmetry and musical performance, Science, 189:68-69.

Kimura, D., 1964, Left-right differences in the perception of melodies, Quart. J. Exp. Psychol., 16; 355-358.

Sparks, R.W., and Holland, A.L., 1976, Method: Melodic Intonation Therapy for Aphasia, J. Speech Hear. Disord., 41:287-297.

Tucker, D.M., Watson, R.T., and Heilman, K.M., 1977, Discrimination and evocation of affectively intoned speech in patients with right parietal disease, Neurology, 27:947-950.

---

* Vocal sounds illustrating this paper are presented in the recording included with this book (see Appendix for details).

Chapter IX

PERCEPTION AND PERFORMANCE OF MUSICAL RHYTHM

Alf Gabrielsson

Department of Psychology
Uppsala University
Uppsala, Sweden

INTRODUCTION

Rhythm is often said to be the most fundamental element of music in any culture of the world (see, for instance, Gaston, 1968). In spite of this there is still very much confusion about the concept of rhythm, both on the empirical and on the theoretical side. Many rhythm phenomena have proved to be elusive for analytical and/or empirical approaches, and the attempts at theoretical explanations are rather limited in number as well as in scope. Most of the experimental research on rhythm does not directly refer to rhythm in connection with music - there are some outstanding exceptions, however. For historical reviews of rhythm research see Gabrielsson (1973a, 1979).

GENERAL DEFINITION OF MUSICAL RHYTHM

A simple descriptive model may be useful to survey the phenomena we are dealing with and to formulate some basic questions to be investigated (see Fig. 1).

To the left we have some kind of musical performance, that is, one or more musicians playing or singing. This activity results in sound sequences emanating from the instruments/voices (the middle box), and these sound sequences may give rise to a rhythm response in listening persons (the right-hand box). The performances and the rhythm responses are psychological/physiological phenomena, while the sound sequences as such are acoustical/physical phenomena. Between the sound sequences and the rhythm response(s) there are certain psychophysical relations; that is, the properties of the sound sequences are related to the properties of the rhythm response - in other words, how the music is performed will affect the rhythm response. There is also a feedback from the rhythm response to

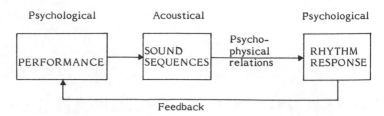

Fig. 1. General framework for empirical research on musical rhythm.

the performance: the performer is a listener, too, and how he himself perceives the rhythm will influence his way of performing (and, of course, the rhythm responses of the other listeners may also affect his performance).

According to this view musical rhythm is thus defined as a response that may occur when one is listening to certain kinds of sound sequences. The rhythm response may further be split up into some different aspects:

(a) experiential aspects, which refer to various perceptual, cognitive and emotional variables (for instance, the rhythm may be experienced as 'rapid', 'dancing', 'complex', 'aggressive');

(b) behavioral aspects, which refer to more or less overt movements like 'beating time' with your feet, swaying of the body, dancing; and

(c) physiological aspects such as changes in breathing, heart rate, muscular tensions

There are, of course, complex interrelations and overlapping between these different aspects. In a real life situation the responding person is usually not aware of different components of his rhythm response, and we should, of course, primarily regard the rhythm response as a spontaneous and undifferentiated 'whole'. However, in a research context such a distinction between different aspects may make it easier for us to find out and invest-igate the many complex questions and relations associated with musical rhythm.

Referring again to Fig. 1, three basic questions for empirical research on musical rhythm may be formulated as follows:

1.   What are the characteristics of a rhythm response as opposed to a non-rhythm response - in other words, what distinguishes rhythm from non-rhythm?

2.   What are the characteristics of different kinds of rhythm responses in connection with music - how can we describe the differences in rhythm between different kinds of music or between different performances of the 'same' music?

3.   What are the psychophysical relationships between the (physical) char-
      acteristics of the sound sequences and the (psychological/physiological)
      characteristics of the rhythm responses - or, slightly reformulated in a
      more musical way, how do musicians play different kinds of music in
      order to bring about the intended/desired rhythm responses in the
      listeners?

      The first question will not be dealt with further here except noting that
some suggested characteristics for rhythm as opposed to non-rhythm are
perceived grouping, perceived accent(s), some kind of perceived regularity,
a limitation in time to 'the psychological present' etc.; see further in
Bengtsson et al. (1972) and Bengtsson and Gabrielsson (1977). The remaining
two questions will be briefly discussed in the following using examples from
the rhythm research made in cooperation between musicologists and
psychologists at Uppsala University.
      Before that, however, let us note that learning may play an important
role in connection with all three questions. By continued experience and/or
by deliberate training (as in much music education) one may sometimes be
able to 'hear' rhythm in a sound sequence that earlier was non-rhythm; or
detect more and more differences in rhythm responses to different kinds of
music, for instance, between different types of dance music; or learn to play
a Vienna waltz as it should be played, to imitate Erroll Garner's way of
rhythm performance etc. And apparently, different listeners may sometimes show rather different rhythm responses to the same piece of music/
performance depending on their earlier experiences. In fact by learning you
may make yourself independent of the sound sequence; you can imagine how
it sounds and get an intensive rhythm response from that (such a case of
'internally generated response' is not directly covered by the model in Fig. 1).

INVESTIGATIONS OF RHYTHM EXPERIENCE

      The second question above - how can we describe the differences in
rhythm between different kinds of music or between different performances
- has been the subject of much writing and discussion in music theory and
related fields. However, there are few empirical investigations. Recently a
series of experiments was done to study the experiential aspects of the
rhythm response. They are described in detail in several papers by
Gabrielsson (1973a, 1973b, 1973c, 1973d. 1974a, 1974b), see also Bengtsson
and Gabrielsson (1977) and Gabrielsson (1979). Here only a very short
summary is given presenting the main ideas, methods and results.
      The starting point for these investigations was the assumption that
experience of musical rhythm is a multidimensional phenomenon, that is,
there is a large number of different characteristics/ dimensions in which
musical rhythms may differ. The purpose of the experiments was therefore
to find out relevant dimensions in musical rhythm experience. It was hoped
that these dimensions could constitute the rudiments of an adequate description system for musical rhythms as they are experienced.
      Some twenty experiments were peformed with musicians and some non-
musicians as subjects. Three types of rhythm stimuli were used: monophonic

patterns (performed on a drum and tape-recorded), polyphonic patterns (electronic simulations of various dance rhythms by means of a rhythm box like those found in many electronic organs), and real dance music from various parts of the world (taken from phonograph records). The judgment methods used by the subjects were examples of various multivariate techniques, which have been developed for the purpose of finding out fundamental dimensions of complex perceptual/cognitive phenomena, in this case the fundamental dimensions in the rhythm experience of the stimuli mentioned above. In one such method the subjects listen to rhythms presented in pairs and rate the similarity between the respective two rhythms on a certain scale. The ratings are analyzed according to models for multidimensional scaling to find out the fundamental dimensions underlying the similarity judgments. In another method the subjects rate each rhythm against a large number of adjective scales, and these ratings are analyzed by factor analysis. again to find out a limited number of fundamental dimensions in the crowd of adjectives. Free verbal descriptions were also used as a supplement to the more formal methods.

The resulting dimensions from all experiments together could be naturally grouped into three categories. see Table 1. One category of dimensions refers to the experienced structure of the rhythms (dimensions as meter, prominence of basic pattern, simplicity-complexity etc.) and may be said to reflect cognitive-perceptual aspects. A second category of dimensions refers to the experienced motion of the rhythms (tempo, forward motion. dancing-walking, etc.) reflecting perceptual-emotional aspects. Finally a third category refers to the emotional aspects of the rhythms (vital-dull, excited-calm etc.). Detailed examples are found in the abovementioned papers.

The labelling of the dimensions presents certain problems. To give but one label/name for a dimension often seems difficult since it does not convey the whole meaning of the dimension in question. In certain cases. especially regarding the dimensions within the motion and emotion categories, it may even be felt that our ordinary language cannot provide quite appropriate labels for the phenomena in question. For instance, various motion characters probably reflect relatively unconscious sensory-motor processes for which we have no well developed terminology in language. This also suggests that non-verbal response techniques would be an interesting alternative to study rhythm experience. A related observation is that when rhythm is discussed in music theory, and when rhythm is trained in music education, the emphasis is usually laid on the structural aspects. This is apparently also the case for various rhythm tests which appear in so- called musicality tests.

Of course, the schema in Table 1 does not represent a final result, rather a set of working hypotheses for continued research. It should also be noted that it is limited to the experiential aspects of the rhythm response. Their relations to behavioral and physiological aspects present a fascinating challenge to rhythm researchers.

Table 1. Suggested dimensions in musical rhythm experience.

STRUCTURE	MOTION	EMOTION
Meter	Rapidity	Vital - Dull
Accent of first beat	Tempo	Excited - Calm
Type of basic pattern	Forward motion	Rigid - Flexible
Prominence of basic pattern; Clearness/ Accentuation	Motion characters (Dancing-Walking, Rocking-Knocking, Solemn-Swinging, etc.)	Solemn - Playful
Uniformity - Variation Simplicity - Complexity		
Duration pattern at different beats		
Cognitive/Perceptual	Perceptual/Emotional	Emotional

INVESTIGATIONS OF RHYTHMIC PERFORMANCE

The third question above - how do musicians play different kinds of music to bring about the intended/desired rhythm responses in the listeners - has also been the subject of much discussion but of very little empirical investigation (partly due to technical difficulties in making registrations of musical performance). It is generally known that "you don't play exactly as the notation tells you", and it is often found difficult or even impossible to transcribe performed music (for instance, certain kinds of folk music, jazz music) into the conventional musical notation. Usually this refers especially to the durations of the tones/sound events or, more specifically, to the relationships between the durations of different sound events. It is also fairly common hypothesis that the duration factors are of special importance both for performance and for experience of rhythm (see, for instance, Fraisse, 1956, 1978).

Bengtsson et al. (1969, 1972) hypothesized that live performance of musical rhythm is usually characterized by certain systematic variations as regards the durations of the sound events (SE) in relation to strict mechanical regularity. In the conventional musical notation the duration of each SE is given by its note-value (half note, quarter note etc.) in combination with a tempo designation. The names of the note values indicate (among other things) the relations between the corresponding durations: a half note is twice as long as a quarter note, four times as long as an eighth note etc. A performance in strict adherence to these relations would mean that the duration of each SE designated by a half note should be exactly twice the duration of a SE notated by a quarter note, four times the duration of a SE notated by an eighth note etc. Such a case would probably never occur with human performers - but it does appear in the rhythm boxes found in many electronic organs. Considering human performance the above mentioned duration relations have to be understood in an approximate sense, to be interpreted with considerable freedom depending on the musical context.

However, mechanical regularity could be a convenient frame of reference for comparing different performances. It may be thought of as a rational-mechanical norm, and the characteristics of different real performances could be described in terms of different types of deviations from this norm. Of course, there are always a certain amount of random variations in any performance. However, the hypothesis about systematic variations (SYVAR) refers to consistent/recurring deviations from the mechanical norm. The general hypothesis is that there are different types of SYVAR in the performance of different types of music, and that these different SYVAR are important factors to bring about the intended/desired rhythm character of the music in question. A well-known example is that the Vienna waltz is performed with a short first beat and a long second beat, while the mechanical norm derived from the notation would say that all three beats in the measure should be of equal duration. This was demonstrated, as well as other SYVAR examples, in pilot studies (Bengtsson et al., 1969, 1972· Bengtsson, 1974; Bengtsson and Gabrielsson, 1977).

Extensive registrations have been made of the performances by six musicians playing 28 different pieces of music. A detailed description of the analysis methods as well as of their applications for one of the melodies is given in Bengtsson and Gabrielsson (1980), and further papers will follow. Some very brief glimpses of this work are given here to illustrate the methods and some results.

Consider the simple example given in Fig. 2. It refers to a well-known Swedish tune ("Sorgeliga saker hända") usually notated in 3/4 time as in the figure. The six musicians performed this melody, once or twice (in immediate succession), under different conditions: playing by heart, playing when given the notation in 3/4 time, and playing with two other notations, one in 6/8 time and one absurd notation in 4/4 time. They played the piano, the clarinet and the flute.

All performances were recorded on tape, from which registrations of all durations were made by means of special equipment. Duration means here the time from the onset of a tone/SE to the onset of the next SE. The duration data are analyzed by a special computer program SYVARD (Bengtsson et al., 1978) to study the deviations from the mechanical norm. As seen in Fig. 2 all measures but two contain a half note followed by a quarter note. The mechanical norm derived from this notation would thus say that each SE notated by a half note should be twice as long as each SE notated by a quarter note - in other words, there should be a 2:1 relationship between the two SE within each measure (and the dotted half note in measure no. 8 should be three times as long as the quarter note duration).

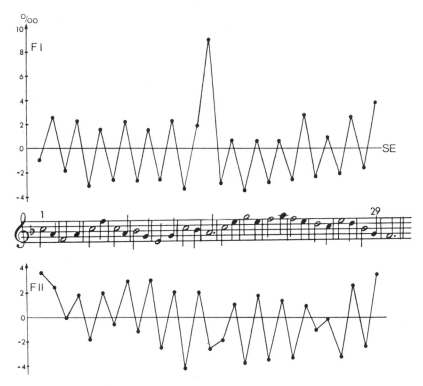

Fig. 2.   Deviations from the mechanical norm for each of the 29 SE in the notated melody (the last SE omitted), see further in text.

As expected, none of the performances followed this mechanical rule. The majority of the performances showed a very pronounced and consistent type of SYVAR illustrated in the upper part (marked F I) of Fig. 2. The mechanical norm is represented by the straight line in the middle (marked O). A deviation upwards from this line means that the duration of the corresponding SE is longer than what it should be. Conversely, a deviation downwards tells that the duration of the corresponding SE is shorter than what the mechanical norm would prescribe. The deviations are expressed in per mille of the total duration of the tune. Most performances had a total duration of 15-20 seconds, and thus one per mille corresponds to 15-20 milliseconds. There is a characteristic zig-zag SYVAR around the middle. It is seen that all SE notated by half notes are shortened, while all SE denoted by quarter notes are lengthened. There is also a marked lenghtening of the single SE in measure no. 8, that is, at the end of the first half period of the tune. The relationship between the two SE within each measure is thus not 2:1 but considerably lower, averaging about 1.75:1.

However, not all performances conformed to this pattern. To get a condensed survey over all different performances (38 in all) factor analysis was applied to the deviation data of all performances. Three factors accounted for 74% of the total variance, and these three factors can be inter-

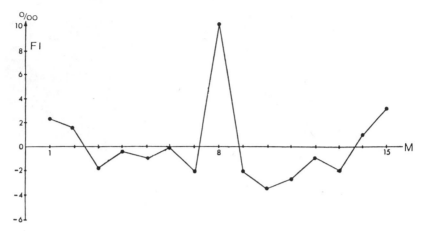

Fig. 3.   Deviations from the mechanical norm at measure (M) level, see further in text.

preted as three different ways of performing the tune. The first of these was actually the case described above (F I). The second way is shown in the lower part of Fig. 2, marked F II). The zig-zag pattern is apparent here, too, but there are two obvious differences against F I: there is a slow start (both SE in the first measure are lengthened), and the dotted half-note in measure no. 8 is shortened instead of lenghtened as in F I. The third way of performance (not shown here) was markedly different and occurred for certain performances of the absurd 4/4 notation.

The above analysis refers to SYVAR in the durations of the single sound events. It is also interesting and enlightening to perform analogous analyses at higher levels, that is, for measures, groups of two measures etc. An example is given in Fig. 3. It shows the dominating way of making SYVAR at the measure level in the same tune as in Fig. 2. According to the mechanical norm all measures (M) should, of course, be equally long. However, most performances show a lengthening of the first two bars (slow start). a marked lengthening at the end of the first half period (measure no. 8), and a lengthening of the last two bars (ritardando towards the end). Consequently all other measures are more or less shortened. (The very last measure is not included in the analysis, since the duration of the final SE cannot be adequately measured.)

The profile in Fig. 3 is reminiscent of what could be called the articulation of the overall form of this melody. Similar or analogous profiles appear for many other melodies in the investigation.

Although the above description is very short it may be sufficient to demonstrate the two main ideas, namely to study systematic variations of durations in relation to a mechancial norm and to find out different types of

performances by means of factor analysis. In the following some preliminary results are sketched without giving the complete context.

The finding that the the half note - quarter note sequence within each
measure of the tune in Fig. 2 was performed in a proportion considerably
less that 2:1 is not unique for that tune. The same phenomenon appears in
several other melodies notated in 3/4 time and even if measures of this type
are embedded in a context of measures with different duration patterns, for
instance, in the example in Fig. 4a (average proportion value 1.8:1). An
analogous result is found for melodies in 6/8 time but then with regard to
the proportion between quarter note and eighth note as, for instance, in the
well-known beginning of Mozart's Piano Sonata in A major, see Fig. 4b. The
quarter note - eighth note sequence appears there once in each of measures
no. 1, 2, and 4, and twice in measure no. 3. In the performances the corresponding proportion values mostly lie somewhere between 1.6:1 and 1.9:1.

Another common pattern in musical notation is the sequence consisting
of a dotted eighth-note followed by a sixteenth-note as in the examples c
and d in Fig. 4. According to a mechanical norm the production between the
corresponding SE should be 3:1. In practice, however, it can vary very much
depending on the musical context. In the Swedish folk tune notated as in
Fig. 4c this proportion value tends to be rather 2:1 instead of 3:1 as played
by the present performers. In many cases the proportion is actually less
than 2:1. On the other hand the proportion value actually approaches 3:1 in
the performances of the march given in Fig. 4d. It seems apparent that the
different 'motion characters' of these two examples call for quite different
performances of the dotted eighth note - sixteenth note pattern (among
other things).

It should be emphasized that detailed analyses of the last-mentioned

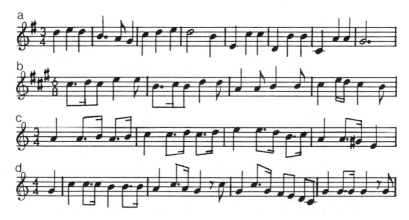

Fig. 4.   (a) Swedish tune, "Flicka Fran Backafall"; (b) The theme in
Mozart's Piano Sonata in A major (K.331); (c) Swedish tune,
"Varvindar friska"; (d) March, "Finska rytteriets marsch".

examples reveal constantly changing features in the performances, between different performers as well as within the same performer. Average values as some of those given above have limited value in themselves - they must be related to the details of the actual context.

We can conclude that timing in music is a highly variable and complex phenomenon of which we still know very little when it comes to details. We know, in a general way, that there are large discrepancies between the conventional musical notation (when dogmatically interpreted) and real performances. However, we are still only in the beginning of the empirical research of these questions, which hopefully will give us a much more detailed knowledge and understanding of musical performance in relation to rhythm responses. The consequences for music theory and musical training might be far-reaching. A better knowledge of timing in music may also contribute to more enjoyable examples of synthesized music by applying information about deviations/systematic variations instead of rigid mechanical regularity which is now very often the case.

SUMMARY

A descriptive model for musical rhythm is proposed with 'performance', 'sound sequences', and 'rhythm response' as the main components. Musical rhythm is defined as a response that may occur when listening to certain sound sequences. It may be separated into experiential, behavioral, and physiological aspects. Three basic research questions are identified:

1.   What distinguishes rhythm from non-rhythm?

2.   What distinguishes different rhythms from each other? and

3.   How do musicians play to bring about the intended rhythm response?

The last two questions are illustrated. Rhythm experience was studied by multivariate techniques resulting in a set of dimensions which referred to the experienced structure, experienced motion, and to emotional aspects of the rhythms. Rhythm performance was studied with regard to systematic variations of durations in relation to strict mechanical regularity, and a striking example of such systematic variations is described. Such studies of musical timing may have wide consequences for music theory and musical training.

REFERENCES

Bengtsson, I., 1974, Empirische Rhythmusforschung in Uppsala, Hamburger Jahrbuch fur Musikwissenschaft, 1:195-220.

Bengtsson, I., and Gabrielsson, A., 1977, Rhythm research in Uppsala, in "Music. Room and Acoustics," Royal Swedish Academy of Music, Stockholm.

Bengtsson, I., and Gabrielsson, A., 1980, Methods for analyzing performance of musical rhythm, Scand. J. Psychol., 21 (in press).

Bengtsson, I., and Gabrielsson, A., and Gabrielsson, B., 1978, RHYTHM-SYVARD, A computer program for analysis of rhythmic performance, Swedish. J. Musicol., 60:15-24.

Bengtsson, I., Gabrielsson, A., and Thorsen, S.M., 1969, Empirisk rytmforskning (Empirical rhythm research), Swedish. J. Musicol., 51:49-118.

Bengtsson, I., Tove, P.A., and Thorsen, S.M., 1972, Sound analysis equipment and rhythm research ideas at the Institue of Musicology in Uppsala, Studia instrumentorum musicae popularis, 2:53-76.

Fraisse, P., 1956, "Les structures rythmiques," Publications Universitaires de Louvain, Louvain.

Fraisse, P., 1978, Time and rhythm perception, in "Handbook of Perception," Vol 8, E.C. Carterette and M.P. Friedman, eds., Academic Press, New York.

Gabrielsson, A., 1973a, Similarity ratings and dimension analyses of auditory rhythm patterns, I, Scand. J. Psychol., 14:138-160.

Gabrielsson, A., 1973b, Similarity ratings and dimension analyses of auditory rhythm patterns, II, Scand. J. Psychol., 14:161-176.

Gabrielsson, A., 1973c, Adjective ratings and dimension analyses of auditory rhythm patterns, Scand. J. Psychol., 14:244-260.

Gabrielsson, A., 1973c, Studies in rhythm, Acta Universitatis Upsaliensis: Abstracts of Uppsala Dissertations from the Faculty of Social Sciences, 7.

Gabrielsson, A., 1974a, Performance of rhythm patterns, Scand. J. Psychol., 15:63-72.

Gabrielsson, A., 1974b, An empirical comparison between some models for multidimensional scaling, Scand. J. Psychol., 15:73-80.

Gabrielsson. A., 1979, Experimental research on rhythm, Human. Assoc. Rev., 30:69-92.

Gaston, E.T., 1968, Man and music, in "Music in Therapy," E.T. Gaston ed., Macmillan, New York.

NEUROBIOLOGIC FUNCTIONS OF RHYTHM, TIME, AND PULSE IN MUSIC

Manfred Clynes and Janice Walker

Music Research Center
New South Wales State Conservatorium of Music
Sydney, Australia

INTRODUCTION

Rhythm means reiteration - in space, or in time, or in both. We shall be concerned with rhythms in time, and, in particular, rhythms encompassed on a time scale in which music has grown. We will attempt to inquire into aspects of how such rhythms are produced, perceived, imagined, experienced, and expressed in sound and in movement, and how these functions may be related.

Gabrielsson (this volume) has noted the relative paucity of recent scientific studies of musical rhythm, among which his work (Gabrielsson, 1973, 1979) and that of Fraisse, (1956, 1978) is notable. Much past work has focused on the auditory property of hearing evenly spaced distinct sounds as grouped into 2, 3 or 4, and on how accent and duration in uneven groups influence our choice of beginnings, ends and perceived relative proportions of iterated patterns (Jones, 1978; Boring, 1942; Handel and Yoder, 1975). But the subtle functions of variously shaped sound pulses at a given repetition frequency have received little attention. Yet these features are essential to the vitality of rhythmic experience.

Although the nervous system control of repetitive movement is being studied to a considerable extent in recent years (Kristan, 1980; Delcomyn, 1980), especially in animals and to a lesser degree in man, the neurobiologic and psychobiologic phenomena of musical rhythm have received little attention. In animals it has been increasingly evident that rhythmic behavior such as found in flying, swimming, and running for example, is controlled by central nervous system programs whose timing and commands drive the output; that is the timing and form is centrally controlled by specific neuronal networks (Bentley and Konishi, 1978; Grillner and Wallen, 1977). In Delcomyn's words:

Evidence presented over the last two decades overwhelmingly supports (the) general principle: that the central nervous system does not require feedback from sense organs in order to generate properly sequenced, rhythmic movement during repetitive behaviors such as locomotion.

Such patterns become more modifiable as evolution proceeds, and in man they can be linked with imagination. How the sensing of time and the process of imagination, and in particular motor imagination, interact is of central concern in investigating the phenomena of musical rhythm. Theoretical studies (Simon, 1972; Greeno and Simon, 1974; Restle and Brown, 1970) of how the brain may process various patterned sequences in performing tasks discuss the levels of complexity involved but do not deal with the specific dynamics of how perceived sound forms entrain motor output dynamics.

How time is experienced clearly underlies the experience of musical rhythm. Conversely, experiencing rhythm can tell us about how time is experienced. Through studying phenomena of musical rhythm, as we shall see, one can document the existence of an extraordinarily stable psychobiologic clock - stable to one part in 500 or better over decades. This stability appears to exceed evidence of the stability of other rhythmic behavior patterns, e.g. speech patterns, although they, too, can show a remarkable degree of stability.

A second essential brain function contributing to musical rhythm is memory. Reiteration of a temporal pattern implies participation of memory. Study of the function of memory in the creation and experience of rhythm and musical rhythm led us to identify a specific short term memory function called 'time-form printing' (Clynes, 1977b, 1980), some detailed aspects of which are described in the following.

The power of musical rhythm to generate moods, shades of feeling, attitudes, and various types of mental and physical energies - in short, the psychic function of rhythm - is seen to relate to the way in which sound patterns are transduced by the nervous system to modulate the neural driving patterns that, in imagination, or actually as in dance, control the form of movement.

How musical rhythms induce and modulate patterns of movement relates to how musical rhythms affect our feeling states and energies. We need to understand how the central nervous system and the neuromuscular system transform a musical rhythm into a movement pattern - in effect, how different types of musical rhythms would necessarily lead to correspondingly different kinds of dance - actual or mental. One can relate the character of the movements, as in the studies of expressive touch (Clynes, 1973), to the qualities of experience. This approach is also in line with a concept of music phrased by Roger Sessions (1970):

It is the quality and character of the musical gesture that constitutes the essence of the music, the essential goal of the performer's endeavors...
We experience music as movement and gesture...
One must emphasize that a real gesture is in its very nature

organic. It takes precise and characteristic shape by virtue of its own energy, its own inherent laws, its goals, its own curve and direction. There is nothing whatever fortuitous about it.

In order to study the relationship between rhythmic sound patterns and the type of movements which they tend to induce we have used the sentographic method previously developed for the study of the expression of emotion through touch (Clynes, 1969a, 1973, 1975). Using this method, a subject presses rhythmically with the pressure of a finger on a pressure transducer sensitive to both vertical and horizontal pressure. The seated subject as it were 'dances' or 'conducts' on his finger, keeping the finger in touch with the transducer all the way through however, so that the rhythmic impulse is expressed as a pressure impulse produced by the arm. In this way pressure pulse contours are obtained that relate to specific sound rhythms; providing improved dynamic information over earlier studies of aspects of rhythm by Fraisse et al. (1953, 1958); Fraisse (1966).

The substitution of dynamic pressure for a larger movement does not appear to alter the character of the rhythmic experience - small movements do in fact necessarily accompany the pressure generation. As in the study of the expressive forms of emotions, pressure is produced in this method mainly in a plane comprised by the vertical, and the horizontal direction away or towards the body, but not to the left or right.

To probe the relationship between rhythmic sound and movement, as input-output, we have studied:

(1)   Arbitrary rhythmic sound patterns.

(2)   Specific rhythmic pulses of popular music including various forms of rock.

(3)   Specific rhythmic pulses of ethnic music including Hungarian, Polish, Scottish, Spanish, French, Roumanian, Viennese rhythms as well as examples of American square dance, Indian, South American, Pygmy and Ethiopian music.

(4)   The special phenomenon of rhythmic generation developed in Western classical music during the eighteenth and nineteenth centuries in which the composer's intimate personality appears to control other aspects of the tonal proportions, and which we have called the 'inner pulse' (Clynes, 1969a, 1974, 1977a).

The investigations also led to observations and experiments concerning time stabilities of rhythmic generation, and of musical thought.

Other experiments investigated auditory sensitivity to small changes of shape in the dynamic amplitude envelope of sound pulses.

These studies are steps toward clarifying the transfer function between sound rhythm and rhythmic movement, and its inverse. Such a transfer function (as a form of non-linear differential equation) could predict what form of movement an arbitrary rhythmic sound would produce and, in consequence, aspects of its qualities of experience.

For rhythmic experience of sound, on the time scale of musical rhythm, largely is not under voluntary control - we are driven by it (as we all sense), and it would be good to know how.

I. WHAT IS THE NATURE OF RHYTHM?

1. Rhythms of Nature and of the Body

In the physical world, rhythm is fundamental to existence. A photon cannot exist without its frequency; an electron cannot abjure its orbital rhythm around a nucleus. Both of these rhythms or frequencies involve space as well as time. The photon has a wavelength, the orbit of the electron a particular shell size.

Curiously, however, nature treats these two frequencies differently: with the expansion of the universe the frequency of the photon decreases, its wavelength lengthens - as may be seen from the photons remaining from the initial Big Bang - while the frequencies and orbital distances associated with other particles, which do not move at the velocity of light, do not change with the expansion of the universe. On a very fundamental scale the universe thus provides an interplay of rhythm - the changing rhythms of the free photons and the unchanging rhythm of the electrons in captivity.

The macroscopic rhythms of the planets, stars, galaxies, are in part reflected in our experience on earth: ice ages, summer and winter, day and night. To some of these we have entrained bodily functions - for example the sleep and wakefulness cycle. These rhythms do not have the infinite precision of those of the elementary particles but have their own varying degrees of 'rubato', as it were, departures from even, mathematically ordained iteration. In rhythms we can observe directly, such as the waves of the ocean, and of the organic rhythm of flying wings, of breathing, of running and walking, of the beating of the heart, of speech, and of music we find interaction between dynamic elements that create the rhythm, and slower, non-rhythmic (or sometimes rhythmic) agencies that modulate the rhythm.

2. Rhythms of the Mind

In that region of time where the nature of our nervous system and neurobiologic function permit us to recognize individual events, as well as their immediate temporal relationship with neighboring temporal events, we find the phenomena of musical rhythm. This region is approximately from 0.1 Hz to 8 Hz. In this region, human perception involuntarily includes temporal relationships. Slower temporal relationships are viewed through voluntary acts of comparison in which imagination, or deliberately evoked memory, must come to our help. Within this region of frequencies perception of rhythm is immediate, involuntary, and a function of the proportions of the temporal patterns encountered. (Similarly, on a clock, we see the second hand moving, but the minute and hour hands are known to move only through memory.)

Rhythms faster than those to be found in music tend no longer to be perceived as rhythms, by us. First, at an event frequency faster than 0.2 seconds per cycle one is aware of the pattern of change but no longer relates to it as a rhythmic cycle, but only as a member of a group which constitutes the cycle. Still faster regular iterations are experienced as vibration through the sense of touch, flicker in vision, and, through our auditory sensors, as sounds. Of course, with increasing rapidity frequencies are no longer sensed at all (exception: the ability to experience color, a narrow region of photon frequencies of about one 'octave').

The rhythms more rapid than 8-10 per second which we can experience are experienced not as composed of individual events but as continuing sensation, that is, as a particular kind of integral of their dynamic characteristics. This includes the perception of tone. Thus in musical rhythms there is a hierarchical organization of experience of frequency: the frequency of the tones, experienced as imperfect integrals of their frequencies (i.e. as pitch), and the superimposed frequencies of the organization of the tones.

3. Imaging Rhythm

Conscious perception of rhythm in this bandwidth seems to relate to the ability to conceive of voluntarily initiated alternating movement. Whether this ability to conceive alternating movement is congruent with our ability to perceive rhythm is not clear, a priori. Certainly it is possible to imagine rhythms that contain no movement at all, such as for instance a rhythmic alternation of colors on a particular spot, or alternation of hot and cold at a particular place on our body. One can even imagine a rhythm devoid of any sensory quality such as mental alternation of "yes, no", of "more alert, less alert", "more hopeful, less hopeful" and so on. (This ability is important in understanding the phenomenon of the 'inner pulse' of specific composers.)

Note how remarkable this property is that we have: our faculty to be able to imagine rhythm!

We can imagine rhythm in many different sensory modes. But consider, can we imagine rhythms without sensory attributes? And how precisely (reproducibly) can we imagine rhythms?

In imagining a rhythm we generally take recourse to imaging some motor pattern - at times in a subliminal way, perhaps as silently thought words can subliminally activate the vocal apparatus. However, just as it is possible to think words on a faster scale than spoken rhythms without corresponding subliminal muscular motivation, as for example in speed reading, so it is also possible to image rhythms without the use of real time motor images, over a range of time scales.

In imaging rhythm one is quite aware whether one is imaging in real time or on some other time scale. In composing one might, for example, image on a faster time scale, in 'shorthand', knowing well that the rhythm is meant to 'go' at a quite different rate in real time. Even so certain characteristics of the rhythm remain available to the understanding. These elements comprise not just the proportions but the evocative character. It seems, thus, that many phenomena of rhythm can exist mentally without necessary realtime motor representation.

II. MOTOR EXPRESSION OF RHYTHM: TIME-FORM PRINTING

Expressed rhythm involves movement: in the human production of musical rhythm (not computer produced) movement is essential (Dainow, 1977; Stetson, 1905; Woodrow, 1909; Christiani, 1885). Motor output involves agonist and antagonist muscle groups. We may ask, does the expression of rhythm involve alternation between a period of muscular activity, and a rest interval, more or less like the action of a marker pen on a moving strip chart?

In our earlier studies of some aspects of rhythm (Clynes, 1969a) we implicitly considered it to be like this. We measured properties of rates of repeated tapping, with the implication that the tapping events were like marked points on a linear time scale and an intervening period of rest occurred between successive taps. It turned out, however, (Clynes, 1977b, 1980) that this conception was wrong, that the iteration of a rhythmic pulse in general represents a unitary event preprogrammed not as an alternation of activity and rest, as musical notation implies, but as a replication of a single dynamic form accurately stored in memory.

Stability of Tapping Rate

If a subject is asked to tap at a constant rate it was found (Clynes, 1969a) that

(1) The rate of tapping showed a long term drift, generally becoming somewhat faster (of the order of 5% per 500 taps).

(2) Fluctuations of the period from one tap to the next tended to be self correcting so that a well defined mean rate was maintained in the intermediate term.
The departures from this mean rate, or 'errors', could be considered unevennesses of individual tap execution, while the mean rate corresponded to the 'idea' of how fast the tapping rate was at that particular time. The long term drift thus corresponded to a drift in the 'idea'.

(3) It was observed that by replacing an arbitrary rate of tapping with the mental imaging of a particular section of a piece of music so that the imaged beat of the music governed the rate of tapping, the long term drift was abolished. The 'idea' now became stable (Fig. 1).

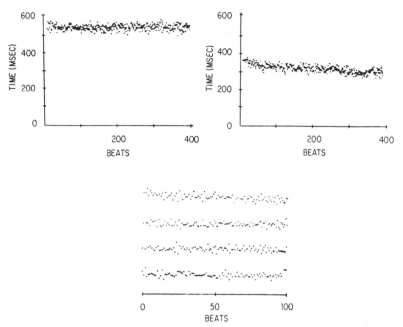

Fig. 1   Distribution of intervals between consecutive beats when required to tap a constant even rhythm (top right) and when tapping according to a steady musical rhythm (Beethoven Waldstein Sonata) (top left) showing a gradual drift in the direction of faster beating in the absence of a musical thought and greater stability of the mean beat frequency with a musical thought. Lower portion of the figure illustrates detail of 400 beats showing deviations from the mean tend to be self correcting rather than cumulative. (Reprinted from Clynes, 1970, by permission of McGraw-Hill Book Co.)

(Recent experiments concerning this stability are described in Section III.)

Although the stability of tapping rates under these conditions was noted, it was not observed at the time that the stability included not only the rate of tapping but the complete spatiotemporal form iterated. Later experiments showed that the memory function which conserves the rate of tapping also conserves the 'wave shape' of the iteration (which may be quite complex). The initial mental command which begins a train of repetitions specifies not only the time period but also the form of the repeated pattern. Thus, for example, in a repeated movement of the hand one may decide to move in an approximately elliptic path, triangular path, square path, or in a rectilinear path at a given angle. The initially chosen shape will tend to maintain itself throughout the repetitions without further command or specific attention.

The repetitions are then performed 'automatically' until further notice, that is until a specific command to stop, or to modify, is given. Or, the initial command may contain a limit instruction: it may specify an integral number of repetitions (2, 3, 4), but generally less than 10 times (except for some complex Indian Tals). For greater numbers, however, an 'unlimited' command is given, (and counting may be required, singly, or in groups), and a separate 'stop' command must be given in order to stop.

The stability behavior of the shape is analogous to the stability behavior of the rate. It may exhibit a long term gradual drift over several hundred repetitions, along with self correcting short term fluctuations, or 'errors'. There is also an analogous stabilizing effect as noted above for rate on the wave form, if this form becomes a musical beat.

The time-form pattern of a beat is printed out repeatedly without further specific attention unless a special modifying command is given. In a musical pattern such commands correspond to rubato, sometimes fermatas, or particular accents, or the end of a piece or major section. We may think of this as the modulation of a basic repetitive 'beat' pattern.

Space-form printing is a memory function of the brain which allows a musical beat to be initially created and then continuingly produced throughout the remainder of the particular music*. The continuation of this beat form may influence the fabric of the music in a number of ways. These include emphasis, articulation, accentuation, timbre changes, and above all microtemporal structure which necessitates deviations from the musically notated metric.

Time-form printing can be a transduction of iteration in various modalities, not only of sound. Also, it can play a role both in creating sound, and in responding to it: it is involved in the transform of rhythmic sound to rhythmic movement and its inverse. If not expressed as movement, the form can still be experienced in an internalized manner.

Some of the properties of time-form printing will be considered further in this section and in Section III of this chapter.

Multimodal Time-Form Printing

Rhythms may be created in which different parts of the pattern are portrayed in different sensory modalities. For example, such a pattern might consist of a succession of three sounds followed by a light, or a touch followed by two sounds and then a light, and so on. Such multimodal rhythms have been little studied but are of considerable interest since they require a different kind of mental imaging and time-form printing. Audiovisual synthesizers permit such rhythms to be readily created. Evoked brain potentials to multimodal rhythms are of particular interest also.

---

* In a good performance the beat is often created mentally or gesturally even before the beginning of the music.

THE BEGINNING OF A RHYTHMIC PATTERN

Where is a beginning to each repeated preprogrammed pattern in time-form printing and what is its significance? Let us consider where in the cycle the repeated initiation or 'trigger' takes place as follows: If one executes a circular repetitive movement with the hand and forearm (at a rate say between 1 and 2 repetitions per second, the hand moving in a vertical plane) one mentally experiences a place of initiation (or trigger) at a specific place on that circle. Depending on where the point of initiation is along the circle, the pattern feels differently. A right-handed person performing clockwise circles will tend to place the point of initiation (or 'trigger') somewhere along the downward path of the circle. He may shift his attention, however, and deliberately place the point of initiation on the upper portion of the circle. The motion will then feel differently, having an 'upward swing' rather than a 'downward swing'. In either case the circular movement, beginning from the point of the initiation and terminating with it is programmed and experienced as an entity. <u>At the location of the trigger beginning the pattern a (small) degree of effort is experienced.</u> Other portions within the pattern are not experienced in the same way.

This property of time-form printing also relates to how a number of sounds in a sequence are mentally grouped together.

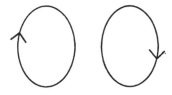

UP BEAT AND DOWN BEAT

When such a rhythmic movement pattern is associated with a rhythmic musical pattern mentally, it becomes a 'beat'. Consider the problem of the initiating trigger for a musical beat.

In a simple up and down beating pattern, where along the pattern is the beginning of the main musical tone to be?* As an orchestra follows the conductor, no one knows 'officially' the precise point along the path of the beat where the main tone (generally the first tone of the bar) should begin. (In fact that point tends to be different for different composers.) The phase of the beat where the main tone begins and where it is experienced is not quite the same. It takes some time for the tone to be built up and to be experienced, as Vos (1981, this volume) has studied, and these two points are separated in time. Moreover, the experienced beginning of the sound and the 'center' where the 'point of rhythmic gravity' (Morton et al., 1976) of

---

*   A beat is considered here as a single repetitive phenomenon, not as a portion of a larger conducting pattern involving all the beats of a bar.

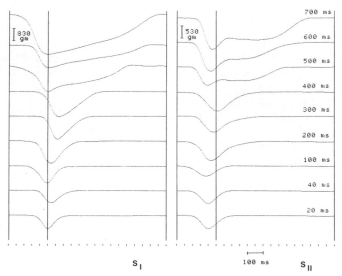

Fig. 2   Relation between motor pulse form and beginning of the sound
          pulse (vertical line) for rectangular sound pulses of durations
          20ms - 700ms, at a repetition rate of 1/sec, for subjects S_I and S_{II}
          (each trace is an average of 100 pulses, stand. dev. of time for
          max. pressure (t max) 30 - 35ms). Carrier frequency was 400
          Hz. Note systematic shift of t max with increasing pulse width,
          though starting from a different degree of anticipation; this
          degree is a specific characteristic for each subject. (Note also
          the change in shape form 'impulse' to square wave' at 500 ms, i.e.
          50% duty cycle.)

sound is experienced are not the same for sounds with longer rise times (e.g.
0.2 sec). This 'point of gravity' has been called the 'P center' by Morton,
Marcus and Frankish (1976). (Note that the P center as defined by Marcus,
is not identical with the perceptual onset, as measured by Vos, except for
relatively fast rise times.)

The Down Beat is the Up Beat

In relation to these questions we measured sentographic responses to
repeated single sound pulses of various rectangular pulse widths. In such a
situation the bottom of a beat (measured as pressure) tends to somewhat
anticipate (40msec) the perceptual beginning of a tone (less so for longer
pulse widths).* But in general, for a main tone of 0.3 seconds duration say,
this tone will be <u>heard</u> during the returning, or upward portion of the

---

* cf. findings of anticipation by Fraisse and others in synchronization
  experiments in which subjects tap 'synchronously' with repeated clicks.

beat (Fig. 2). The musical upbeat (anacrusis), however, is heard on the downward phase of the beat.

The musical up beat tends to be experienced mostly as congruent with the beginning of the initiation trigger phase, and the beginning of the musical down beat completes this phase. (For actually the trigger 'point' experienced in a cycle of time-form printing entails a finite region, and that region generally falls within the temporal space between the up beat and the main beat.) In those instances the function of the music up beat is to start the trigger of the movement time-form printing cycle.

Thus we appear to have the paradoxically sounding relation: the up beat is the down beat and the down beat is the up beat! It appears less Zen-like, however, phrased as: the 'musical up beat' begins the 'movement down beat', and the 'musical down beat' begins the 'movement up beat'.

(Different composers may favor different rates of initiation of tone* and so the place where the tone is heard as 'centered' along the path of the beat may tend to vary with each composer. Thus, for example, in relatively sustained (cantabile) passages, the tone tends to peak later in Beethoven than in Mozart - it tends to have a longer rise time, being governed by a more 'massive' pulse).

III. MENTAL STABILITY OF TEMPO OF MUSICAL RHYTHM

1. Long Term Stability of Peformance Times

Modern techniques of recording have made it possible to examine the temporal stability of musical rhythms over a period measured in years. The most stringent conditions of stability involve examination of performances of specific pieces by the same artist over a long period of time.

The concept of a particular work of music varies with different artists and the tempo chosen varies accordingly. (The meaning of a particular piece of music is not invariant with changes of tempo. Even relatively slight changes in overall tempo (say 2 - 3%) noticeably affect the qualities of the music. Bartok specified the tempo of his compositions to within one third of the usual metronomic subdivisions, that is to within $\pm 1\%$ approximately.) There appears to exist a stability, however, that seems even to exceed the limits of the just noticeable difference (jnd) of tempo. This becomes strikingly evident in comparing specific performances of the same artist at widely different times, many years apart.

In such performances of the same piece separated by a number of years, a remarkable stability can be observed in a number of cases studied (if the concept of the piece has not clearly changed). Toscanini's performance of the Brahms Haydn Variations Op.56 are analyzed in Fig. 3 and Table 1 (Clynes, 1969a). A recent timing analysis of a number of variations from Bach's Goldberg Variations and Beethoven's Diabelli

―――――――

* related to their pulse form.

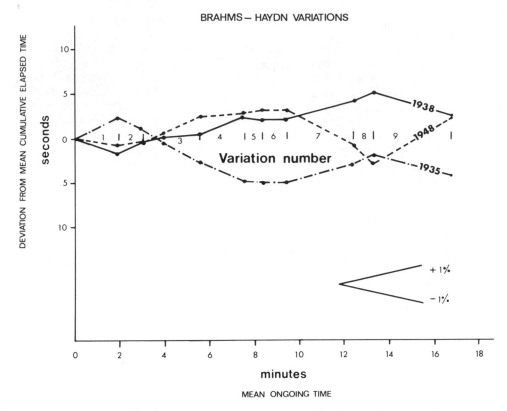

Fig. 3   Comparisons of three performances of the Brahms Haydn
            Variations Op. 56b by Arturo Toscanini as in Table 1 showing the
            course of each performance. The fork on the bottom right
            indicates a slope of 1%: a difference in tempo of 1% from the
            mean. Thus when lines of different performances are parallel
            they indicate the same tempo. Note the great similarity of the
            courses of the 1935 and 1938 performances from Var. 5 onwards
            and the similarity of performances of 1938 and 1948 from the
            beginning to the end of Var. 6. Total duration of the 1938 and
            1948 performances is closely maintained.

Variations recorded by M. Clynes between 1965 and 1981 is given in Figs. 4
and 5 and Tables 2, 3 and 4*. For this piece the greatest stability was
observed for the faster variations. In these the fingers and hands execute a
continuing rhythmic motion comprising a steady number of notes per beat.

---

* Tape recordings of these public performances can be obtained from the
  authors.

Table 1   Timings of three performances of the Brahms Haydn Variations Op. 56b by Arturo Toscanini and the NBC Symphony Orchestra in Studio H in 1935, 1938, and 1948 respectively. A great similarity exists in the sections from theme to variation 6 in the last two performances, total time 9:28 and 9:29 respectively, while the sections from variations 5 to 9 are very similar in the first two performances, being of total time 9:18 and 9:18 respectively. The differences in the timings in the other variations are considerably greater and indicate a change in concept. Variation 7 has two time markings, the second one for a repetition. The changes in variations 7, 8, and 9 of the last two performances are mutually compensating so that the total time of the performance differed by less than 0.5 sec. Accuracy of the timing system was about two times greater than this deviation. (from Clynes, 1969a)

	1935		1938 Feb.26		1948 Feb.21	
Theme		1.56		1.52		1.53
Var.1	Cumulative Time 3.04½	1.08½	C.T. 3.03	1.11	C.T. 3.03	1.10
2	3.56	.51½	3.56½	.53½	3.57	.54
3	5.29	1.33	5.32	1.35½	5.34	1.37
4	7.26	1.57	7.33	2.01	7.33½	1.59½
5	8.14	.48	8.21	.48	8.22	.48½
6	9.21	1.07	9.28	1.07	9.29	1.07
7	12.23	2.01 / 1.01	12.30	2.03 / .59	12.25	1.58 / .58
8	13.18	.55	13.25	.55	13.17	.52
9		3.26		3.25½		3.33½
Total		16.44		16.50.6		16.50.3

(Timings from original masters in minutes and seconds)

The stability observed is greater than the jnd. It is not easy to give a justifiable explanation for the existence of a psychobiologic clock of such stability, although it would be possible to posit theories involving macromolecular vibrational properties - but not enough is yet known about cellular function to provide the basis for a sensible theory. (Even the clock for embryonic development is not known although it also has considerable stability.) But we do see that time-form printing, when combined with musical significance, can lead to extremely stable temporal form - extremely stable, that is, when compared to other known organic rhythms.

The second property that appears from these observations is that often the total timespan of a work of music appears to be a mental entity - mentally defining the 'size' of the piece - and that changes in different parts of the music tend to compensate, so as to maintain that total 'size'.

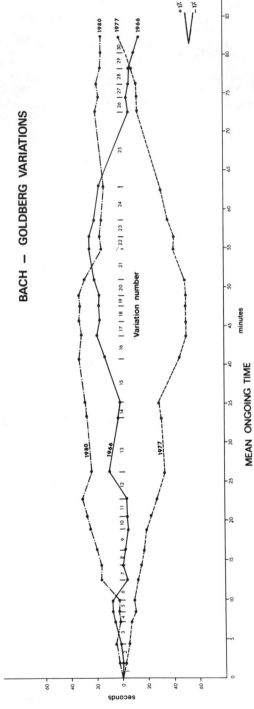

Fig. 4   Course of three recorded performances of Bach's Goldberg Variations by M. Clynes in 1966, 1977 and 1980 (aria not illustrated). Times include pauses between variations. Note the tendency of changes in the tempo of individual variations to compensate conserving the overall duration. Total time for all variations (without the Aria): 1966, 81 min 57.3 sec; 1977, 82 min 12 sec; 1980, 82 min 26 sec.

Table 2   Timings of the faster variations of Bach's Goldberg Variations of five different recorded public performances by M. Clynes. Each variation has two parts of 16 bars, and both parts are repeated. Timings are from the beginning of the first note to the beginning of the first note of the following part, except for the last repeat, where they end with the end of the last note. Because of this, and the difficulty at times to obtain an accurate timing of the end of the last note, the timing for the last repeat for each variation is shown in parenthesis, being not quite comparable. A further consideration is that ritards may occur at the end of the second repetition. Consistent timings are notable for all the examples covering a time span of more than 14 years. Var. 19 is particularly noteworthy. The performances were in different halls and environments and on different Grand pianos. These variations mostly have continuous, running motion.

Var. 14	Part A	Repeat	Part B	Repeat		Var. 17	Part A	Repeat	Part B	Repeat
Feb 1966	28.8	28.5	29.0	(29.8)		Feb 1966	27.1	27.7	28.0	(29.6)
18 Nov 68	28.0	27.8	28.4	(30.1)		18 Nov 68	27.8	28.1	27.9	(30.8)
Sep 1977	28.3	29.4	29.0	(30.9)		Sep 1977	27.7	28.3	28.8	(31.6)
12 Sep 78	28.9	29.2	29.3	(30.9)		12 Sep 78	27.7	28.5	28.9	(31.5)
9 Sep 1980	28.6	29.0	29.3	(32.2)		9 Sep 1980	28.4	29.0	28.5	(32.0)

Var. 19						Var. 20				
Feb 1966	18.3	18.5	18.9	(21.4)		Feb 1966	27.9	28.0	30.2	(30.8)
18 Nov 68	18.0	18.6	19.0	(21.6)		18 Nov 68	27.2	26.7	29.2	(30.9)
Sep 1977	18.1	18.7	18.8	(20.9)		Sep 1977	28.4	28.6	30.4	(32.0)
12 Sep 78	18.2	18.3	18.7	(21.3)		12 Sep 78	28.1	27.9	29.8	(32.0)
9 Sep 1980	18.3	18.5	18.8	(21.5)		9 Sep 1980	27.6	27.9	30.2	(32.2)

Var. 23						Var. 26				
Feb 1966	27.9	28.0	29.2	(29.7)		Feb 1966	30.4	29.5	28.6	(29.3)
18 Nov 68	28.1	27.8	28.9	(30.2)		18 Nov 68	27.7	27.9	26.8	(27.8)
Sep 1977	27.9	28.6	30.3	(30.4)		Sep 1977	29.1	29.3	28.5	(30.6)
12 Sep 78	28.8	29.1	30.1	(30.8)		12 Sep 78	28.6	29.2	28.1	(29.4)
9 Sep 1980	28.9	28.9	30.5	(30.6)		9 Sep 1980	28.3	29.0	28.1	(28.9)

Var. 27						Var. 28				
Feb 1966	23.8	24.2	24.3	(25.1)		Feb 1966	29.9	30.5	30.4	(31.4)
18 Nov 68	23.4	24.8	24.7	(25.9)		18 Nov 68	30.5	31.1	31.8	(32.8)
Sep 1977	24.2	24.6	24.6	(25.9)		Sep 1977	30.9	31.0	32.3	(32.7)
12 Sep 78	24.2	25.0	25.0	(26.4)		12 Sep 78	30.4	30.6	31.8	(32.6)
9 Sep 1980	24.9	24.9	25.1	(25.8)		9 Sep 1980	29.7	29.9	30.3	(30.4)

Var. 29	Part A	Repeat	Part B	Repeat
Feb 1966	29.1	29.5	27.8	(30.7)
18 Nov 68	28.8	29.6	27.8	(31.1)
Sep 1977	28.5	29.4	28.2	(35.3)
12 Sep 78	28.7	29.5	27.7	(35.8)
9 Sep 80	28.3	29.0	27.5	(35.6)

Table 3   Examples of slow variations from the same performances as in Table 2. In contrast to those of the faster variations these timings show a tendency for progressive slowing over a number of years, and a greater fluctuation, as did other slow variations, as well as the aria. This indicates a change in interpretation, as it is not indicative of a change in the timing of slower pieces in general over those years. (See Table 4)

	Part A	Repeat	Part B	Repeat		Part A	Repeat	Part B	Repeat
Var. 24					**Var. 25**				
Feb 1966	55.4	59.9	64.7	(67.5)	Feb 1966	132.9	131.3	140.9	(141.7)
18 Nov 68	56.8	57.9	61.6	(66.6)	18 Nov 68	122.1	114.2	124.9	(135.7)
Sep 1977	59.1	63.4	65.8	(70.0)	Sep 1977	134.9	139.5	138.0	(155.7)
12 Sep 78	62.1	64.4	70.3	(77.1)	12 Sep 78	137.3	142.3	147.9	(163.4)
9 Sep 1980	56.4	61.6	65.2	(69.9)	9 Sep 1980	132.4	137.4	144.0	(156.3)

Table 4   Timings of two performances of Beethoven's Diabelli Variations Op. 120 eleven years apart, by M. Clynes. Cumulative times include pauses between variations in this table. Some timings show a considerable stability in both fast and slow variations. Others deviate, however deviations tend to compensate mutually, so that a stable overall time is observed. Thus changes of interpretation tend nevertheless to maintain overall duration. (See also Fig. 5)

		1966	1977	1966	1977
				Cumulative	
Theme		51.1	47.8	56.3	49.8
Var.	1	1 : 52.0	1 : 35.2	2 : 51.9	2 : 25.8
	2	58.4	58.9	3 : 51.9	3 : 24.6
	3	1 : 40.3	1 : 45.0	5 : 33.6	5 : 09.4
	4	1 : 11.9	1 : 08.0	6 : 47.2	6 : 18.0
	5	57.5	1 : 03.3	7 : 47.4	7 : 22.3
	6	1 : 58.4	1 : 51.8	9 : 49.5	9 : 14.1
	7	1 : 04.0	1 : 04.6	10 : 56.9	10 : 20.8
	8	1 : 40.4	1 : 50.3	12 : 40.8	12 : 11.6
	9	2 : 12.6	1 : 54.6	14 : 56.3	14 : 08.6
	10	33.2	35.3	15 : 33.6	14 : 45.9
	11	1 : 30.8	1 : 41.6	17 : 05.6	16 : 27.9
	12	58.8	51.3	18 : 06.2	17 : 20.3
	13	59.5	1 : 07.2	19 : 10.2	18 : 34.2
	14	4 : 34.3	4 : 47.3	23 : 47.4	23 : 23.6
	15	32.6	32.4	24 : 20.4	23 : 58.1
	16	57.4	56.5	25 : 17.9	24 : 54.6
	17	57.1	58.8	26 : 17.7	25 : 56.8
	18	2 : 04.3	2 : 19.1	28 : 24.6	28 : 16.6
	19	46.1	48.1	29 : 13.3	29 : 09.2
	20	2 : 19.9	2 : 29.1	31 : 44.1	31 : 44.6
	21	1 : 05.4	59.6	32 : 53.2	32 : 46.3
	22	46.6	50.6	33 : 42.8	33 : 40.4
	23	50.1	50.8	34 : 36.9	34 : 34.4
	24	3 : 18.3	3 : 24.4	38 : 01.2	38 : 01.3
	25	41.7	42.5	38 : 44.3	38 : 45.9
	26	1 : 17.5	1 : 25.4	40 : 03.6	40 : 12.1
	27	57.5	56.2	41 : 03.8	41 : 09.2
	28	52.4	46.8	42 : 00.2	42 : 00.1
	29	1 : 35.5	1 : 40.8	43 : 37.9	43 : 41.4
	30	1 : 55.6	1 : 52.4	45 : 36.4	45 : 34.3
	31 (Largo)	6 : 23.4	6 : 28.8	52 : 01.4	52 : 05.6
	32 (Fugue)	3 : 06.4	3 : 07.8	55 : 13.4	55 : 16.0
	33 (Minu.)	1 : 52.6	1 : 49.3	57 : 05.3	57 : 06.0

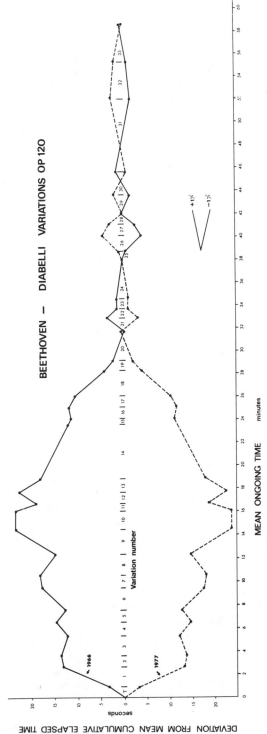

Fig. 5   Two performances of Beethoven's Diabelli Variations Op. 120 by M. Clynes in 1966 and 1977 showing a considerable change in interpretation of the first part of the composition up to Var. 20 and a high degree of stability from Var. 21 to the end. Note again the tendency for interpretive changes to compensate, preserving the total duration.

2. Stability of Tapping with Mentally Imagined Music

Recent experiments were carried out with tapping series of several thousand taps under various conditions. (Between series the subject generally continued to tap for 50 - 100 taps that were not measured.)

Results show that tapping stability by a musician between runs of 1000 taps when imaging Mozart's C major piano concerto K467 (first 16 bars) was .5110 sec + .0026 during 4000 taps and .5109 sec + .0007 the following day with 3000 taps (same subject). (No temporal cues were given in either experiment. Excerpts from a recording of the concerto (Artur Schnabel with the London Philharmonic Orchestra) had been played in a different test three times 3 weeks before the test.)

Results typically show an improvement by a factor of 5 in medium term stability (30 minutes) when a musical piece was repeatedly thought by a musician as compared with a verbally imagined phrase such as "Saturday, Sunday", and a further factor of 3 when compared with tapping without mentally repeated image. Results further show that mean short term 'errors' for the music image series were 10 times larger than the longer term drift - the 'errors' between successive 1000 series. Short term errors (beat to beat) were of similar magnitude in all series. They appear largely like noise introduced inside the control loop.

Results are summarized in Table 5.

Experiments are being conducted to test this stability over a long time span to determine over which time span maximum stability occurs.

3. Comparison of the Tempo of Imagined and Performed Rhythm

We may compare the durations of thinking a musical rhythm, as in actual performance - thinking the music at the rate at which we would perform it in real time - with that of an actual performance by the same person, on the same occasion. (In imaging on a real time scale subliminal motor activity of a glottal, tongue or palatal nature is almost unavoidable.) Experiments in which pieces or portions of pieces of music less than 1 minute long are executed (1) mentally only, (2) conducting, (3) playing (particular pieces are executed five times for each condition by each of 8 musician subjects* - with a total of 240 trials) show the following: (a) mean standard deviation for each piece performed by a given musician is 1.92% for playing, 3.48% for thinking; (b) a consistently slower mental execution (mean 8.9%, p <.0001)(Table 6).

Conducting seemed to produce timing intermediate between thinking and performing; but the difference between conducting and performing was significant only at p .01. The consistency of the results was such that of 65 trials of thinking of the 'slower thinking' musicians in only 6 out of 65 trials was thinking not slower than the slowest of the playing times for that piece by the same subject.

---

* 3 pianists, 2 violinists, 1 cellist, 1 organist, 1 guitarist.

Table 5   Increased stability with increasing number of taps is shown by this table. Although individual taps typically show errors of several centiseconds larger tap groups show an increasing stability. Thus it seems that the idea of the tempo of the music is more stable than the ability to execute taps in accordance with it. Errors of individual taps tend to compensate each other showing presence of a higher hierarchical control. Improvement of errors with larger groups is only 3 dB less than the theoretical signal/noise improvement ratio for a perfectly stable signal in the presence of noise equivalent to the tap to tap errors.

Stability of Tapping
While Thinking Mozart Piano Concerto K 467
(First 16 Bars) Repeatedly

	June 25	June 26
Number of Taps	4000	3000
	Means (seconds)	
Entire Run	.5112	.5092
First 1000	.5117	.5086
Second 1000	.5109	.5092
Third 1000	.5085	.5099
Fourth 1000	.5137	

Stability Analysis of Run of 4000 Taps

	1	10	100	Per Groups of 200	500	1000
mean error	.0128	.00529	.00338	.00283	.00172	.00150
standard dev.	.01936	.00610	.00416	.00378	.00285	.00216
Examples of Consecutive Individual Values		Consecutive Means				
	.5010	.5174	.5154		.5122	.5117
	.5313	.5189	.5117		.5113	.5109
	.5155	.5181	.5122		.5099	.5085
	.5002	.5227	.5106		.5119	.5137
	.4757	.5234	.5110		.5056	
	.4990	.5168	.5131		.5114	
	.4853	.5133	.5096		.5113	
	.5189	.5098	.5127		.5160	
	.4992	.5110	.5126			
	.5077	.5071	.5080			
	....	....	....			
	....	....	....			

Slope of line of best fit for 4000 taps: less than   −0.1 microsec/tap
                                                            −0.2 microsec/sec

Table 6   Timings of Playing and Thinking portions of various musical pieces of 1/2 - 1 minute duration, by different musicians. (Referred to 100 as mean playing time, for each musical example.)

SUBJ. & PIECE	PLAY			THINK			p
	Duration - 5 performances	Stand. Dev. %	Mean	Duration - 5 'performances'	Stand. Dev. %	Mean	
GB1 Mozart Rondo in D Haffner Serenade (violin)	98.5 100.4 99.9 101.3 99.9	1.02	100	111.9 113.5 111.4 111.4 113.3	1.03	112.3	< .001
GB2 Kreisler Tambourine Chinois	101.2 100.2 98.4 100.7 99.6	1.08	100	106.2 108.3 108.5 110.5 111.3	2.01	109.0	< .001
MM1 Chopin "Berceuse"	102.8 103.4 99.9 94.8 99.1	3.43	100	103.8 102.6 105.9 104.8 101.6	1.71	103.7	< .01
MM2 Schubert Dance D820 No.6	99.1 98.7 100.6 101.6 100.0	1.16	100	106.6 100.4 102.7 101.8 105.0	2.48	103.3	< .01
RO1 Schumann Kinderscenen "A Great Event"	101.7 99.0 98.3 99.8 101.1	1.42	100	112.7 102.3 107.6 103.8 104.8	4.10	106.2	< .02
RO2 Mozart Sonata in C K.330 (1st mvt.)	98.9 98.6 97.1 103.8 101.7	2.69	100	98.2 116.8 111.4 110.9 112.4	6.96	109.9	< .02
QG1 Chopin Mazurka in G minor	96.5 99.3 106.2 96.8 101.2	3.97	100	108.0 114.4 127.1 117.8 119.4	6.99	117.3	< .001
QG2 Beethoven F minor Sonata Op.2 No.1 (1st part, 1st mvt.)	97.9 103.0 97.1 101.0 100.9	2.44	100	123.9 133.9 131.1 128.1 132.0	3.90	129.8	< .001
IV1 "Home on the Range" (violin)	101.5 97.7 99.6 100.0 101.2	1.51	100	101.2 106.2 104.2 107.5 105.4	2.39	104.9	<.01
IV2 Traditional Square Dance Tune	101.1 100.2 99.2 99.2 100.2	0.80	100	119.9 123.2 125.6 121.4 119.5	2.52	121.9	<.001
IV3 Handel Allegro from E major Sonata for violin and piano	101.4 99.5 101.4 99.5 98.2	1.39	100	91.1 104.6 109.1 111.0 104.0	7.77	104.0	<.02
AL1 J.S. Bach from Anna Magdalena Notebook	96.2 98.3 100.4 100.4 104.7	3.15	100	117.5 115.4 113.2 116.5 117.5	1.80	116.0	< .001
AL2 "Un Pezzino", composer - subject's own composition	94.8 101.9 100.7 101.9 100.7	2.97	100	110.2 122.0 118.5 118.5 122.0	4.82	118.2	< .001
MV Bach Minuet (cello)	102.7 100.4 98.3 97.7 100.9	2.03	100	102.0 101.2 99.0 97.7 101.7	1.88	100.3	NS
FO1 Carulli Rondo in D major (guitar)	100.0 100.4 100.6 99.6 99.3	0.54	100	96.0 95.0 94.5 95.2 96.0	0.65	95.3	< .001
FO2 Sor Study No.3 in A major (guitar)	99.1 98.9 100.2 101.5 100.4	1.06	100	84.5 95.5 90.5 93.1 85.8	4.69	89.9	< .002

All musicians tested are consistently either slower (7) or faster (1), in their thinking than in their playing (p < 0.005) and their thinking/playing time ratio is specific for the music selected.

If we combine the observation of the stability reported in the previous sections with the finding that purely mental experience of the rhythm, without physical execution, appears to have a slightly slower tempo, then it follows that the deviation from 1 of the mental/performed rhythm transform ratio may itself be a stable function for that music, and musician.

We must inquire to what extent this ratio depends on auditory feedback as compared with kinesthetic feedback, before we can attempt to formulate a theory for this apparently paradoxical finding: that in a musical piece the experience of thought rhythm, alone, for most musicians is consistently slightly slower than when it executes the movement it thinks.*

IV. SIGNIFICANCE OF THE REPETITIVELY EXPERIENCED BEAT FORM

The specific form that is timeform-printed gives the rhythm its character. This precise form of the beat may govern the time proportions of note patterns and to a degree the relative accentuation. To these, the musical notation is an approximation. Exact 3:1, 4:1 temporal ratios are hardly ever found, not because of laxness of execution, but because the beat (and, in a different way, other expressive influences; see Clynes and Nettheim, this volume) constrains a different, numerically non-simple ratio, by the timing of the initiations of elements of the motor pulse. These ratios may display stability within one performer for a given piece, but also across performers (cf. Gabrielsson, 1979, this volume) for specific ethnic and 'popular' beats, and for particular expressive functions to be explored.

Different pulse forms affect the state of the subject differently. The subtlety of form may give rise to peaceful or energetic, joyful or sexually exciting, enthusiastic or placid, matter-of-fact or excited conditions, and many shades in between. Because of its repetition its effect is hierarchically on a different level than other meaningful structures of music. It represents a frame of reference around which the music is built. Minsky, Jackendoff and Lerdahl, Deutsch, and Pribram (this volume) in different ways note the importance of repetition in musical structure. The form of the beat is the most obvious and primary repetitive phenomenon that music has to offer. Pribram's contention that repetition in music is accompanied by a lowered awareness of what is repeated (habituation) may seem to apply prima parte to the pulse (and to some avant-garde music, where slight variation becomes the focus of attention) more than to the hierarchically higher structures with which he, and Bernstein (1976), are concerned.

---

* Current experiments with a silent keyboard suggest that auditory feedback can be excluded as a significant factor in the phenomenon.

In those repetitions of sequences and phrases in music contributions to symmetry generally overrule diminution of interest due to repetition; in a good composition repetition of up to three (or in some cases perhaps, four) times may be felt as giving added significance, the whole is more than the sum of its parts; beyond this however it generally tends to become irritating, boring, and is mostly shunned by good composers.* Musical symmetry (repetition combined with function and anti-function, which may be a harmonic sequence, for example) functions with the help of short term memory of what has preceded, and with expectations of what is to follow; it is a highly important musical function: its proper use gives Mozart's music much of its greatness. Like the synthesis of opposites, it appears to heighten awareness, and its effects remain to be studied from a neuropsychologic point of view - relating the phemonema of symmetry in time with those of symmetry in space. In looking at a hexagon, we do not find it boring that every line turns through the same angle at every corner - we enjoy the overall form, mainly because we can see all lines simultaneously. In good music a balance has been found to allow us to experience both sequentially and simultaneously together: i.e. simultaneously!

With the beat, however, symmetry applies only within metric divisions; overall the beat is printed out relentlessly, without concern for yesterday or tomorrow**. Yet by varying its tempo, and relative emphasis it is subject to influence from the higher hierarchical musical powers. Thus repetition (Zajonc, 1968) and variation work together in creating significance in the musical beat.

Pulse forms of ethnic music often show a strong relationship to the rhythms of the corresponding language. The rhythms of poetry as adumbrated by Jakobsen (1956) correspond primarily to the pulse form in music. Poetic pulse forms had been identified by Sievers (1875-1915) and Becking (1928) even before the pioneering work of Becking with the specific pulse form of composers.

But analysis in terms of 'strong' and 'weak' alone (Jackendoff and Lerdahl, 1980; Cooper and Meyer, 1960) cannot do justice to the great subtleties of relative timing, accent and the details of form of the pulse, which determine its actual character. This is an inherent weakness of analysis based in the written score only (and not based on realized music) since the indication of the score is limited by the capacity of music notation. This weakness is of much lesser concern in harmonic, contrapuntal and structural analysis, but becomes severe in rhythmic analysis, and also in expressive analysis.

Although repetitive time forms do not excite by novelty after a certain number of repetitions, still they represent an attitude. According to Zajonc,

---

* For further consideration of the effects of repetition on the mental state and emotional intensity, see Clynes and Nettheim (this volume) and Clynes, 1980.

** Although, of course, it can itself express qualities of longing or hope, for example.

we often tend to get to like repeated patterns, i.e. the attitudes implied - at least temporarily. However, the 'hypnotic' aspect of repetitive sound, the aspect of feeling that the rhythm takes us over, relates to the time-form printing property that requires only one initial decision for the generation of the beat - thereafter no further conscious decision is required: in listening even this initial decision is taken away from us! While time-form printing takes place without further conscious attention to the rate and shape, both are elements of an attitude that persists throughout the repetition. What the nature of that attitude is in various popular, ethnic, and classical music will be examined in more detail later.

V. STUDY OF THE RELATIONSHIP BETWEEN SOUND PULSE AND MOTOR PULSE

In order to study the relationship between the rhythm of music and corresponding motor form (beat) we conceive of replacing the music by its sound pulse form, and define the sound pulse form of a particular music to be that form which will produce the same rhythmic motor form as the original music.

This concept allows us to study aspects of the rhythmic character of actual pieces of music apart from melodic and harmonic superstructure.

A further way to study the relationship between sound pulse and movement pulse is to introduce various arbitrary test sound pulses and observe the motor pulses that correspond to them - as part of a dynamic control system analysis.

We may formulate our approach as follows:

(1)   A specific (non sound) time-form exists which gives rise to the character of the musical rhythm.

(2)   This time-form can be represented as amplitude modulated tones of a single sinusoidal frequency, the sound pulse.

(3)   The sound pulse thus created should produce the same movement patterns or motor pulse as the music which it represents, to be regarded as correct.

(4)   The relationship between the correctly extracted sound pulse form and the motor pulse it produced can be studied in order to determine the general relationship between time-form printed sound and its movement correlate.

(5)   By studying a sufficient number of pairs of sound pulses and motor pulses we may gradually establish a transfer function between sound pulse and motor pulse - i.e. we can predict that a particular form of sound pulse will produce a particular motor pulse.

(6)   By relating specific motor pulses to a number of dynamic expressive forms studied in the expression of emotion (see Clynes and Nettheim,

this volume) we can derive a degree of understanding of the qualities and particular psychic energies inherent in the specific motor pulse forms and thus in turn in the specific sound pulses.

(7)   How a particular sound pulse form originates mentally can be studied through the inverse transfer function, where this may be applicable. For example, we may ask what type of musical pulse would correspond to a particular type of dance pattern.

We need to recognize, however, that sound pulses may also originate without corresponding motor images, as discussed earlier. Such types of sound pulses are not encountered in either ethnic or popular music. They can be found in the inner pulses of some composers as distinct from specific rhythmic patterns displayed in their music, a distinction which we shall describe later.

In the following we shall first consider the relationship of the sound pulse to the motor pulse for (1) arbitrarily created sound pulse forms, (2) pulse forms extracted from popular music and ethnic music.

(A) ARBITRARY PULSE FORMS

160 different rectangular sound pulse pair combinations of constant frequency were tested. In these studies as well as those in the following sections, two sound pulses were used to constitute the iterated pattern. Studies with single sound pulses, and preliminary studies with a greater number of pulses appeared to show that two-pulse patterns would yield the most highly differentiated analyzable motor pulse forms. This choice also parallels the musical concepts, up beat and main beat. (When considering shaped musical pulses, however, i.e. not merely rectangular, single shaped pulses may sometimes suffice for characterization.) Pulses are produced by amplitude modulating a sinusoidal carrier by rectangular wave forms (rounded off by a 2 msec time constant to avoid 'flapping'). In producing a pair of such pulses there are 7 variables to control:

(i)   repetition rate of the pattern;
(ii)   duration of the first pulse;
(iii)   duration of the second pulse;
(iv)   interval between the first and second pulse;
(v)   relative amplitude of first and second pulse;
(vi)   frequency (pitch) of the pulses;
(vii)   the overall loudness.

For this study three variables were kept constant: (a) the repetition rate was 1 per second for all patterns, (b) the frequency (pitch) of both pulses was chosen to be 392 Hz, (c) the mean loudness was chosen 50 dB above threshold.

The other four variables were varied in a systematic fashion producing 160 different combinations. (Amplitude ratios selected were - 1,1, 1,1/3, 1/3,1, 1/9,1. Pulse widths of either pulse - 3,10,20,35,50 centiseconds. Interval durations between the two members of a pulse pair - 2,6,10,14,21,30 centiseconds. The combination of these parameter choices results in 120 trials. 40 additional trials used intermediate values of pulse widths and durations.

The experiment is conducted as follows:

A person seated in standardized position (Clynes 1975) responds to sound from a speaker by rhythmically pressing on the finger rest of a sentograph as the sound pulse is repeated 70 times (finger contact is maintained throughout). The motor pulse forms recorded as finger pressure are averaged using a Minc MNC digital computer. As in the experiments for

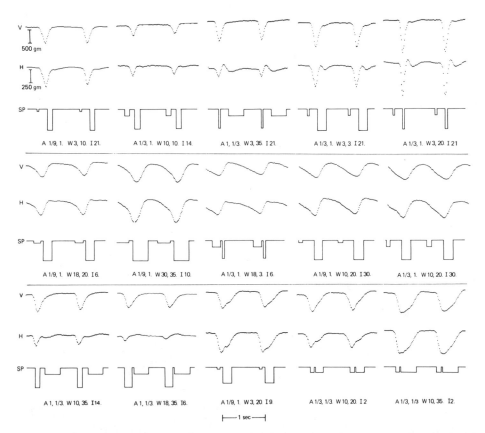

Fig. 6   Types of motor pulses. Varieties of Type I – top left: simple unmodulated pulse; top right: accelerated simple pulse; middle group: slowed fall time; bottom group: slowed rise time. Each record shows the vertical component of pressure as the top trace (V); horizontal component, middle trace (H); and sound pulse (S), bottom trace. The relative amplitudes (A) and the sound pulse widths in 100ths/sec (W) and the interval between the two pulses (I) in 100ths/sec are given under each record. Each record is the average of 30 sweeps and shows two motor pulses. Repetition rate of the pulse pairs is 1/sec.

measuring the expressive forms of emotions, motor pulse forms are measured in a plane including the vertical and a horizontal direction away or toward the body. Pressure in a left-right direction is not normally measured. The pressure pulse appears to be largely contained in the measurement plane, although, depending on the larger scale bar rhythm, occasional submultiple left-right swaying (comprising several beats) may be additionally encountered. The first 10 sound pulses are presented before

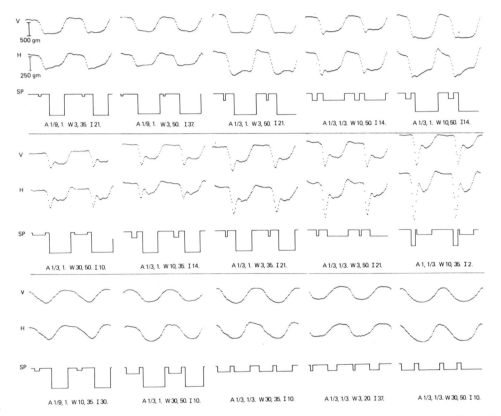

Fig. 7   Types of motor pulses. Varieties of Types II and III - as in Fig. 6. Examples of (a) square wave like motor pulses (top group, Type II); (b) square wave with overshoot type (middle group); (c) Type III, rounded type (lowest group) - note absence of fast response component. Type II 'square wave' shows the presence of two dynamic components that add to give the observed shape (1) an under damped fast response, present mostly for the downward phase; (2) a component with slower time constants.

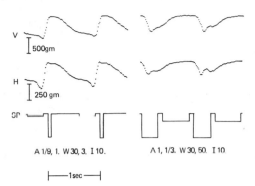

A 1/9, 1. W 30, 3. I 10.   ∧ 1, 1/3. W 30, 50. I 10

Fig. 8   Examples of motor pulses having shapes different from the five
basic patterns described. These shapes are not commonly found
in music but can be seen to be analyzable in terms of the
components of the other forms presented.

measurement begins in order to permit the subject to become adjusted to
the pattern, and let his motor responses become synchronous with the sound
patterns. (A number of pulse patterns need to be heard to establish the
pattern in short term memory so that the response includes the anticipation
of the next pattern, or beat. The synchronizing effect generally takes
place within a few beats, and itself is an interesting phenomenon. This has
been studied in various experiments by Fraisse, 1966.)
    Results show the following:

(1)   Response patterns fall into the following different types (Figs. 6, 7, 8) –

    (a)   Simple impulse.

    (b)   Impulse with slowed or accelerated fall time.

    (c)   Impulse with slowed or accelerated rise time.

    (d)   'Square wave form' with varying degrees of overshoot (mainly in
        the downward direction). This is the result of a subdivision of the
        beat into a separate down and up phase.

    (e)   Rounded wave-like forms.

    In addition the forms can be characterized by the ratio of vertical to
horizontal components, that is, by the angle of pressure.

(2)   The subject mentally chooses one of the two pulses of the pair as the
main pulse. The choice is influenced primarily by the loudness of the pulse –
the louder one being chosen as the main beat. This choice is counterweighed

secondarily by the duration, however, so that a longer pulse will be chosen as the main pulse in preference to a shorter one of equal loudness, and greater duration will outweigh a somewhat reduced loudness (as was already found by Boring, 1942, for sequence of clicks; cf. iambic and trochaic grouping also, in diction and poetry).

There is thus also a region of uncertainty where either of the pulses may be picked as the main one, and will be chosen so at different times by the same subject. The region of the ambiguity occurs when both pulses are of equal amplitude and duration, and also when increased duration of one pulse is counterbalanced by an appropriate degree of increased loudness of the other.

(3) (a)   Within a region of influence, the pulse before the main pulse (the auxiliary pulse) will tend to govern the beginning of the down phase of the motor pulse. That is, the closer in time the secondary pulse is immediately before the main pulse (up to a point of maximum effect at approximately 60 msec at a repetition rate of 1 pair per second), the faster the motor 'down beat'. As the auxiliary pulse moves away from the main pulse, the motor down beat becomes slowed, until the secondary beat moves out of the region of influence (with respect to its initiation); at which point the down beat reverts to its unmodified character (i.e. its form without the auxiliary pulse). This occurs at approximately 25% of the duty cycle or 0.25 seconds, at the repetition rate chosen (1 per second).

(b)   The upward phase of the motor pulse is slowed down with longer main sound pulses so that its completion tends to coincide with the end of the main pulse. Thus for longer main pulses the beat rises during the entire main tone.

(c)   For longer main pulses quite close coincidence of the bottom of the beat with the beginning of the main pulse tends to occur and the anticipation effect is gradually eliminated.

(d)   If the auxiliary beat is near the mid point of the cycle, it can give rise to the 'square wave' form motor pulse, in which the beat is subdivided, giving rise to two separate 'step function response' movements instead of a single 'impulse response', in control system terms.

(e)   The auxiliary or secondary pulse has little effect on the motor pulse if it follows the main pulse rather than anticipates it, unless it is relatively close to the main pulse in time. In this case it acts as a 'brake' causing an increase of tension in the beat (eliminating 'bounce') which slows 'forward momentum' and can also become quite unpleasant (and thus is not so frequently used in music).

(4)   If both main and auxiliary pulses are prolonged rounded beat forms result.

(5)   The sensitivity of relative temporal displacement of the main and secondary pulse is greatest when (a) the two pulses are close together, and also (b) when they are nearly evenly spaced in time. In both of these regions small changes in the timing have a greater effect than in the intermediate region. Also, with a longer main pulse the auxiliary pulse has to be slightly displaced in time in order for it to be perceived as evenly spaced.

(6) Relatively loud and prolonged main pulses will tend to accentuate the outward horizontal component of pressure (that is, the direction of pressure becomes horizontal, and outward). A prolonged and very soft main pulse can tend to cause the horizontal component of pressure to become negative, that is, inward towards the body.

Although the 160 patterns tested cannot fully explore the ranges of the four variables tested - to do that a much larger number of patterns would be necessary - they show that appropriate pair combinations of amplitude modulated pulses of a single frequency can produce a systematic and wide range of motor output patterns. Among these may be found forms that resemble actual motor pulse forms observed for various types of popular music and ethnic music, as well as inner pulse forms of a number of classical composers.

The motor pulses shown in Figs. 6, 7, 8 are from the same subject. Motor pulses of different subjects for the same sound pulse show variation in the relative amount of the dynamic components of the motor pulse, but generally do not vary in the type of pulse. Such variations in the relative components is to be expected as subjects differ in arm weight (inertia/force ratio), and in the degree of relaxation. (The amount of overshoot in square wave type motor pulses, for example, is influenced by these factors, as well as, to some extent, the relative slowing or acceleration of rise or fall times.) However, the relationship between the motor pulse responses for various sound pulses appears to bear the same general features for different subjects. (For comparisons for three subjects see Fig. 14, Section V.)

A study of the degree of fluidity of different subjects in the ability to readily produce a variety of motor pulse forms is being conducted. (Fluidity improves with practice, and its cultivation may in fact have some mental therapeutic value.)

(B) TEST PROBE FOR DYNAMICALLY NONLINEAR AMPLITUDE SHAPE SENSITIVITY

In the previous section we examined motor response patterns to rectangular sound pulse forms. While these gave many varied and specific forms it is clear that actual music does not use rectangular pulse forms.

In order to arrive at transfer functions between the sound pulse (input) and the motor pulse (output), it is not sufficient to study rectangular inputs (impulse and step function inputs) but dynamic relationships should be tested with various shapes of input to investigate essential nonlinearities. One has reason to search for these: (a) small differences in time relationships may have strong and specific effects. (For a sound pulse made from two (unequal) component pulses forming a pair, the jnd of the relative timing of the two component pulses was of the order of 1msec, when thought of in relation to music - with component pulses being as much as 200 ms apart. This is less than the jnd found by Michon, 1964; Abel, 1972; Lunney, 1974, in non-musical contexts.)

(b) the sign of an amplitude increment and its relative placement in the transient shape both strongly affect the result in ways that might not be expected.

In order to examine the relative importance of different types of changes of the details of a pulse form a series of tests was devised using shape probes. These tests on pulse amplitude envelope shapes were conducted by using 'standard' rounded and triangular pulse envelope forms of 0.80 seconds duration and superimposing a small local change, a probe disturbance which could be either positive or negative, and had the form of half a cycle of a sinusoid. This 'blip' was typically 10% of the amplitude of the pulse and one tenth its duration, but could be varied in relative amplitude and duration (Fig. 9). (In effect, one studies the sensitivity to relatively sustained positive and negative second derivatives at different levels of the first derivative, and of amplitude. Corners (discontinuities of slope) of the amplitude envelope are not perceived. The second derivative must be sustained through about 15 msecs to be perceived.)

In studying the sensitivity of hearing perception to changes in the shape of a sound pulse by means of this probe, it was found broadly that:

(1) The regions of a single pulse-form most sensitive to small changes in form were the last two thirds of the rising phase of the pulse. Less sensitive was the first half of the falling part of the pulse. The beginning, end and top of the pulse (for a rounded pulse) were of lower sensitivity.

(2) A change in the shape in the direction of locally first decreasing the amplitude was generally more noticeable than a corresponding local initial increase. Thus a negative 'blip' was generally more effective than a positive 'blip' in the same position on the standard pulse. This means that if the amplitude slope is first reduced and then increased it is more effective than if it was first increased and then reduced.

We may consider these findings to suggest aspects of unidirectional rate sensitivity of the amplitude envelope (unidirectional rate sensitivity is a general dynamic function of biologic communication and control systems, Clynes, 1961, 1962, 1969b).

These findings suggest that there is a different sensitivity for changes from a dynamic condition compared with changes from a static condition of the amplitude envelope. The implication of this dynamic sensitivity at a given frequency for the analysis of speech sounds, musical sounds, and to the design of hearing compensation is notable.

(C) EXTRACTION OF BEAT FROM THE MUSIC

The best test of the relation between sound pulse and motor pulse is provided by the sound pulses corresponding to actual music.

We therefore tried to extract, as far as possible, the actual pulse form shapes contained in various pieces of music. We did this by designing the shapes with the aid of a computer program - shaping the pulse forms so that they sounded just right to the ear, as representing the actual pulse form of

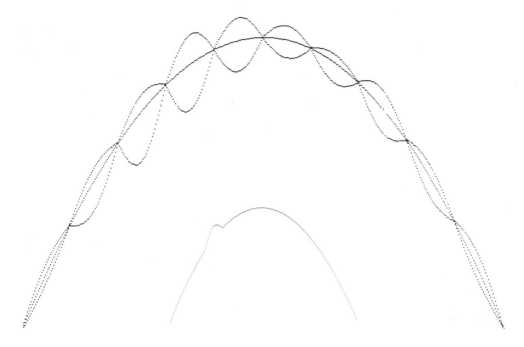

POS AND NEG BLIPS

Fig. 9   <u>Inset</u>: Test shapes for measuring the sensitivity to change of <u>shape</u> of the amplitude envelope of the sound pulse of carrier frequency of 234 Hz, consisting of a mean rounded form described by $x(1 - x)$, for x between zero and 1, of duration 0.8 seconds; plus a 'blip'. The blip was chosen to be 10% of the amplitude of the main form, and 10% of the duration (80 msec). The test consisted of comparing the sound pulse with and without the blip. The blip could be shifted to any position on the main rounded form, and could be either positive or negative.

<u>Main</u> figure shows the relative sensitivity, measured by rating scale scores, at various blip positions illustrated by the size of the blip drawn (both positive and negative). Greatest sensitivity is for negative blips in the fourth position. Blips near the beginning, near the end, and on the falling part of the main form are less audible. A second test form used a triangular form in place of the rounded blip form, also 0.8 sec in duration, on which the blip would be positioned in a similar manner. Trapezoidal test forms 2 and 3 sec long were also used. Experimental determination of jnd-s for the same positions, by varying the amplitude of the blips showed sensitivity patterns generally similar to those illustrated here.*

*Masking effects--forward, backward, and automasking--cannot explain these findings.

the music, i.e. until no conflict could be heard between the artificially produced pulse form and the actual music. As before we restricted ourselves to using a single sinusoidal carrier frequency and only two sound pulses per beat.

In simulating the sound pulse forms we found it convenient to use our Beta-function dynamic simulation program (Nettheim and Clynes, 1982). This method makes it easy to create a wide variety of suitable dynamic forms, as envelopes. The Beta-function is a function of the form

$$y = (x)^A (1-x)^B \quad \text{for } 0 \leq x \leq 1$$

(called the Beta density function in statistics – but will be called Beta-function for short in this context). The interval can be chosen to correspond to any interval, or portion of the interval on the time scale on which a pulse is to be shaped. By choosing appropriate parameters A and B (any positive values), a wide variety of shapes can be created from a single Beta-function; shapes which rise and fall in various ways and return to the baseline. It has the advantage over conventional exponential rise and fall (with or without overshoot) in that it dispenses with discontinuities between rise and fall, and with 'inactive' plateaus and can conveniently represent a convex ending. Using only 2 parameters, it can also approximate exponential rise and fall. Several Beta-function trajectories may be added, in various proportions moreover, to create the pulse form.

When the sound pulse shape was correctly formed for each music sample, it was found that the sound pulses when played simultaneously with the music on a separate audio channel reinforced the musical experience rather than detracted from it. The latter occurred if inappropriate pulse shapes were used. The rightness of a particular sound pulse depended on a highly selective choice of parameters.

(D) SOUND AND MOTOR PULSE FORMS FOR ETHNIC AND ROCK MUSIC

With the appropriate sound pulse forms thus created for the various musical samples under study, a three track test tape was made which synchronously combined the actual music samples (65 beats long) with the corresponding computer generated sound pulse forms (also 65 beats) on a second track. In order to achieve this, trigger pulses were recorded on a third track (by pressing on a button-switch in time with the music) following the beat to beat fluctuations of the tempo of the music. From these trigger pulses a timing file was created on the computer which stored all consecutive time intervals from trigger to trigger (beat to beat) with a resolution better than 0.1 msec. This allowed the computer to generate the sound pulse sequence with exactly the same tempo fluctuations as the music. The sound pulse track (track No. 2) produced by the computer was then recorded in precise synchrony with the music.

When tracks 1 and 2 were simultaneously played the music and the pulses could be heard together, seemingly reinforcing one another. (If a music sample was played with a pulse belonging to another music excerpt, a strong disagreeableness, conflict, even a ludicrous effect was generally observed even though the pulse and the music were properly synchronized.)

An interesting effect is provided by the possibility of selectively turning the volume control on either channel so that either the music or the pulses can at times be made to dominate and provide the sense of continuity.

In the experiments either the music or the pulse sequences alone were played to the subject, in turn. The subject produced motor pulses on the sentograph and in each run they were recorded and averaged as described in the previous section.

Thirteen ethnic music samples, each about 1 1/2 minutes long, were played to the subject, and nine rock and blues samples. The corresponding thirteen and nine sound pulse sequences were also played to the subject, in a random order of presentation. At the end of the experiment, the averaged motor pulse forms for the music sample and its sound pulse were graphically compared (Figs. 10, 11).

Since the music and the pulses were played at the same tempo and with the same nuances of beat to beat tempo fluctuations, and the identical trigger timing pulses were used for averaging, the results are directly comparable. The figures show a generally good comparison between the motor pulse form generated by the music itself and generated by the computer programmed sound pulse form.

Where correspondence was faulty, more careful attention to the musical qualities generally would result in an improved version of the sound pulse, giving a better correspondence. Comparison between the motor pulse of the actual music and that of the sound pulse in fact provides feedback to improve the sound pulse form. Mostly, however, the initial sound pulse form created by using one's careful hearing perception was sufficiently accurate.

The motor pulse forms for these ethnic and popular examples observed from these experiments clearly fall into one of the types found in the responses to the 160 test patterns described in the previous section. For each type, the quality of expression varies with the subtleties of the form observed. Different states of tension of the muscles producing the motor pulse, however, might sometimes result in a superficially similar form - the product of different degrees of simultaneous tension in the agonist and antagonist muscle pairs. Experiments in which EMGs will be measured in the appropriate muscles groups should further improve differentiation.

Using shaped sound pulses rather than rectangular ones gives us a better understanding of the relationship between sound pulse and motor pulse. Comparing their graphs it may be seen, analogously to the transformation from touch into sound discussed in Clynes and Nettheim (this volume), that an aspect of the transformation of sound pulse to motor pulse displays a tendency to follow the dynamic character of the sound pulse, given the initial choice of the main pulse, but unlike for the slower (essentic) forms of the expression of specific emotions, the time constants of the motor pulse response are not sufficiently fast for it to be able to follow the shape of the sound pulse form accurately. The resulting dissimilarity of form between the sound pulse and motor pulse is not felt as disturbing, however. The relative system sluggishness in tracing out aspects of the sound pulse form is experienced as an integral part of the rhythm experience. We may pose the question, if a less sluggish motor output were possible such as perhaps the tongue, could a more acute rhythmic experience ensue?

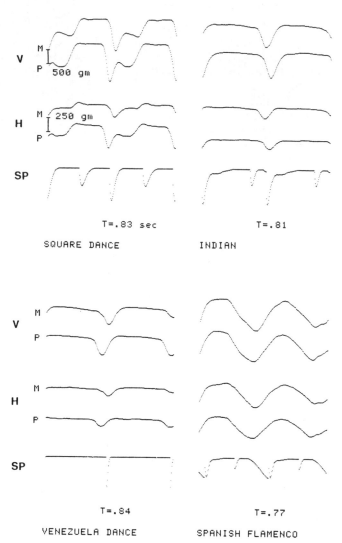

Fig. 10   (a) & (b) Motor pulses (M) to music compared with motor pulses
(P) to the sound pulses extracted from the music. Results are
shown both for the vertical (V) and horizontal (H) components of
the motor pulses. The bottom trace shows the sound pulse
amplitude envelope used (SP), generated by the computer. The
time scale for the beat is given for each example. The order of
the experiments was randomized and comparisons printed out by
the computer after all experimental runs were complete. Each
trace is the average of 25 sweeps. The sound pulses were played
with the same beat by beat timing as the music. Generally good

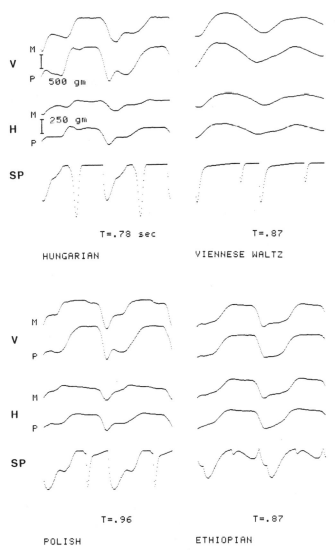

correspondence between the motor pulses to the music (M) and those to sound pulses (P) show that the sound pulses were appropriately shaped. An unexplained phase shift between (M) and (P) may be related to incorrect estimation of the p center in the formulation of the sound pulse. Note also that the motor pulse shapes found in these experiments belong to the categories described in Section V(A). These forms can be related to the attitudes and feelings they embody (see text). (Recordings of music examples used are listed at the end of References)

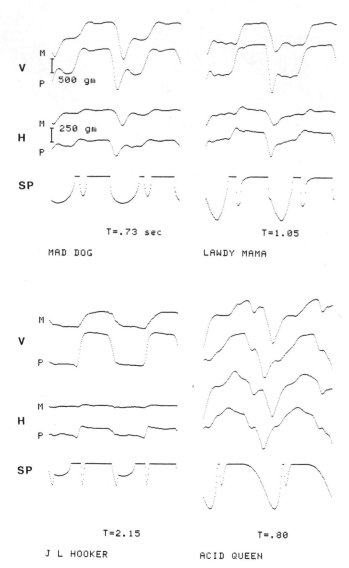

Fig. 11   As in Fig. 10 but for rock and blues (Hooker). Generally good
           correspondence is observed here also. The "Acid Queen" example
           shows a strongly marked sexual quality of the motor pulse form
           (prominent horizontal component); the blues pulse is tinged with
           sadness (cf. Clynes and Nettheim, this volume, for comparison
           with emotionally expressive forms).

(E) SOME QUALITIES OF EXPERIENCE AND MENTAL ENERGIES RELATING TO THE TYPES OF MOTOR PULSE

A few examples of how different sound pulse and motor pulse forms represent different attitudes will be given. These descriptions are, of course, not exhaustive; there are many shades of expressiveness to be found that remain to be described, if indeed they can be described.

The simple pulse form with slight modification can be akin to the expressive shape for joy (see Clynes and Nettheim, this volume). Thus it lends itself to joyous expression as in the Indian music (Fig. 10), or in a different way in the Viennese Waltz. The joyous energy can be ecstatic as in the Indian example. Or, it can contain excitement and some tension making it more exuberant and aggressive, with slight sexual overtones, as in the Venuzuelan example of South American music, or, the joyous element can become subordinated to an agressive impulse, as in the American square dance, or, it can contain elements of vigorous self-assertion, as in the Scottish bagpipes. All of these examples have in common that they partake in joyous energy, in varying degrees either mixed or unmixed with other qualities. (The 'lightness' of joy is related to the paradoxical effortless upward return of a downward impulse movement - this displays a quasi-elastic 'bounce'; (Clynes, 1981.)

A completely different kind of energy production is found in the square pulse form and its varieties. In this form the movement is divided into a separate down and up phase, the down phase frequently with overshoot. In this category, we may distinguish (a) a type of beat as in Rock producing aggressive outgoing energy with a sequence of relaxed movements. Each up and down phase terminates in a relaxed condition but displays considerable energy. (b) A similar subdivided type pulse may be seen in the Hungarian pulse but here each subdivision does not end in relaxation but remains tense, supplying the beat an added quality of energy, or 'temperament'. The aggressive energy is coupled with enthusiasm (or 'fighting stance') which keeps the tension, as opposed to the rock beat whose energy is without enthusiasm. A similar subdivision may be found in the Polish Mazurka beat but it is part of a triple not duple subdivision (which is rare for this type of beat). The quality of the energy here is less vehement, acquiring a greater measure of elegance and grace while maintaining a degree of enthusiastic involvement. (c) When this type of beat has a large horizontal component it displays overt sexual qualities (cf. the expression of sexual qualities of touch, with its large horizontal component, Clynes and Nettheim, this volume). This may be strongly seen in the Acid Queen example (Fig. 11). The Flamenco example (Fig. 10) also illustrates a sexual aspect of aggressive energy.

A more detailed analysis of these factors in various types of ethnic music made possible by these methods is in preparation.

(F) COMPOSER'S INNER PULSE

The third class of time forms studied comprises the phenomena of the inner pulse of composers (Clynes, 1969a, 1977). This distinctive iterative phenomenon appears mainly in eighteenth and nineteenth century Western music. With composers of that period the inner pulse is a personal dynamic signature. Some general remarks concerning the nature of the inner pulse may be appropriate here. First described qualitatively by Becking (1928) as an outgrowth of the work of Sievers (1885-1915), its existence can be demonstrated strikingly if one selects a particular musical passage from a piece of one composer and considers it to have been composed by another. It is best to choose a bar or two which might possibly have been composed by either composer. If one now conducts the piece one will invariably stumble in the beat when it comes to the bar concerned, even though it is the same note for note, because the form of the beat is necessarily quite different. (We can see why this stumbling occurs now in terms of time-form printing.)

There appears to exist a pulse form characteristic of a particular composer and this pulse form is a kind of dynamic signature of his works. We could even suggest that the good composers of that period succeeded in stamping their works with this dynamic key to their own distinct personal point of view - a means for intimate portrayal of a unique person: as previously different ethnic pulses identified ethnic groups so now composers discovered their own individual indentity in the form of a dynamic pulse. Unlike the ethnic pulse which is generally related to the rhythm of language (though both may possibly share a deeper common origin) the composer's own inner pulse does not necessarily seem primarily to correspond to a purely motor pattern. Nor does it in any way relate to the loudness or softness or to the special accents of a unique piece. The inner pulse continues undiminished in a complete rest within a piece and does not wax or wane with increasing and decreasing loudness; it is as clear in a pianissimo passage as in fortissimo and is perhaps most clearly perceived in the silence of a rest, at the end of a piece, or before it begins. One finds the inner pulse continuing at the end of the piece like a damped oscillation for a small number of beats. The more highly damped pulses such as Mozart continue for a considerably shorter duration than a pulse with greater inertia such as Beethoven's. (A perceptive audience starts to clap when the inner pulse has died down and thus there will often be a few beats silence after the last note of a Beethoven composition, and a shorter pause after a composition of Mozart.) Before a piece is begun a good conductor will often make the pulse shape known from his movement before the first tone is begun.

Previously measurements of the inner pulse were described by Clynes (1969a, 1970 and 1977a). In this present study we try to show that it could be possible to portray the inner pulse as a sound pulse, to extract a sound from the music in a manner similar to the way in which we extracted the ethnic sound pulse from ethnic music as shown in the previous section, while fully recognizing that the inner pulse is not a sound. We did this because it seemed clear that the inner pulse is represented in the score implicitly in

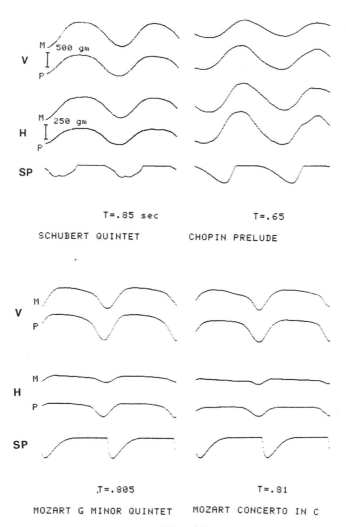

Fig. 12

Figs. 12 & 13

Motor pulse to music (M) and to the sound pulse (P) for vertical (V) and horizontal (H) components of pressure for various examples of classical composers. The same sound pulse (SP) is used for all the examples of a particular composer. Note the similarity of the motor pulse to music to that produced by the sound pulse, and also that various pieces by the same composer

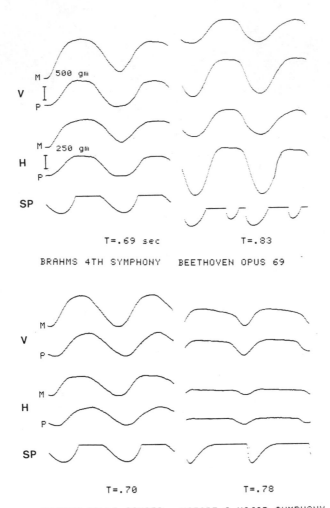

Fig. 13

have similar shaped motor pulses, corresponding to the inner pulse of that composer. Although the inner pulse was represented here by a sound pulse the nature of the inner pulse is non-sound since it propagates during rest equally well. The illustration also shows that the inner pulse can be represented as a single pulse as well as a pulse pair.

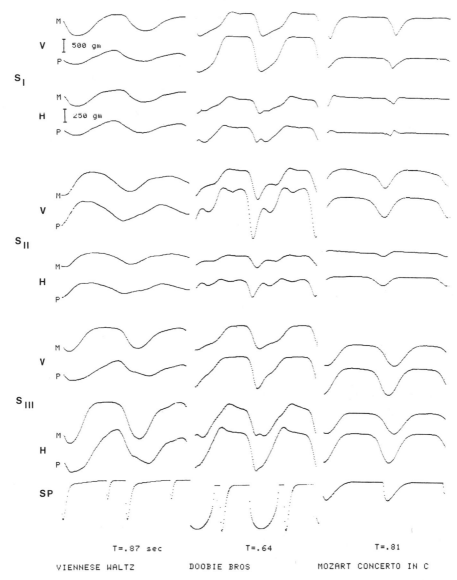

Fig. 14   Comparison of the motor pulses of three different subjects to the same music and sound pulses. All subjects show a good match between their own motor pulses to the music and to the sound pulse but vary more from one another. Variations among subjects however result from the effect of different parameters within the same type of motor pulse rather than from a choice of different types. Thus the response to the Doobie Brothers shows various degrees of overshoot; no overshoot is present in any of the responses to the Mozart Concerto. Differences in the relative amplitudes of the vertical and horizontal components are also found across subjects.

some way and that the first step in being able to extract the inner pulse directly from the score would be to demonstrate what the inner pulse (previously measured as a motor pulse) would appear like as a sound pulse.

In this process we were greatly aided by the concept of time-form printing which made it clear that once a particular pulse form was established it would then carry through across relatively un- differentiated parts of music such as, for example, a scale passage - passages which might well have been written by one or another composer. We appear to get our intuition of the inner pulse from certain key sections of the music, where it is most clearly spelled out. It then carries through, by time-form printing across the entire piece and puts its stamp on all the otherwise undifferentiated parts. In this way the simplest scale passage or repeated note motif acquires an authentic character. We recognize the presence or absence of Beethoven in the way such a part is played. We feel disappointed and as it were vacant if the pulse form should temporarily disappear. Thus one of the requirements of an authentic performance is continued presence of the inner pulse form.

We selected a number of musical examples by each composer. As for the ethnic pulses, we constructed sound pulse forms which appeared to clearly fit the composer. These pulse forms were then tested sentographically to see whether they produced the same pressure pulse form as the various music examples. A number of results are shown in Figs. 12, 13. As before, these pulses were created from a a single sinusoidal carrier frequency by amplitude modulation.

Although the present studies were not designed to probe individual differences in transduction of sound pulse to motor pulse, a comparison of responses of three subjects is shown for the same music and pulses in Fig. 14. These illustrate that within an overall transfer function, individual differences can be described as differences in particular functional parameters rather than in the structure of the process.

SOUND EXAMPLES

Sound examples of shaped sound pulses of specific music, recorded synchronously with the music, are given in the record included with this book, and are listed in the Appendix.

CONCLUSION

We have looked at some properties of rhythm: repetitive function in thought, sound and movement. Relationships between them were investigated. Repetition occurs without continuing attention once the form of the beat is begun, so that attention may be focused on other aspects of the music yet it forms a partially aware and partly subconscious basis to the music. Sensitivity to changes in the form of the pulse invokes a special kind of aural sensitivity, different from the known static sensitivities. Each sound pulse form has its own qualitative character, and in its repetition becomes an attitude, which may have feeling or emotional significance. This character in turn can be expressed only by the appropriate dynamic form. Thus individual note beginnings and durations need to relate to the specific dynamic form rather than to simple numeric ratios to be appropriately and characteristically expressive. The proper musical timing can be related to the initiation and termination of motor phases implied by the form. Detailed shaping of the sound pulses is governed by the specific attitude that is implied. The experiments we have described are designed to provide data for obtaining a mathematical description of the dynamic brain processes that transform sound rhythm to motor rhythm.

SUMMARY

Musical rhythm is studied in relation to Central Nervous System function: (1) in terms of temporal stability (2) in terms of the transduction by the nervous system of sound pulse to motor pulse. Stability is a function of the brain process of time-form printing, which iteratively produces a spatiotemporal form decided on initially, without further selective command. Long term stability of the order of 1-2 parts in a thousand is shown to be possible with musical thought in this brain-clock function. Mentally imaged rhythm of the same music surprisingly is generally slightly slower than when performed. The transduction of sound pulse to motor pulse is dynamically analyzed in relation to the 'beat' (a) with 160 rectangular sound pulse pair patterns of varying duration and amplitude showing the prevalence of several types of motor pulse; (b) with 22 rock popular and ethnic music selections; (c) with examples from Mozart, Beethoven, Schubert, Brahms and Chopin. Characteristic sound pulse forms are extracted from the music, and generated by computer. Pulse forms are considered to be correct when they result in the same motor pulse forms as the music. Aural sensitivity to changes in the pulse shape is shown to be markedly affected by the region of the pulse where the change occurs, a finding that appears to have relevance to understanding the aural analysis of sound in general. The results are useful towards finding a general transfer function for transforming sound pulses into motor pulse by the CNS (to enable one to predict the motor pulse resulting from any arbitrary sound pulse). Various feeling qualities, or attitudes pertaining to the sound pulses are related to their specific forms.

ACKNOWLEDGMENT

The help of Nigel Nettheim and Brian McMahon in preparation of this paper and its critical discussion is gratefully acknowledged. Special appreciation goes to Dorothy Capelletto for assistance with the manuscript. This work was aided in part by a grant from the Commonwealth Education Research and Development Committee of Australia.

REFERENCES

Abel, S.M., 1972, Discrimination of temporal gaps, J.Acoust.Soc.Am., 52: 519-524.

Becking, G., 1928, "Der Musikalische Rhythmus als Erkenntnisquelle," B. Filser, Augsburg.

Bentley, D., and Konishi, M., 1978, Neural control of behavior, Annu.Rev. Neurosci., 1:35-59.

Bernstein, L., 1976, "The Unanswered Question: Six Talks at Harvard," Harvard University Press, Cambridge MA.

Boring, E.G., 1942, "Sensation and Perception in the History of Experimental Psychology," Appleton, New York.

Christiani, A.F., 1885, "The Principles of Expression in Pianoforte Playing," Harper & Brothers, New York and London.

Clynes, M., 1961, Unidirectional rate sensitivity: a biocybernetic law of reflex and humoral systems as physiologic channels of controls and communications, Annals N.Y.Acad.Sci., 92(3): 946-969.

Clynes, M., 1962, The nonlinear biological dynamics of unidirectional rate sensitivity illustrated by analog computer analysis, pupillary reflex to light and sound, and heart rate behavior, Annals N.Y.Acad.Sci., 98(4): 806-845.

Clynes, M., 1969a, Toward a theory of Man: Precision of essentic form in living communication, in: "Information Processing in the Nervous System," K.N. Leibovic, and J.C. Eccles, eds., Springer, New York.

Clynes, M., 1969b, Cybernetic implications of rein control in perceptual and conceptual organization, in: "Rein Control, Or Unidirectional Rate Sensitivity, A Fundamental Dynamic and Organizing Function in Biology," M. Clynes, ed., Annals N.Y.Acad.Sci., 156(2):629-671.

Clynes, M., 1970, Toward a view of Man, in: "Biomedical Engineering Systems," M. Clynes, and J.H. Milsum, eds., McGraw-Hill Book Co., New York.

Clynes, M., 1973, Sentics: Biocybernetics of emotion communication, Annals N.Y.Acad.Sci., 220(3): 55-131.

Clynes, M., 1974, The biological basis for sharing emotion, Psychol.Today, 51-55.

Clynes, M., 1975, Communications and generation of emotion through essentic form, in: "Emotions - Their Parameters and Measurement," L. Levi, ed., Raven Press, New York.

Clynes, M., 1977a, "Sentics: The Touch of Emotions," Doubleday/Anchor Press, New York.

Clynes, M., 1977b, Space-time form printing by the human central nervous system, Society for Neuroscience, Los Angeles, abs.

Clynes, M., 1980, The communication of emotion: Theory of sentics, in: "Theories of Emotion," R. Plutchik, and H. Kellerman, eds., Academic Press, New York.

Clynes, M., and Walker, J., 1980b, Sound pattern and movement: introduction to a neurophysiologically based theory of musical rhythm, 10th International Acoustics Congress, Sydney abs.

Clynes, M., 1981, Paradoxical effortlessness in rebound lifting: Programmed absence of sensation of effort by the nervous system, Nature.

Cooper, G.W., and Meyer, L.B., 1960, "The Rhythmic Structure of Music," University of Chicago Press, Chicago and London.

Dainow, E., 1977, Physical effects and motor responses to music, J.Res.Mus.Ed., 25: 211-221.

Delcomyn, F., 1980, Neural basis of rhythmic behavior in animals, Science, 210(4469): 492-498.

Fraisse, P., Oléron, G., and Paillard, J., 1953, Les effets dynamogéniques de la musique - Etude expérimentale, L'Année Psychologique, 53: 1-34.

Fraisse, P., 1956, "Les Structures rythmiques," Publications Universitaires de Louvain, Louvain.

Fraisse, P., Oléron, G., and Paillard, J., 1958, Sur les repères sensoriels qui permettent de controller les mouvements d'accompagnement de stimuli périodiques, L'Année Psychol., 58: 321-338.

Fraisse, P., 1966, L'anticipation de stimulus rhythmiques - vitesse d'établissement et précision de la sychronisation, L'Année Psychol., 66: 15-36.

Fraisse, P., 1978, Time and Rhythm perception, in: "Handbook of Perception," Vol.8, E.C. Carterette, and M.P. Friedman, eds., Academic Press, New York.

Gabrielsson, A., 1973, Similarity ratings and dimension analyses of auditory rhythm patterns, Scand.J.Psychol., 14: 138-176.

Gabrielsson, A., 1979, Experimental research on rhythm, Human.Assoc.Rev., 30,1/2: 69-92.

Greeno, D.J., and Simon, H.A., 1974, Processes for sequence production, Psychol.Rev., 81: 187-197.

Grillner, S., and Wallen, P., 1977, Is there a peripheral control of the central pattern generators for swimming in dogfish? Brain Res., 127: 291-295.

Handel, S., and Yoder, D., 1975, The effects of intensity and interval rhythms on the perception of auditory and visual temporal patterns, Quart.J.Exp.Psychol., 27: 111-122.

Jackendoff, R., and Lerdahl, F., 1980, "A Generative Theory of Tonal Music," MIT Press, Cambridge, MA (in press).

Jakobsen, R., 1956, Two aspects of language and two types of aphasic disturbances, in: "Fundamentals of Language," R. Jakobsen, and M. Halle, eds., Mouton, The Hague.

Jones, M.R., 1978, Auditory patterns: Studies in the perception of structure, in: "Handbook of Perception," Vol. 8, E.C. Carterette, and M.P. Friedman, eds., Academic Press, New York.

Kristan, W.B., Jr, 1980, Generation of rhythmic motor patterns, in: "Informal Processing in the Nervous System," H.M. Pinker, and W.D. Willis, Jr, eds., Raven Press, New York.

Lunney, H.W.M., 1974, Time as heard in speech and music, Nature, 249:592

Marcus, S.M. 1976, "Perceptual Centres," unpubl. Fellowship Diss., Kings College, Cambridge, Eng.

Michon, J.A., 1964, Studies on subjective duration 1. Differential sensitivity on the perception of repeated temporal intervals, Acta Psychol., 22: 44-450.

Morton, J., Marcus, S., and Frankish, C., 1976, Perceptual centers, Psychol.Rev., 83(5): 405-408.

Nettheim, N., and Clynes, M., 1981, The Beta Function, a versatile tool for modeling convex pulse forms, Computers in Biol. and Med.

Restle, F., and Brown, E., 1970, Organization of serial pattern learning, in: "The Psychology of Learning and Motivation: Advances, Research and Theory," Vol. 4, G.H. Bower, ed., Academic Press, New York.

Sessions, R., 1970, "Questions About Music," Harvard University Press, Cambridge, MA.

Sievers, E., 1875-1915, "Collected Works," Stuttgart.

Simon, H.A., 1972, Complexity and the representation of patterned sequences of symbols, Psychol.Rev., 79: 369-382.

Stetson, R.B., 1905, A motor theory of rhythm and discrete succession, Psychol.Rev., XII: 250-270, 293-350.

Vos., J, and Rasch, R.A., 1981, The perceptual onset of musical tones, Perc. and Psychophys. (in press).

Woodrow, H., 1909, A quantitative study of rhythm, Arch.Psychol., XIV: 1-66.

Zajonc, R.B., 1968, Attitudinal effects of mere exposure, J.Personal.Soc. Psychol., 9(2):2.

Music illustrated in Figs. 10, 11, 12, 13 and 14 is taken from the following recordings

Zambra Moia	NPL 18 000
Bialy Mazur	PRONIL - SXL 1205
The Blue Danube	MGM 3110 018
Ragupati Ragava	FOLKWAYS/NY FW 6911
Venezuela: Dance	FOLKWAYS/NY FE 4507
Buffalo Gals	FOLKWAYS/NY FA 2001
A menyasszany szépvirag	HUNGAROTON SLPX 18033
Introduction of a Man to a Woman (Ethiopian)	FOLKWAYS FE 4353
Acid Queen	POLYDOR 2625 028
Stampede (Doobie Brothers)	WARNER BROS INC.
I Fall to Pieces (Mad Dog)	DECCA/EMI
Blues Way (John Lee Hooker)	ABC BLS 6023
Mozart C Major Symphony no.36 "LINZ" K.425, 1st Movt. - Casals	COLUMBIA ML 5449
Mozart Piano Concerto No.21 in C Minor K.467, 1st Movt. - Schnabel	ANGEL COLH 67
Beethoven Sonata No.3 in A Major for 'Cello & Piano Op.69, 1st Movt. - Casals; Serkin	RCA VICTOR LCT 6700
Schubert Quintet in C Major Op.163, 1st Movt.	COLUMBIA M5 30069
Brahms F Minor "Cello Sonata Op.99 No 2, 3rd Movt. - Casals; Horszowski	COLUMBIA M5 30069
Brahms 4th Symphony, 1st Movt. - Bruno Walter	CBS S 75 091
Chopin Prelude Op.28 No.8 - Ivan Moravec	SUPRAPHON 111 2139

Chapter XI

THE JUDGMENT OF MUSICAL INTERVALS

Horst-Peter Hesse

Musicological Institute of the University of Hamburg
Federal Republic of Germany

INTRODUCTION

According to the general doctrine of music theory prevalent today there is a basic rule which reads as follows: "The musical note has four elementary properties; pitch, volume, timbre and duration." Traditional music theory holds that these properties are valid as independent dimensions of sound perception; they are held to be quantities each one of which can be altered at will while keeping the others constant.

There exists. however, a profusion of observations incompatible with the concept of independence of pitch and timbre - observations known to practically every musician - but which are generally dismissed as being musically insignificant acoustic illusions. I am referring to the deceptiveness of octaves.

It is well known that a low, whistled note - for example D5 according to the American standard - can be perceived as being equivalent in pitch to the piano's D4 or to the D3 of a male voice. It is equally possible to confuse D3 as sung by a man with D4 as sung by a woman (Ritsma, 1966; Hesse, 1972).

Similar phenomena can be observed in instrumental music. In the instrumentation of a melody, where consecutive sections are to be executed by various instruments one must take into account the deeper sound of the darker timbres - say that of the flute against that of the oboe. If in the performance of a melody various instruments alternate, so that single motifs are taken over by different instruments, then one must transpose certain passages an octave in order to avoid the effect of breaks in the melodic line. This rule has grown up over the years in musical practice, and is mentioned as early as 1863 by Gevaert in his textbook on instrumentation (Gevaert, 1863).

217

I.   EXPERIMENTS ON INTERVALS CONSISTING OF TWO NOTES WITH
DIFFERENT TIMBRES

After the above observations were confirmed by means of various pilot
tests, the correlations were tested in an experiment (Hesse, 1978) that could
be evaluated statistically.   With the aid of a synthesizer, tones of five
typical timbres were produced.   For each of the five different types of tone
every degree of the chromatic scale from C4 to D-flat 5 in the equally
tempered system could be produced.

The sound spectra of the individual types of sound can be described as
follows (Fig. 1):

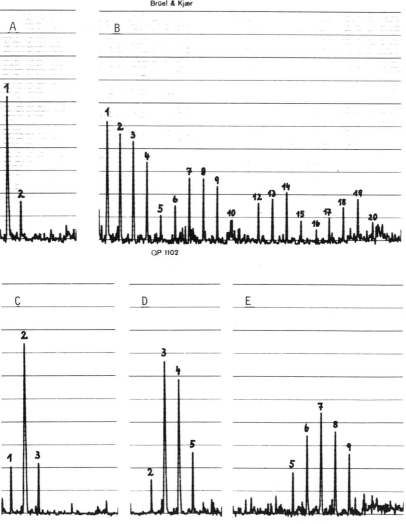

Fig. 1.   Sound spectra of A4 of the five types of sound labelled A to E.

The spectrum of the first type is characterized by a marked line of the fundamental frequency, which is complemented only by the considerably weaker second harmonic;

Spectrum B comprises in addition to the fundamental frequency a large number of harmonic vibrations of gradually diminishing intensity;

Sound types D and E are residual sounds - they lack the fundamental frequency (Schouten, 1940).

The next step was to form intervals, each consisting of two notes in different timbres. The two notes, each of which lasted a second, were always played one after another. All the intervals from the unison to the octave - both upwards and downwards - occurred equally often. These sounds were presented to 27 music students. A detailed description of this experiment and the statistical procedures are given in Hesse, 1978.

The result of the test can be summarized as follows: the experiment showed that the sound spectrum has a statistically highly significant influence on the estimation of the musical octave position. The octave position to which the listener estimates a note belongs, is not determined merely by the fundamental frequency - a leading role is also played by the brightness of the sound, the latter being dependent upon the structure of the spectrum. In spite of the same fundamental frequency a note can be estimated as being higher than another if its brightness substantially exceeds that of the other. A melody in which certain individual notes - indicated by an asterisk - were played with a considerably brighter timbre, was evaluated by the subjects as follows (Ex. 1):

Example 1:

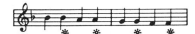 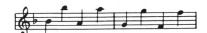

It can be seen that jumps of an octave were heard.

If the brightness of one note of an interval be altered to a certain degree, then the musical impression switches over to that of the complementary interval; for example, a downward leap of a fourth becomes an upward leap of a fifth, or, conversely, an upward leap of a seventh becomes a downward leap of a second, which results in a completely different meaning as far as musical expression is concerned.

In the following example, the melody is made up of notes with two different kinds of timbre. Those indicated by an asterisk are brighter. The octave-jumping effect transforms this melody into the following (Ex. 2):

This effect can completely alter the musical character of a melody; it occurs when subsequent sections or even subsequent notes of a melody are transmitted by means of greatly differing timbres - for instance, when the former are distributed amongst various instruments. It is also of consequence for harmonic structures. For tonally homogeneous ensembles there are no problems as far as the judging of pitch is concerned, and thus also the

Example 2:

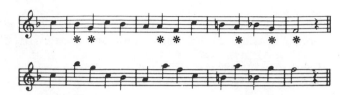

partwriting - the introduction of dissonance, and its resolution - is unproblematic. However, since the Romantic Era in music the large orchestra has acquired a considerably enhanced wealth of color, and this gives neighboring musical pitches a more extensive and potentially ambiguous relationship to one another. Because of this a freer treatment of dissonance is also allowed for, and the possibility of novel harmonic complexes and of chords arranged in multitone layers is promoted due to the fact that the sounds of the individual notes stand out against each other by virtue of their differing brightnesses - almost as if stretched out into "open position". Consequently, chords such as these can be perceived as articulated sound structures, whereas a sound uniform in character - in "closed position" as it were - would make the chords fuse into undifferentiated tone clusters.

To what extent this relationship between pitch and timbre follows natural law cannot as yet be formulated unequivocally, because hitherto no one has done detailed research into the following question: what quantifiable relations exist between physically determinable structural factors of sound and the perceptive dimension "brightness"?

Lichte in experiments on the attributes of complex tones concludes that "complex tones have, in addition to pitch and loudness, at least three attributes. These are brightness, roughness, and one tentatively labelled fullness" (Lichte, 1941, p.479). "Brightness is a function of the location on the frequency continuum of the midpoint of the energy distribution" (p.472).

Our experiments showed that pitch and brightness are not independent, but brightness is one component or dimension of pitch. At this time it has been established that there are three ways of altering the sound so as to increase the brightness:

1. A "brightness series" arises when the complete spectrum is shifted into higher frequency belts, while keeping the interrelations of its components constant. The limiting case with the simplest sound spectrum structure is sinusoidal sound. This is the classical requirement for a rise in pitch - the brightness changes in proportion to the position of the sound's fundamental frequency.

2. A second "brightness series" arises when one enriches a sound vibration with additional partial frequencies of higher and higher orders, while keeping the fundamental frequency constant. In the present experiment this method - which in classical terminology is described as an alteration of timbre - was applied by contrasting sound types A and B.

3. Furthermore, an increase in brightness occurs when one shifts a for-
    mant belt from the lowest partial frequencies in the sound spectrum to
    the highest, i.e. when one intensifies the relative intensity of the higher
    frequency components. In the present experiment this requirement was
    also realized.

Thus we see that pitch as dependent on brightness is a function of the
fundamental frequency as well as of the energy distribution within the
frequency continuum. Terhardt (1974) and Roederer have pointed out that
"even an elementary percept such as the subjective pitch of a single musical
tone is the result of a complex context-dependent pattern recognition process involving higher operations in the cognitive system" (Roederer, 1979).

II. EXPERIMENTS WITH "MELODIES" COMPOSED OF GRADED CHROMALESS NOISES

In a further experiment it was shown that brightness can also occur in
music as an independent dimension - that it has a musical meaning not only
in association with the second pitch component, namely chroma. Chroma is
the tonal property held in common by all notes an octave apart, and it
manifests itself in that these notes are named with the same letter
(Bachem, 1950; Hesse, 1972).

For this experiment, noises graded according to their brightness were
used - noises which had no chroma, i.e. could not be allotted to any degree
of the musical scale. In each case continuous noise spectra with a formant
region around 2000 Hz were used, and keeping the lower frequency region
steady the brightness was increased by broadening the spectrum in the
direction of the higher frequencies. Thus the brightest sounds had the
widest spectrum (Fig. 2). These sound processes were provided with an
amplitude modulation profile, so that they were perceived as varyingly
bright pulses - somewhat like the clapping of hands. According to the
judgment of a group of test subjects - 60 musically-trained students of
musicology - the degrees of brightness of the sounds were so closely
adjusted to one another that 75% of the subjects were able to specify the
direction of a change immediately.

When it is possible to create the same sort of brightness change in a
succession of sounds through several degrees, one mentally forms an index
of direction to assess that change of sound: there also arises in addition to
the sense of direction the impression of larger or smaller gaps - of varied
spacing. When a diastematic structure such as this is combined with the
rhythmic articulation, there arises a "melody" - a brightness melody.

Such melodies were created and tape recorded in the manner set out.
These melodies are played for test subjects repeatedly, in order to accustom
them to the strangeness of the sounds. The listeners were instructed to
write down the melodies they heard in continuous linear form. The result
showed that the melodies were specified by all the listeners as having
unambiguously recognizable dynamics and progression, despite the absence
of discrete spectral lines with which to guide the perception of an interval.

The next thing was to examine whether these melodies are really
qualitatively articulated entities as defined by the gestalt theory, that is,

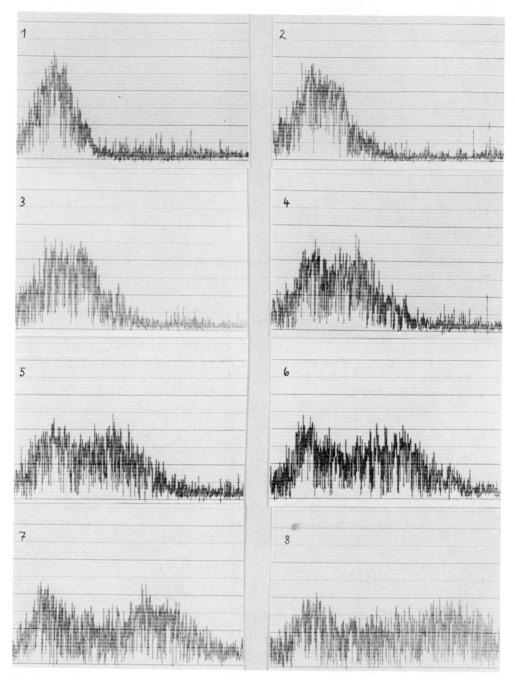

Fig. 2.   The sound spectra of one of the brightness scales used in the experiments showing the energy distribution on the frequency continuum from zero to 10,000 cps.

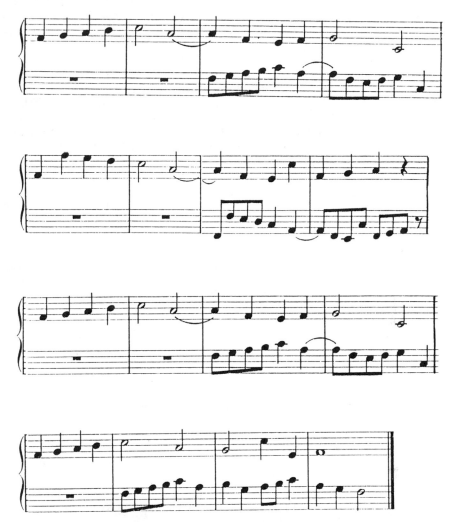

Example 3:   Canon by diminution composed of graded noises.

entities which fulfil the requirement of being transposable. In several
two-part studies which made use of various imitative polyphonic techniques
- for example canon by diminution (Ex. 3) - the unequivocal compre-
hensibility of polyphonic structures made up of chromaless brightness
melodies could be shown.

The musical example shows a canon by diminution used in the experiments. The melodies consist exclusively of graded noises, and are transcribed in note form on a musical staff without a clef at the beginning of the
staff; the notes indicate only the relative position of the graded noises on a
brightness scale.

This experiment shows that using apparently insignificant non-tonal sounds, one can not only form static expanses of sound, or juxtapose these sounds as alternatives and give them rhythmic structure, but also - as with the traditional stock of musical sounds - form sequences of unquestionable direction and energy.

Contemporary music tends towards replacing the classical parameters - like pitch and interlinked harmonies - with ones hitherto usually considered as accessories. Through the interchange of fixed and free parameters, the domain of the "consonantal" color valences (which are usually dismissed as being noises) unfolds itself. I consider it feasible that further experiments with sound will make accessible to the organizing powers of science those hitherto scarcely surveyable multiplicity of timbres, and furnish the basis for a future non-tonal theory of music, complementary to the traditional one - a theory embracing far more acoustic dimensions than is possible today.

SUMMARY

The octave position to which the listener assigns a note is not determined merely by the fundamental frequency - a leading role is also played by the brightness of the sound, the latter being dependent upon the structure of the spectrum. If the brightness of one note of an interval is altered to a certain degree, then the musical perception switches over to the complementary interval. With noises lacking in the property of chroma, brightness also occurs as a separate dimension. This is demonstrated in polyphonic structures made up of chromaless brightness melodies. Such structures exhibit sequences of direction and energy - as does tonal music - and can contribute to a basis of a future non-tonal theory of music complementary to the traditional one.*

REFERENCES

Bachem, A., 1950, Tone height and tone chroma as two different pitch qualities, Acta Psychol., 7:80-88.

Gevaert, F.A., 1863, "Traité général d'instrumentation, exposé méthodique des principes de cet art dans leur application à l'orchestre à la musique d'harmonie et de fanfares, etc.", Gand.

Hesse, H.P., 1972, "Die Wahrnehmung von Tonhöhe und Klangfarbe als Problem der Hörtheorie", Arno Volk, Cologne.

Hesse, H.P., 1978, Experimente zum musikalischen Intervallurteil, Jahrbuch des Staatlichen Instituts für Musikforschung, Berlin, 72-87.

Lichte, W.H., 1941, Attributes of complex tones, J. Exp. Psychol., 28:455-480.

---

*   Sounds illustrating this chapter are presented in the recording included with this book (see Appendix for details).

Ritsma, R.J., 1966, The 'octave deafness' of the human ear., IPO Annual.
    Prog. Rep., 1:15.
Roederer, J.G., 1979, The perception of music by the human brain, Human.
    Assoc. Rev., 30:11-28.
Schouten, J.F., 1940, The residue, a new component in subjective sound
    analysis, Proc. Konl. Nederl. Acad. Wetenschap., 43:356-365.
Terhardt, E., 1974, Pitch, consonance and harmony, J. Acoust. Soc. Am.,
    55:1061-1069.

Chapter XII

AFFECTIVE VERSUS ANALYTIC PERCEPTION OF MUSICAL INTERVALS

Scott Makeig

University of California at San Diego
La Jolla, California, USA

INTRODUCTION

When I see an apple, what do I experience? Of course I see it at a certain place in space, and of a certain size - both with respect to my body, and with respect to other things in its environment. But at the same time, I see and experience some of its qualities - its shape, its color, etc. And from these, I may get an imagination of its taste.

This, however, depends on my interest, If I am hungry at the time, I may feel, "Ah, a tasty apple!" But if I am not at all hungry, I might feel, "Oh, just a little apple . . . " In short, the quality of my experience depends on how seeing the apple relates to me personally, or, how I imagine that it relates to me. For instance, even if I were to see a plastic apple, I might still experience seeing what I imagine to be a delicious real apple.

Now, while I might have some particular handicap or personal impression of apples which could alter or distort my experience - for instance, if I were nearly blind, or had once been poisoned with an apple - normally, in our culture at least, ripe apples are more or less relished as tasty, healthful food, and this is quite compatible with the biological fact that for most people, apples are both healthful and tasty. And this fact we understand as being due to our common genetic and physiological heritage.

Now, musical intervals are like apples, in that what we experience when we listen to a musical interval - like what we experience when we see an apple - depends on what kind of interest, motivation, and imagination we bring to the perception.

Meher Baba, the contemporary spiritual author, has described the human mind as having two aspects - the 'inquiring and reflecting' aspect, which pertains to thoughts, and the 'impressive and sympathetic' aspect, which pertains to feelings (Meher Baba, 1955). These are commonly referred to as 'mind and heart' but are, I believe, indissoluble aspects of the

227

human mind and of human experience - though they may be found in differing balance and harmony in different individuals.

Now, when we hear a musical interval, we certainly can hear its relative pitch-height and size, and we can also hear its physical qualities - its timbre, loudness, consonance, etc. But our whole experience of the interval depends on how we imagine that the interval relates to us personally.

If we are thirsty to hear music, in order to satisfy some emotional need or desire, we may feel, "Ah, what a beautiful chord!" On the other hand, if we were to listen to the same interval as simply a physical sound, with a motive only to analyze or judge its physical properties, we would no doubt have a very different experience, and might think, "Yes, an interval of about four semitones, of complex timbre, . . ." and so on.

The interest of psychophysicists has usually been in this last way of experiencing sounds, as physical sensations. And they have discovered that, excepting various individual variations, limitations, and degrees of sensitivity, most sounds are heard rather the same by most people - and this is understood again to be a reflection of common genetic and neurological heritage.

However, for me and I believe for most of the world, the usual and deepest motive for experiencing music is mainly for the sake of emotional experience. It is important therefore for music psychology and science to consider closely the emotional or affective experience of musical intervals.

If our judgments of the size and pitch of musical intervals are more or less due to our similar neurophysical make-ups, why should not our affective experiences of some intervals be also more or less the same?

RATIOS AND AFFECTS

It is my belief that there exists a particular set of integer-ratio musical intervals which do tend to qualitatively affect our affective imaginations in consistent ways; that is, when we listen to harmonic musical intervals while imagining that they are expressing some feeling, we then tend to agree about what feeling each interval expresses.

On what do I base that conviction?

1. On my own experience as musician and composer;
2. Reading many of the references to qualities of intervals from the Western literature through the centuries;
3. Having experimented for some time with finely tuned intervals;
4. Asking others for their affective impressions of the same intervals;
5. On the results of a pilot experiment which supports the idea that certain musical intervals, even outside of any explicit musical context, tend to effect consistent qualitative changes in the imagination of listeners, when those listeners listen to those sounds as expressions of human personality or feeling.

Some Historical Evidence

1.   A second millenium B.C. Babylonian tablet has recently been deci-
phered which instructs musicians in tuning a diatonic scale by ear, tuning by
consonances (4/3 fourths).   After tuning seven consecutive fourths, the
tablet notes, the seventh and first strings will make a dissonant interval (the
tritone) (Kilmer, Crocker and Brown, 1976).   This establishes that the
so-called 'Pythagorean' scale of Boethius and medieval tuning theory was in
use at least a millenium before Pythagoras, and that experience of physical consonance has been taken as a basic music principle for at least 3,000
years.   In fact, the scale of the Babylonian tablet is the first historical
example of what I call a tone-group (see below).

2.   The first Western medieval reference to the (5/4) just major third
called it more sweet or 'suave' than the then-traditional (81/64) Pythagorean
third (Gut, 1976).   Helmholtz (1862), who devoted the final but often overlooked chapter of his monumental book on the experience of music to the
differences in feeling of just, Pythagorean, and equal-tempered tuning systems, wrote:

> The later interpreters of Greek musical theory have mostly
> advanced the opinion that the differences in tunings which
> the Greeks called 'colorings' (chroai) were merely speculative
> and never came into practical use . . . But it seems to me
> that this opinion could never have been entertained or adv-
> anced by modern theorists, if any of them had actually
> attempted to form these various tonal modes and to compare
> them by ear.
>
> It is not at all difficult to distinguish the difference of a
> comma (81/80 or 1.25%) in the intonation of the different
> degrees of the scale, when well-known melodies are per-
> formed in different 'colorings', and every musician with whom
> I have made the experiment has immediately heard the diff-
> erence.
>
> Melodic passages with the Pythagorean thirds have a strained
> and restless effect, while the just thirds make the same pass-
> ages quiet and soft. (Helmholtz, 1862, p. 407-408).

Note the agreement of Helmholtz' nineteenth century subjects with the
medieval manuscript cited by Gut.   The small (enharmonic) pitch differences
in the just and Pythagorean variants of the intervals of the Western scale
have been all but forgotten since the establishment of the compromise
system of equal temperament.   At the same time, belief in innate connections between intervals and affects has been replaced with widespread
skepticism.   However, the apparently systematic connection of interval
affect with interval ratio referred to here by Helmholtz is a most interesting phenomenon.

3.   Again, Boomsliter and Creel (1963), repeating Helmholtz' experiments with melodies, found that musicians almost always hear such small (enharmonic) pitch shifts as differences of 'color', i.e. timbre or feeling, rather than as pitch differences - unless they are specifically asked to list for pitch shifts.

My Own Work

My experiments have shown me that the way such small pitch differences among integer-ratio intervals are experienced depends on what listeners imagine they are hearing. An extremely small change in pitch of a complex tone will give rise to a distinct impression of vowel shift when listeners are asked to imagine a vowel sound in the tone. When I ask listeners to imagine that they are hearing musical expressions of personality or of feeling, they hear small differences in tuning of a musical interval as distinct differences in feeling or expression. Moreover, in a pilot experiment (Makeig and Evans, 1979), the feeling experienced for each interval, or more exactly, the qualitative effect of each of several intervals on the imaginations of listeners seemed to be significantly consistent among listeners. The method of projective imagination has rarely been consciously used in psychoacoustic research, but deserves to be more so.

Sensitivity to Ratios

Listening for the feeling of an interval instead of for its size dramatically increases one's sensitivity of feeling to small tuning differences, especially for many integer ratio intervals and their mistunings. As Erv Wilson, the tuning theorist, recently remarked*, the more in tune an (integer-ratio) interval is, the more one wants to hear it in tune. This has been the spontaneous remark of several musicians to whom I have demonstrated the affective results of tuning variations of musical intervals.

However, intervals which are exactly tuned to integer-ratios take on, as Wilson notes, a (beat-free) 'glassy' quality which sounds unlike ordinary music. It is not the feeling quality of the integer-ratio intervals which sounds 'un-natural', but the physical sound-texture. This would seem to indicate that the musical feeling quality of an interval is separate in experience from its physical consonance, pitch register, or timbral quality. This fact is the basis of the practice of musical transposition. Although variations in register, timbre, or sound-texture certainly can alter the overall feeling experienced, there is yet some quality of an interval by which musicians recognize and identify it (as noted, for example, by Siegel and Siegel, 1977).

Modern experiments to define the feeling associated with various intervals have generally not been successful (Maher, 1979). However, the

---

*   at a Partch Foundation Symposium at San Diego State University, July 1980.

technique of projective imagination, combined with multi-dimensional scaling of responses appears to be a most promising technique for objective study of this phenomenon.

Recent Evidence for Parallel Affective and Analytic Perception

That the feeling of a musical interval may be a separate experience from the experience of the pitch-height of the tones of the interval and may even be mediated by different neural information processing has been suggested by the psychoacoustician Evans (1978) on the basis of recent neurological and psychoacoustic evidence. Evans suggests that recognition of musical intervals is based on periodicity ('time') information, whereas pitch-height and physical consonance is most likely supplied mainly by 'place' information. Goldstein (1978) points out that the accuracy of pitch judgments is greater than would seem to be physiologically possible using either place or time information, but is within the range of expectation if both kinds of information are in fact used in some integrated manner. Both de Boer (1976) and Evans (1976) have commented that lack of attention to the 'subjective' experience of the various psychoacoustic phenomena associated with 'pitch' has created confusion in the field, for not all experiences of pitch share a common subjective or objective nature. A similar confusion is seen in aesthetic research which attempts to measure aesthetic experience with a one-dimensional measure ('preference'), rather than analyzing the significant dimensions on independent ranges of variability in the experience.

Evans' theory of the dual nature of pitch seems in accord with the phenomenology of experience of small pitch variations. When we hear a singer sing a note 'flat', we mainly experience a note that feels 'sour', rather than experiencing (or before experiencing) the same note as being 'too low'. Musicians may feel that their most immediate experience is of the note being 'too low'. However, the reaction-time experiments of Balzano (1978) show that even advanced music students know that a minor third for example is 'some kind of third' before they know that it is a minor third (or 'flat' third). Similarly Siegel and Siegel (1977) showed that musicians have extreme difficulty in judging whether a fixed out-of-tune interval is too sharp or too flat. This fact is common knowledge among musicians who must tune their own instruments, and find it easier to do so by varying the pitch steadily until the quality of the interval is recognized most clearly.

Kunst-Wilson and Zajonc (1980) have found that under certain circumstances, persons exposed to brief flashes of random octagon shapes can better recognize which shapes they have seen before by asking themselves, "Do I seem to like this shape?" than by asking the more analytic question, "Do I recognize this shape?" This is only one of several memory experiments referred to by Kunst-Wilson and Zajonc which show that access to prior experience may be more direct through attention to affective association than through conscious analytical inquiry. The following analogy shows, I believe, the value of using affective as well as analytical abilities in a process of on-going perception.

Imagine two kinds of speedometer displays. In one, the speed of the vehicle is displayed on the front window of the vehicle in numerical form. In the second, speed is shown by tinting part or all of the window with a color whose wavelength (i.e. hue) is proportional (or inversely proportional) to the speed of the vehicle. It is possible that this second display would be much more useful in high-speed maneuvering, where attention to the displayed information in the first example, would tend to interfere with attention to rapidly changing details of the environment. The hue-coded speedometer might come to be experienced by the driver (or pilot) much like an affective sense or feeling of the speed of the vehicle, without interfering with his or her attention to the world outside the vehicle.

I do not mean to imply by these arguments that the major function of affective experience is to increase perceptual efficiency. Through feelings, we are able not only to better know ourselves, but also to better know and be able to identify with others. Through affective experience of art and music, we are able to deepen our knowledge through feeling, not only of the artist or composer, but also of ourselves and our relationships to others. I believe that such experience is for most people the primary and deepest appeal of music (see Meyers, 1927).

The Left-Right Dichotomy

The much-explored differentiation in function between the right and left hemispheres (in 'normal' right handers) may possibly be characterized as a differentiation between sequential, rapidly varying perception and cognition, and 'held', more slowly changing, global spatial and affective processes (Pribram, 1978; Smith and Tallal, 1980; Polzella et al., 1977). In particular, results of many of the dichotic pitch recognition experiments show a small right-ear (left hemisphere) advantage for trained musicians (especially on more difficult tasks (Shannon, 1980). 'Non-musicians' usually show no such ear advantage, or more commonly show a left-ear advantage.

However, the idea that musicians experience music more with their left brain while non-musicians experience music more with their right brain has recently been shown to be unrealistic. Gordon (1978) found a right-hemisphere advantage for musicians in a major chord recognition task. Moreover, recently Sidtis (1980) has claimed that the right hemisphere is specialized for complex pitch perception, as opposed to pure tone frequency following. Most interestingly, Shannon found that hearing a harmonic (simultaneous) octave in the right ear allowed musicians to respond quicker, "Not an octave!", whereas heard with the left ear they responded quicker, "Yes, an octave!" This suggests there is more than one way to recognize an octave, and that each side of the brain may work on the task differently, perhaps according to different modes of listening which may be concurrent.

It is plausible that some 'left-right' polarization might be found for 'affective' and 'analytic' aspects of pitch perception as well. Interval quality (and timbre) might be better perceived using the right hemisphere, whereas rapid and accurate pitch-trajectory tracking might be better performed using the left hemisphere. In a recent review, Brust (1980) refers to evidence that this may be the case. However, to my knowledge, no experiment has specifically inquired into how 'affective' listening alters the left-right balance, and to what extent.

The Experience of Musical Consonance

Terhardt (1977) has pointed out the difference between the experience of physical consonance based on sensation of roughness at 'places' on the basilar membrane, and the experience of consonance of musical intervals (in Western tonal music at least) which seems to be based on the same principle of 'harmonic template matching' which is apparently used by the nervous system in deriving fundamental pitch from a complex harmonic or inharmonic sound.

Beament (1977) has suggested in some detail how presence of periodicity within the auditory nervous system at submultiples of spectral frequencies generates an array of subharmonics which could be used by the nervous system for recognition of integer-ratio musical intervals. The often-noted presence of a range of subharmonic periodicities for each of a range of harmonics of a normally harmonic musical sound implies the existence within the nervous system of a harmonic/subharmonic network of activity, which in the case of integer-ratio musical intervals becomes an interrelated array of information.

Goldstein (1976) has suggested that the periodicity information may be

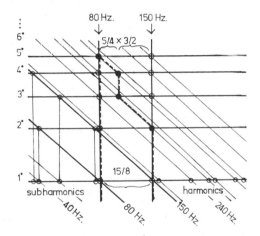

Fig. 1.   Schematic tonotopic planar array capable of factoring ratios into their lowest prime factors, (also capable of signalling fundamental frequency of a complex harmonic or near-harmonic tone). Oblique stripes represent spectrum - here, fundamental frequencies of two tones (80 and 150 Hz.) related by the interval (frequency ratio) 15/8. Horizontal thick lines represent successive harmonics (here 1-5 only). Vertical lines 'collect' harmonics of a single frequency. Information about the higher tone's frequency spreads out along the vertical lines wherever an oblique frequency stripe intersects a harmonic line. One most direct path from the higher to lower tone is shown in dotted lines. The prime factors of the ratio are determined by the number of vertices of such a direct path which occur on each harmonic stripe.

translated at the brainstem level into a central tonotopic or 'place' representation of pitch. Figure 1 shows how such a central tonotopic tract might hypothetically be arranged so as to signal (1) fundamental frequency, and (2) the component prime factors of an interval which approximates an integer-ratio interval.

The harmonic lattice of fifths and thirds recently illustrated by Longuet-Higgins (1978) has been used to plot musical tuning systems since the time of Mersenne. Now, if harmonic intervals were represented at some stage in the nervous system within some such a tonal harmonic array, and if our emotional nervous system were connected in some orderly way to such a neurological representation, we might expect that the structure of our affective experience of intervals which are in or are close to integer-ratios might be similar to the underlying structure of pitch relations among the intervals themselves.

Neurologically, this is mere speculation. However, psychologically this does seem to be the case. It is remarkable that the theory of ratio-interval affect which I shall outline in this paper, though seemingly far from the concerns of psychoacousticians and auditory neurologists seems very much in harmony with latest trends in the theory of pitch perception.

Both Evans (1978) and de Boer (1976) have pointed out that in psychoacoustic tests of frequency discrimination more than one kind of experiential cue is normally used by subjects, for residue pitch and fine frequency discriminations particularly. While this even seems to be the case in isolated psychoacoustic experiments, affective perception is much more important in the process of normal music listening, in which the stream of sonic events is much too dense and complex to be 'understandable' without use of affective perception. Although some highly trained musicians may claim to follow musical activity purely 'analytically', experiments such as Balzano's (1978; this volume) show that they do not in fact do so.

In any case, highly analytical listening is not a possibility for that large majority of music lovers whose analytical abilities to label, retain, and identify musical pitch and time relationships are undeveloped, and, as beginning music theory teachers know, are often surprisingly poor. For example there have been unpublished reports of many untrained listeners being unable to recognize major and minor triads as 'different'. Yet the affective difference between major and minor triads is one of the principal means used by composers to manipulate the feeling of popular songs and melodies. Its efficacy is indirectly attested by the extreme commercial success of such music.

A really valuable science of music must, I believe, include a detailed understanding of the experience of music which I have been calling affective experience. Helmholtz (1862, p.410-411) himself ended his book on music with the request that others in the future take up and carry on the study of musical affects which he had begun. With the availability of present computer synthesis, multidimensional scaling, and psychoacoustic measurement techniques the time for such study seems to have come.

Definition of Affective Quality

I define the affective quality of a musical interval to be its consistent tendency to qualitatively influence the imagination of listeners particularly, but not limited to the imagination of personal feeling.

The physical variable which I propose to isolate is pitch ratio. To do this, I assume all other physical parameters - timbre, dynamics, register, rhythm - are:

1. made musically normative
2. held constant, and
3. made as affectively neutral as possible.

I am therefore isolating only a small part of the affective experience of music itself. However, I believe that this modest approach accurately reflects the state of current knowledge, or I might say, of current ignorance of the subject of musical affect in general. I further believe that intensive study of one aspect of musical affect may be of greater use than the method (widespread in the music education literature) of studying the affective experience of recordings of excerpts of various complex musical performances. Furthermore, the affects of individual musical intervals and harmonies is not at all an inconsequential subject, since harmonies and consonances play such an important structural and affective role in Western tonal music.

THE BASIS OF THE WESTERN HARMONIC SYSTEM

If, as I have suggested, the structure of our affective experience of harmonic musical intervals is based on the structure of the pitch relationships among the harmonic intervals - what is this common structure? I take as my musical example common-practice Western tonal music with octave equivalence.

The Hierarchy of Harmonic Contexts

The Western tonal harmonic system may be modelled as a self-embedded hierarchy of harmonic contexts, namely the central tonic, the tonic-fifth duality, the triad, the 5-tone or pentatonic scale, the 7-tone or diatonic scale, and the 12-tone chromatic scale system (see Fig. 2). These six harmonic contexts are the most basic reference contexts used in Western tonal music.

Tone-Groups

Now, what is their common structure? Each of these contexts (excepting the triad) can be modelled as strings of consecutive fifths - that is, as nearly 3/2 pitch ratios. But all of them have an important additional property. Each of the strings of fifths comes very close to forming a circle of fifths. That is, the interval from the last tone to the first tone of each

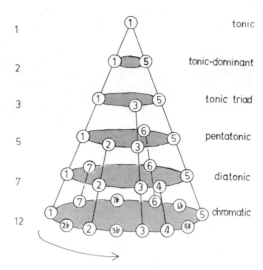

1

2

3

5

7

12

tonic

tonic-dominant

tonic triad

pentatonic

diatonic

chromatic

Fig. 2.   The six hierarchical harmonic contexts of common-practice Western tonal music. In each figure of this article, the numbers
within the tone-circles refer to degrees of the major diatonic
scale, possibly modified by sharps or flats.

string of fifths is in each case almost itself another fifth (see Fig. 3).

Here 'almost' a fifth means in particular that the difference between
this closing interval and a perfect (3/2) fifth is an interval which is not
larger than any interval occurring between any two tones of that level in the
hierarchy. Such near-circles of a single generating interval I call one-
dimensional TONE-GROUPS, and in particular, CONSISTENT tone-groups.

One dimensional tone-groups can unambiguously be considered to be
one-dimensional cyclic groups by identifying each tone with all of its
octaves. Members of a tone-group are then often said to be 'pitch-classes'
or 'chromas', under the assumption of 'octave-equivalence' (see Balzano,
1978, Shepard, in press)*.

The triad, however, (either major or minor) cannot be modelled satisfactorily as a one-dimensional tone-group. It can, however, be modelled as
a two-dimensional tone-group generated by a 3/2 fifth and a 5/4 just major
third. It turns out that consistent two-dimensional tone-groups, generated
by the same two intervals, can model each of the six hierarchical levels very
well. The structure of a two-dimensional tone-group can best be pictured in
three dimensions as a torus or doughnut.

_____

* Topologist Michael Freedman has given me the following mathematical
definition - tone-groups are the fundamental domains of approximate
quotient groups of finitely-generated rational or real commutative free
groups modulo the octave.

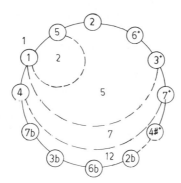

Fig. 3.   Near-circles of fifths forming consistent one-dimensional (Pytha-gorean) tone-groups (under octave equivalence).   The closing 'near-fifths' are shown using dashed lines.

Figure 4 shows a still larger, so-called enharmonic, 53-tone consistent tone-group of perfect fifths and just thirds*. It contains both the one-dimensional (so-called Pythagorean), and the two-dimensional, (so-called just), tone-group hierarchies. In a two-dimensional tone-group, there are several closing intervals, each almost equal to one or the other of the generating intervals.

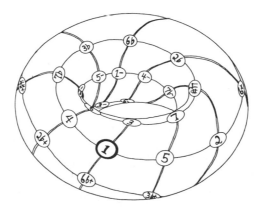

Fig. 4.   Extended-just 53-tone tone-group as a web-of-fifths-and-thirds formed into a torus by identifying tones separated in pitch by schismas (0.1%) and emmas (0.3%).   This tone-group contains all the smaller tone-groups belonging to both the Pythagorean and the just tone-group hierarchies (Makeig, 1979a).

---

*   The schisma (about 0.1%) is the difference between five octaves and eight fifths plus a just third. I have coined the word 'emma' for the difference (about 0.3%) between an octave and five fifths less six just thirds.

Now, I believe, we have modelled the harmonic basis of the Western tonal musical system as a hierarchy of self-embedded consistent one- or two-dimensional tone-groups. It turns out, most significantly, that these are the only such hierarchies generated by the intervals 3/2 and 5/4. Note also that tone-groups generated by 3/2 and 5/4 could in another sense be said to be generated by the whole set of intervals 2/1, 3/2, 4/3, 5/4 and 6/5 - by octave and group inversion. That is, these are the only consistent tone-group hierarchies generated by compounds of frequency ratios occurring among the first six linear harmonics of a harmonic complex tone.

Further, the basic chords (major, minor, sevenths) and modes (major, minor Dorian, etc.) found in Western music in fact correspond to the different placements of the fundamental domains of the basic tone-groups within the lattice of octaves, fifths and thirds.

The Tonal Harmonic Lattice

Now both of these hierarchies of tone-groups can be represented as hierarchies of the successive consistent sub-groups of the infinite lattice of intervals composed of octaves, perfect fifths and just thirds, which Longuet-Higgins (1978) has recently illustrated following earlier tuning theorists. Longuet-Higgins argues convincingly that diatonic scales and keys are in fact compact subsets of the harmonic lattice, and he discusses the compromises effected by equal temperament. However, he neglects the affective distinctions created by the fine distinctions in tuning which result as one goes farther and farther out from the tonic in the lattice. That is to say, he discusses only the diatonic and chromatic levels in the tone-group hierarchy in relation to the lattice, and neglects the enharmonic.

The two enharmonically equivalent sub-systems of intervals (Pythagorean and just), with respect to a common tonic, generate chromatic (12-

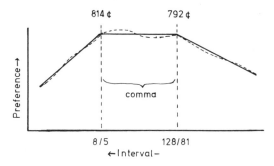

Fig. 5.   Relative percent of 'in tune' judgments (labelled 'preference') for various sizes of minor sixths, as a function of frequency ratio. The dotted line shows the actual data, the solid line Tanner's interpretation of the data. Note boundaries of zone of highest preference, the just (8/5) and Pythagorean (128/81) minor sixths. (From Tanner, 1972).

tones to the octave) scale-systems whose tones differ by only a comma (1.25%). Equal-tempered tuning evolved as a compromise chromatic system, whose tones all lie within the commatic (1.25%) zones bounded by the respective tones of the Pythagorean and just chromatic tone-groups. Tanner (1972) reported that musicians strongly tended to describe as 'in-tune' those thirds and sixths whose ratios were within the commatic zone defined by the Pythagoean and just thirds and sixths respectively, and to describe as 'out-of-tune' thirds and sixths whose frequency ratios did not fall within these so called 'zones of tolerance' (see Fig. 5).

This phenomenon exemplifies the role of a lower (finer) level of the tone-group hierarchy defining pitch categories which are then used in categorical perception of actual musical pitch relations at a higher (grosser) level in the hierarchy. For instance Siegel and Siegel (1977) found that musicians described as 'in tune' those fourths, fifths and tritones whose frequency ratios were within 20 cents (1.25%) of the respective simplest harmonic (3/2) fifth and (4/3) fourth. (Their tolerance for tritones, an interval that has no simple ratio interpretation, was somewhat larger.) The results of Siegel and Siegel were limited by their use of only five different tunings for each interval. Tanner's results showed that, for several degrees of the musical scale, the 'in-tune' zone is actually a comma (1.25%) wide, rather than two commas, as suggested by Siegel and Siegel's results. Tanner (1972, 1976) calls this the zone of 'identification by tolerance.'

Higher and Lower Octaves

If the restriction of formal octave equivalence is dropped from our model then each tone-group can be modelled as a doughnut or circle containing and contained in concentric doughnuts or circles of tones at higher and lower octaves. This gives rise to an inherently five-dimensional model which is similar to that proposed by Roger Shepard (1978). These five dimensions are built up of two dimensions (for circles of thirds), plus two

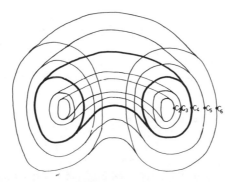

Fig. 6.   Cross-section of a five-dimensional model of extended-just harmonic pitch relationships, collapsed into three dimensions. Only one tone (C4) and its higher and lower octaves are shown.

more (for a circle of fifths), plus one more (for higher and lower octaves). They can be modelled in three dimensions as in Fig. 6.

Shepard generates the same structure as the cross-product of a circle of fifths and a circle of rising chromatic semitone steps. While he overlooks the possibility of the psychological existence of enharmonic varieties of the twelve chromatic scale-steps, his five-dimensional 'double helix of musical pitch' model is structurally homologous to the spatial representation I propose here.

Group Theories of Perception

It seems to me that the tone-group model, and the group structure generated by physical harmonic relationships which it represents, must be an important clue to the understanding of our ability to perceive and experience tonal musical pitch relations - and must be at least part of the reason that Western tonal music has been so long-lived, and is being so well assimilated in other places in the world today.

Note also that its structure seems similar to the systematic and hierarchical structures of:
1. phoneme features in speech,
2. opponent color processes in vision,
3. Western musical meter (which also is built of nested hierarchic cycles, e.g. periods, measures, beats, half-beats, etc.).

An example of group theory in modelling of perception is given by Ermentrout and Cowan (1979), who show that the geometry of visual hallucination patterns can be explained using a group-theoretic model based on known principles of feature detection in the human visual system. In fact, the theories of tone-groups and interval affect developed in this paper are quite similar to the Ermentrout and Cowan work in that both theories model a range of percepts using group theories whose generating elements are primary logarithmic transforms of sensory input to the nervous system (real log frequency transforms in the case of pitch, complex log spatial transforms in the case of vision).

Jairazbhoy (1971) has hypothesized that the evolution of North Indian raga scales is based on cultural evolution of stable Pythagorean tonegroups. Jairazbhoy dismisses the possibility of just or other extended-just ratios forming the basis of scalar structures, but his rejection of this possibility does not seem to be based on personal experience. That the extended-just tone-group is the basis of Indian music and music theory, as well as being the basis for ancient Chinese, Greek and Arabic music theories, is the claim of Daniélou (1978). His historical evidence for this claim is apparently quite debatable (see Bake, 1957 for review). But the theory is essentially a psychoacoustic or pyschoaesthetic theory, and should not be judged on the basis of references in historical music theory.

Other closed, symmetric representations of perceptual ranges have been catalogued by Roger Shepard (1978, 1979), who terms them 'perceptual manifolds'. A recent major and accessible synthesis of more general topological thinking applied to dynamic biological processes is Winfree (1980).

THE THEORY OF INTERVAL AFFECT

The tone-group model for tonal music raises the question whether harmonic perception as well as interval affect might be modelled using a similar structure. The basis for such a model has in fact been proposed for the affective perception of intervals used in classical Indian and other world musics by the French world-music theorist Alain Daniélou (1978).

In essence, according to Daniélou's theory, any musical interval which is composed of a sum or difference of one or a few finely-tuned (2/1) octaves, (3/2) fifths and (5/4) thirds - outside of any particular musical context, but considering the lower tone to be a fixed tonic - has an affective quality which can be modelled, likewise, as the sum or difference of the basic qualities of its constituent upwards and downwards octaves, fifths and thirds. This holds not only at the first six levels of the tone-group hierarchy, but for larger tone-group levels, each composed of sums and differences of (2/1) octaves, (3/2) fifths and (5/4) thirds, out to the 53-tone tone-group which I call the extended-just. This implies that the affective qualities of the octave, fifth and third are distinct or conceptually orthogonal.

Figure 7 shows the 53-tone extended-just 'doughnut' (large tones) un-

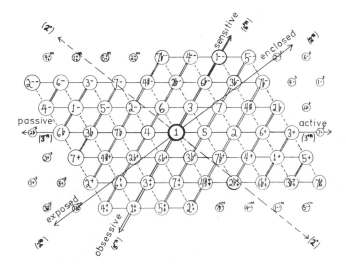

Fig. 7.   The tonal lattice of fifths and thirds (assuming octave equivalence), showing the three affective axes of the theory of interval affect (Daniélou, 1967; Makeig, 1979). The central tone is the tonic. Fifths ascend left to right. Just major thirds ascend lower-left to upper-right. Relative distances of tones from the affective axes reflect the relative powers of 2, 3 and 5 in the integer ratio by which each tone is related to the tonic tone. In this chart each tone is considered to lie in the octave above the tonic. (From Makeig, 1979).

rolled onto a flat surface. Each interval is named according to its upper note, and is thought of as being smaller than an octave. The three 'affective axes' are also drawn on the figure.

For example, the 15/8 just major seventh (the interval from the tonic 1 up to 7 in figure 7), composed of a perfect (3/2) fifth (1 up to 5) and a just major (5/4) third (5 up to 7) - has both the 'sweet, suave, sensitive' quality of the third and also the 'dynamic, active' quality of the fifth. Furthermore, 15/8 has a 'rooted, potent, enclosed' feeling which is the peculiar quality of downward octaves (1/2).

Interval Affect and the Semantic Differential

Note that Figure 7 gives one-word descriptions of the poles of the three affective axes. These simple verbal labels are intended for intuitive interpretation only. I would like to note, however, an apparent parallel between these three dimensions and the three principal dimensions of verbal affective meaning discovered by Osgood et al., (1957).

Specifically, the dimension labelled 'active-passive' (corresponding to positive and negative powers of 3 in ratio) is similar to the semantic differential, 'active-passive' axis. The dimension which I label 'enclosed-exposed' (corresponding to negative and positive powers of 2 in an interval ratio) parallels Osgood's potent-impotent dimension. Finally, the dimension which I label as 'sensitive-obsessive' (corresponding to positive and negative powers of 5 in an interval ratio) parallels Osgood's good-bad dimension.

Osgood (1971) has noted that he began his semantic differential studies thinking he was measuring attitudes, but later felt he was really measuring underlying dimensions of affect. However, Osgood did not go on to rephrase his original scales in terms of purely affective markers. For example, his scale, 'good-bad', has both conceptual (judgmental or 'evaluative' in Osgood's terminology), and also affective connotations.

It is my tentative conclusion, based on intimate experience with the qualities of the intervals, that the three dimensions of interval affect actually represent the purely affective dimensions underlying Osgood's semantic differential results. However, the individual conceptual interpretations which different individuals give to the different dimensions may depend on the person, and their experience. The semantic differential hypothesis may be tested, I believe, by modelling both the semantic differential space and the interval affect space, using multi-dimensional scaling of verbal responses to intervals, in a paradigm which allows free use of projective imagination (imagining that the interval represents affective characteristics of some person's moods or feelings)*.

---

*   The possibility of collecting parallel physiological data for this experiment is suggested by Chapman's evoked potential experiments with the semantic differential (Chapman, 1980).

Objections to the Theory

Those readers who are familiar with the sound of the abovementioned major seventh only in its tempered form may not be able to associate with it the adjectives I have proposed. But note that the tempered major seventh is a whole one-eighth of a semitone higher than the just major (15/8) seventh. And such small differences in pitch can make big differences in affective perception, even (as Helmholtz also noted) in the perception of melodies. While this fact may surprise many modern musicians, in this matter (as again Helmholtz also clearly stated) only persons with personal experience have a basis for judgment. (Some subjective experience is available through the sound examples accompanying this volume.)

Here I feel I should state my view that a certain proportion of recent music psychology literature has been written by persons who attempt to make far-reaching conclusions from limited experiments, without ever having bothered to try to experience critically for themselves the musical phenomena they are writing about. I would say that those who question the idea of 'the beauty of just intervals' without ever having actually listened musically for that beauty under the guidance of someone who appreciates it, are making risky claims, particularly since objective studies of the qualitative effects of musical intervals on imagination of listeners have not been carried out formally.

In such circumstances, the informal studies that have been made by experimenters (e.g. Helmholtz, Boomsliter and Creel) and musicians (Hindemith, 1945; Chalmers et al., 1973-) ought to be given considerable weight. Even if formal objective results were to be presented, it seems to me that, even for a 'theorist', there is no substitute for personal experience, particularly in the case of a little-known perceptual phenomenon.

Why are ratio distinctions not taught?

A stronger objection to the theory of integer-ratios is that musicians are not taught to think or play in terms of ratios, that enharmonic distinctions in ratios are not usually notated, and that most studies of actual tunings used by musicians do not show that they play exact ratios (Ward, 1970). Are these final blows for any integer-ratio theory of music?

The intonation of actual music is a highly complex subject. Tanner (1976) played musicians several 'do re mi' sequences of tones. In some, the interval (frequency ratio) between mi and re, and between re and do were equal; in others, they were unequal. The musicians preferred the tuning by equal steps, even when the equal intervals were not those preferred in isolation. This would indicate that at least two factors enter into musicians' judgements of intonation; 1. the zones of tolerance, which are delimited by, or somehow 'built-on' the tone-group skeleton of extended-just ratios (Tanner, 1972); 2. attention to relative step-sizes, as part of perception of dynamc trajectory of movement within a one-dimensional pitch-height space (Tanner, 1976).

Terhardt (1977) has pointed out a third factor in musical pitch perception, one which makes the results of previous pitch-tracking experiments suspect. Perceived pitch is shifted systematically (up to about 1%) by shifts in timbre, loudness, ear, etc. Thus any theories or studies of preferred pitch which claim to analyze perceived pitch by calculating physical frequency must make psychoacoustic corrections before claiming accuracy to much less than 1%. Until this has been done, there will have been no really accurate studies of how musicians actually play in expressive performance.

Several other faults in previous pitch-tracking experiments may be perceived:

1. 'Musicians' used as subjects may vary in level of talent and musical effectiveness. Averaging over a group of average music students will not necessarily show the same trends in the fine details of tuning, etc., as would studies of best performances by the most effective performers.

2. Averaging over several performances by one group of performers will tend to obscure the ever-present differences in degree of artistic success from one performance to another. At Ossiach (1980), Weinrich suggested having musicians record several performances, asking them to then listen and rate their own performances for correctness and artistic effect, and then weighting the averaging of the results accordingly.

3. Most studies of 'tuning preference' have used the simplistic hypothesis that musicians use either Pythagorean, just or equal-tempered tuning. The broader hypothesis, that both just and Pythagorean tunings form parts of an 'extended-just' system of integer-ratio based intervals which may be used for various musical purposes, has not usually been considered. As a result, uni-modal averaging would distort an inherently bi-modal pitch distribution (see figure 5), and give a false result favoring a 'median' equal temperament.

4. The 'stretching' and 'shifting' of intonation due to considerations of equal steps (as in Tanner's experiment), or pitch-height acceleration (as when string players decrease the size of a trilled semitone) must be carefully minimized or balanced. In other words, in dynamic musical performance, dynamic pitch trajectory or 'vocality' (Meyer, 1929) should be expected to 'pull against' the underlying tone-group framework, and the absolute frequency of the theoretical tonic of the tone-group structure may be expected to adjust itself to preceding pitches and trends.

5. The affective usefulness of dissonant tunings has usually been overlooked in psychophysical research. Do barbershop singers really prefer a beat-free sound texture, as hypothesized by Hagerman and Sundberg, (1980)? Or is the 'glassy' quality of beat-free harmonies contrary to the artistic and affective intentions of performers, as noted by Wilson?

6. The experiments of Boomsliter and Creel (1963) show that even musicians who are used to performing on fixed-pitch equally-tempered instruments maintain, when given a larger fixed set of tuning choices, that they prefer tuning known melodies using intervals which do not lie within any one just or Pythagorean 7-tone group, but which are found to move systematically within the hierarchy of extended-just tone-groups, according to the feeling which the melody is meant to express.

Thus, for example, the opening of the "Marseillaise" tune was preferred by all their accomplished musician subjects with a 27/20 fourth, an interval which is a comma higher than either the perfect 4/3 fourth or the equally tempered fourth. With a perfect fourth, the tune has none of the proud, stirring quality which it is intended to evoke. If one plays this tune on the piano, and listens carefully to the actual pitches of the notes, one will discover a blandness in the ordinary tuning which is usually masked by use of martial rhythmic and dynamic emphases.

Using carefully recorded sine tones, I made a tape of continuous integer-ratio intervals. When I listened to a 27/20 raised fourth, I found that I could easily perceive it as being out of tune, and dissonant. Yet when I actively imagined it as the musical expression of pride or vainglory, it seemed to sound exactly in tune. I have been able to demonstrate this phenomenon to other musicians as well. Thus it appears to be a principle that in isolation from musical context and for Western musical listeners, at least-

> an interval tends to sound in tune when our imagination of the feeling or affective quality of the interval is 'in tune' with the inherent affective tendency of its harmonic composition.

Of course this sense may be altered by psychoacoustic factors, and may require a musical sensitivity not consciously used by all musicians. I state it simply as being in accord with my personal experience to date.

AFFECTIVE VERSUS ANALYTIC EXPERIENCE OF MUSICAL INTERVALS

The theory of interval affect can be seen as simply a working out of the idea that the range of affective qualities of tonal musical intervals is at least structurally similar to the structure of tonal pitch relations, based primarily, it would seem, on three underlying affective dimensions corresponding to the first linear harmonics (numbers two, three and five) of the voice and other natural and harmonic musical sounds.

Affective qualities cannot be visualized as moving points in space as can high and low pitches. They are qualities. This is the primary distinction I wish to make between 'analytic' and 'affective' perception of intervals. Analytic perception of pitch is dynamic perception of pitch contour and location in the one-dimensional space of high/low pitch judgments. My use of the term 'analytic' includes both perception of pure (sine) tone pitch and also perception of residue or fundamental pitch of complex tones (distinguished as analytic and synthetic respectively by Terhardt, 1974, 1977).

My term 'analytic pitch perception' contrasts with 'affective pitch perception', by which I mean perception of pitch relations and changes as qualities - whether of texture, timbre, association, or of feeling.

Listening at Different Levels in the Tone-Group Hierarchy

Normally, in listening to music, affective perception tends to make use of lower (finer) levels in the tone-group hierarchy than analytic perception. For instance, a chromatic semitone shift in an otherwise diatonic melody is apt to be, at least first, experienced by most listeners affectively, rather than analytically. One might say of the experience, "I felt a change, but I didn't follow the pitch going up or down." This fact has recently been demonstrated in experiments by Balzano (1977) (who first introduced me to the idea of using group theory to model tuning theory) and was also confirmed by the Siegels in their provocatively titled paper, "Musicians can't tell sharp from flat" (Siegel and Siegel, 1977).

The same kind of experience holds (as Helmholtz noted) for pitch changes at the enharmonic (commatic, sub-chromatic) levels. Helmholtz (1862, p.407) noted that the Greeks used the word 'colorings' (chroai) to describe small pitch shifts. Boethius said that the musical scale-term 'chromatic' itself originally referred to the breaking up into pieces of the various diatonic scale-steps like broken glass prismatically refracting light into new colors (Bower, 1962). The analogy to color seems a natural one, if by it the Greeks meant that the experience of small pitch steps was largely affective, for color metaphors are very often used to describe affective qualities.

The comments by Rameau (1750) on use of enharmonic intervals in his music show that he was acutely aware of their harmonic and affective natures. Although Rameau was an early champion of equal temperament as a practical method of harpsichord tuning, his comments on the affective qualities of intervals in fact fit the experience of their extended-just, rather than their equal-tempered versions.

The gradually progressive exclusive use of equally tempered tuning in European music during the eighteenth and nineteenth centuries is apparently correlated with the progressive use of more and more complex harmonies. As the affective distinction between enharmonic variations in intervals was less appreciated, harmonic affect came to be suggested by much more extreme harmonic combinations than had been permissible previously. This is the conclusion of several theorists who have experimented both with extended-just and tempered intervals (including Helmholtz).

Nowadays, the atonal music of the twentieth century avant garde is still experienced with discomfort by those who are used to listening to diatonic or mildly chromatic music, but is not necessarily experienced as unpleasant by those who have learned to listen more analytically at the chromatic and enharmonic levels. In turn, the 'simplistic' diatonic music of the sixteenth century sounds dull to singers trained to sing harmonically more complex music, until the original extended-just (or only partially tempered) intervals are used, when the music seems to take on subtle but much-appreciated richness of experience.

Furthermore, the testimony of those who have experimented with composing in different forms of equal temperaments (Darreg, 1975) indicates that tonal music performed in equal temperaments (for example of 12, 19, 22 or 31 tones to the octave) tends to have a characteristic mood which corresponds to the affective qualities of those extended-just intervals which are approximated most closely by intervals in the temperament (Makeig, 1979). I have previously shown (Makeig, 1979) that the characteristic mood of each equal temperament can be calculated as a vector in the space of interval affect, corresponding to the rotation angle of the natural linear mapping from the temperament to the web-of-fifths-and-thirds representation of the extended-just tone-group.

CONCLUSION

Relatively little research has been done since the 1930's on musical affect.* Distinctive among recent work is Clynes' 'sentic' theory of the dynamic and rhythmic expression of emotions (Clynes, 1977, 1980). For the study of the theory of interval affect using projective and multi-dimensional scaling techniques, the following questions and applications suggest themselves:

.   Might music synthesized using tone-group theory be effective in influencing mood?
.   Might use of extended-just ratios either in foreground or in background sound have psychotherapeutic uses?
.   Would the theory of interval affect be validated in field studies of non-Western musical cultures?
.   In what other ways might the affective power of music be explored and refined?
.   How do the static and dynamic aspects of musical affect interact and combine?

Though I have developed and exposed the theory of interval affect in relation to common-practice Western tonal music, it is quite possible that the observations and conclusions may apply as well to other types of known music; they also suggest many compositional possibilities. I believe that the inspirational and also the therapeutic possibilities of music are as yet little understood and rarely put to full use. For this reason I recommend that the detailed study of musical affect be not ignored, but on the contrary encouraged.

SUMMARY

How music suggests or communicates feelings is largely unknown. This paper discusses how the affective experience of tonal harmonies is linked to their objective structure.

In Western tonal music, I maintain, the basic harmonic and modal pitch relations among tones, intervals and chords form a hierarchy of highly structured 'tone-group' relationships which can be considered to be generated by compounding of small-integer frequency ratios. This hierarchy of 'tone-groups', defining successively finer pitch categories, is generated by the interaction of a small number of principles, and also may be modelled spatially.

---

*   Charles Meyers' study (1927) of what listeners report experiencing when they listen to music is a particularly good example of descriptive psychology of that era combined with both personal insight and at the same time objectivity.

The French ethnomusicologist Alain Daniélou has proposed that the range of affective characters of musical intervals can be modelled in a similar way, based on three fundamental affective dimensions, linked to the (2/1) octave, the (3/2) fifth, and the (5/4) major third. This theory is in accord with many longstanding observations on the affective qualities of tonal chords and intervals; it also predicts that their affective characters can be focused or varied through fine-tuning to underlying larger tone-groups of pitch ratios.

I discuss the unity of analytic and affective experience of tonal harmony in terms of, and with implications for present psychoacoustics, psychology, and music theory.

REFERENCES

Bake, A., 1957, Review of Daniélou, 'Traité de musicologie comparée,' Ethnomusicology, 5(3):231.

Balzano, G.J., 1978, "Higher-order Attributes and the Perception of Musical Intervals," Paper presented at the Research Symposium on the Cognitive Structure of Musical Pitch.

Beament, J., 1977, The biology of music, Psych. of Music, 5(1):1.

Boer, E. de, 1976, On the 'residue' and auditory pitch perception, in "Handbook of Sensory Physiology," W.D. Keidel, and W.D. Neff, eds., Springer-Verlag, Berlin.

Boomsliter, P., and Creel, W., 1961, The long-pattern hypothesis in harmony and hearing, J. Mus. Theory, 5:3-31.

Boomsliter, P., and Creel, W., 1963, Extended reference - an unrecognized dynamic in melody, J. Mus. Theory, 7:2.

Briscoe, R.L., 1975, "Rameau's 'Démonstration du principle de l'harmonie (1750),'" Ph.D. diss., University of Indiana.

Brust, J.C.M., 1980, Music and language: Musical alexia and agraphia, Brain, 103:367.

Budden, F., 1972, "The fascination of Groups," Cambridge University Press, Cambridge, Eng.

Chalmers, J., ed., 1973-, Xenharmonikon: An Informal Journal of Experimental Music, Houston.

Chapman, R.M., McCrary, J.W., Chapman, J.A., and Martin, J.K., 1980, Behavioral and neural analyses of connotative meaning: word classes and rating scales, Brain and Lang., 11:319.

Clynes, M., 1977, "Sentics: The Touch of Emotions," Doubleday/Anchor Press, New York.

Clynes, M., 1980, The communication of emotion: theory of sentics, in "Theories of Emotion," R. Plutchik, and H. Kellerman, eds., Academic Press, New York.

Darreg, I., 1975, New moods, Xenharmonic bulletin No. 5, Xenharmonikon 4.

Daniélou, A., 1967, "Sémantique musicale," Hermann, Paris. (2nd ed. 1978).

Ermentrout, and Cowan, 1979, A mathematical theory of visual hallucination and patterns, Biol. Cybern., 34:137.

Evans, E.F., 1978, Place and time coding of frequency in the peripheral auditory system: some physiological pros and cons, Audiol., 17:369.

Goldstein, J.L., 1978, Mechanisms of signal analysis and pattern perception in periodicity pitch, Audiol., 17:421.

Gordon, H.W., 1978, Hemispheric asymmetry for dichotically-presented chords in musicians and non-musicians, males and females, Acta Psych., 42:383.

Gut, S., 1976, La notion de consonance chez les theoriciens du moyen age, Acta Musico., 48:20.

Hagerman, B., and Sundberg, J., 1980, Fundamental frequency adjustment in barbershop singing, Quart. Prog. & Stat. Report, Apr:28-42. Speech Transmission Lab., Royal Inst. Technology, Stockholm.

Helmholtz, H.L.F. von, 1862, "On the Sensations of Tone as a Physiological Basis for the Theory of Music," Peter Smith, New York (1948).

Hindemith, P., 1945, "The Craft of Musical Composition," Book I, (4th ed.), Schott, New York.

Jairazbhoy, N.A., 1971, "The Rags of North Indian Music: Their Structured Evolution, Wesleyan University Press, Middletown, Conn.

Kilmer, A., Crocker, R., and Brown, D., 1976, "Sounds from Silence: Recent Discoveries in Ancient Near Eastern Music, Bit Enki Productions, Berkeley, Calif. (Booklet and long-playing record.)

Krumhansl, C., 1979, The psychological representation of musical pitch in a tonal context, Cog. Psych., 11:346.

Kunst-Wilson, W., and Zajonc, R.B., 1980, Affective discrimination of stimuli that cannot be recognized, Science, 207:557.

Longuet-Higgins, H.C., 1978, The perception of music, Interdisc. Sci. News, 3:148.

Makeig, S., 1979, "Expressive Tuning: The Theory of Interval Affect," Master's thesis, University of South Carolina.

Makeig, S., 1979, The affects of musical intervals (Part 1), Interval, 2(1):18.

Makeig, S., 1980, The affects of musical intervals (Part 2), Interval, 2(2):23.

Makeig, S., and Evans, J., 1980, "Pilot Study Summary of a Projected Test of Interval Affect," paper presented to S. Carolina chapter, American Psychology Association meeting, Myrtle Beach, S. Carolina.

Makeig, S., 1980, The theory of tone-groups (unpublished).

Makeig, S., 1980, "On Fokker's Chinese Bells" (unpublished).

Makeig, S., 1981, Means, meaning, and music: Pythagoras, Archytas, and Plato, ex tempore, 1(1):36-62.

Meher Baba, 1955, "God Speaks: The Theme of Creation and Its Purpose," Dodd, Mead, New York (2nd ed., 1973).

Meyer, M.F., 1929, The musician's arithmetic, in "The University of Missouri Studies," 6(1):5.

Meyers, C., 1927, Individual differences in musical perception, in "The Effects of Music,", M. Shoen, ed., Harcourt-Brace, New York.

Moore, B.C.J., 1980, Neural interspike intervals and pitch, Audiol., 19:363.

Osgood, C.E., 1971, Exploration in semantic space: a personal diary, J. of Soc. Iss., 27(4):5.

Osgood, C.E., Suci, F.J., and Tannebaum, P.H., 1957, "The Measurement of Meaning," University of Illinois Press, Urbana, Ill.

Peretz, I., and Morais, J., 1980, Modes of processing melodies and ear asymmetry in non-musicians, Neuropsych., 18:477.

Polzella, D.J., DaPolito, F., and Hussman, M.C., 1977, Cerebral asymmetry in time perception, Perc. and Psychophys., 21(2):187.

Pribram, K.H., 1978, Modes of central processing in human learning, in "Brain and Learning," Greylock, Stamford, Conn.

Shannon, B., 1980, Lateralization effects in musical decision tasks, Neuropsych., 18:21.

Shepard, R.N., 1979, Individual differences in the perception of musical pitch, in "Perceptual Organization," M. Kubovy, and J.R. Pomerantz, eds., Lawrence Erlbaum Associates, Hillsdale, N.J.

Shepard, R.N., (1978), The circumplex and related topological manifolds in the study of perception, in "Theory Construction and Data Analysis in the Behavioral Sciences," S. Shye, ed., Jossey-Bass, San Francisco.

Shepard, R.N., in press, Structural representations of musical pitch, in "Psychology of Music", D. Deutsch, ed., Academic Press, New York.

Sidtis, J.J., 1980, On the nature of the cortical function underlying right hemisphere auditory perception, Neuropsych., 18:321.

Siegel, J.A., and Siegel, W., 1977, Categorical perception - musicians can't tell sharp from flat, Perc. and Psychophys., 21:399.

Smith, J., and Tallal, P., 1980, Rate of acoustic change may underline hemispheric specialization for speech perception, Science, 207:1380-1381.

Tanner, R., 1971, Le phénomène d'identification par tolérance; le préjuge de la gamme juste, Acustica, 25:158.

Tanner, R., 1972, Le problème des deux tierces (Pythagore ou Zarlino): Sa solution psycharithmétique, Acustica, 27:335.

Tanner, R., 1972, La différenciation qualitative des psycharithmes et des intervalles musicaux, Rev. Mus., Num. Spec.

Tanner, R., 1976, La fonction et la justesse mélodiques des intervalles, Acustica, 34(5):259.

Terhardt, E., 1974, Pitch, consonance, and harmony, J. Acoust. Soc. Am., 54:1061.

Terhardt, E., 1977, The two-component theory of musical consonance, in "Psychophysics and Physiology of Hearing," E.F. Evans, and J.P. Wilson, eds., Acadmic Press, London.

Ward, W.D., 1970, Musical perception, in "Foundations of Modern Auditory Theory," J.V. Tobias, ed., Academic Press, New York.

Winfree, A.T., 1980, "The Geometry of Biological Time," Springer-Verlag, Berlin.

Chapter XIII

TWO CHANNEL PITCH PERCEPTION

Leon van Noorden

Association for the Blind in the Netherlands
Rotterdam, Netherlands

INTRODUCTION

Physiological experiments show that information about frequency of tones is coded in two distinct ways in the auditory nerve. Nerve spikes can be distinguished as to when and where (in which nerve fiber) they occur. It is an old question whether the time or the place information plays a role in pitch perception.

In this paper we speculate that the auditory system uses both kinds of information, resulting in two distinct patterns of behaviour. Comparing results in music psychology, psychophysics and physiology shows that a number of phenomena can be separated into two clearly distinct groups with chroma and low pitch of complex tones tentatively related to time information, and tone height and sharpness of timbre to place information. We propose a psychophysical model of chroma perception that is based on the temporal information in the auditory nerve.

PITCH PHENOMENA

1.1 Two Pitch Qualities

The idea that tones have two different pitch qualities is an old one, referred to, for instance, by Drobisch (1855), and Revesz (1913). Bachem (1937) introduced the terminology 'chroma' and 'tone height'. Chroma was defined as the quality for which the octave relationship plays an important role (expressed through the fact that in music, tones an octave apart have the same name), while tone height was defined as the quality that rises monotonically with frequency. A series of tones that are separated by a whole number of octaves, for example, have the same chroma but differ in tone height. Empirical support (discussed below) for distinguishing two pitch

251

qualities comes from different fields of investigation, such as those concerning absolute pitch, pitch and timbre of complex tones, and pitch scaling.

1.2 Absolute Pitch

Absolute pitch is the capacity of some observers to identify a large number of tones of different frequency, commonly in terms of their musical note name, without a reference tone being presented to them. In literature one can find examples of observers who can make correct absolute judgements of 45 to 70 different tones. (Miller, 1956; Ward, 1953; Attneave, 1959). This large number is at variance with Miller's famous "Magical number seven plus or minus two" (1956), the maximum number of well discriminable stimuli along a one dimensional continuum that can be recognised in an absolute judgement experiment (see also Attneave, 1959; and Garner, 1962). However, Pollack's results (1952, 1953) were in line with the general observation of Miller. His subjects, who were not claimed to be possessors of absolute pitch, were unable to make reliable absolute judgements of more than five equally likely tones (cf. also Fulgosi and Zaja, 1975). A possible explanation for this discrepancy is that observers with the faculty of absolute pitch make use of the two channels chroma and tone height, each with its own limited capacity of about 3 bits, as is suggested by Stanaway, Morley and Anstis (1970). Six bits of information corresponds to an ability to recognize 64 tones without error.

The types of errors that are made by absolute (AP) and nonabsolute (NAP) pitch observers further confirm the explanation. The error distribution of APs is multimodal. The modes have octave relationships, which suggests that the chroma is extracted without error but that there is occasionally an error in the tone height. NAPs show a unimodal distribution that is considerably wider than the main mode in the error distribution of the AP observers (Bachem, 1937; Carrol, 1975). as if NAPs only use tone height.

1.3 Pitch and Timbre of Tones

In pyschophysics pure tones play an important role. These stimuli are easy to describe in physical terms. They seem to have a clearly defined pitch and observers with the best absolute pitch performance can distinguish these tones with about the same precision as tones of musical instruments, like the piano (Siegel, 1972; Stanaway et al., 1970). However, pure tones make it non-trivial to conceive pitch as a two dimensional subjective entity since it is not clear how the variation of only a single physical dimension, i.e. the frequency of the sine-wave, causes the perception of the tone to vary in a two-dimensional subjective space. To tackle this problem we want to argue that pure tones are analyzed by two different perceptual mechanisms of the ear.

Most of the sounds we encounter in daily life are complex tones. Physically these can be described as a superposition of a number of pure tones. In the large class of harmonic (or periodic) tones, the frequencies of these components are multiples of the fundamental frequency. The distribution of the energy over the components is called the spectrum. From psychophysical research it is known that there is a 'low pitch' (cf. Plomp 1976) of complex tones that is connected with the fundamental frequency of the tones (even if the energy of the component of the fundamental frequency is below hearing threshold (Schouten, 1938, 1940a, 1940b). The perceptual quality 'timbre' is determined by the spectrum. Pitch and timbre of a complex tone can be varied independently (within limits) by varying fundamental frequency and spectrum. The spectrum can be varied in many ways. Investigators of timbre (for example: Plomp 1976; von Bismarck, 1974) have shown that as a consequence, timbre is a multidimensional entity. However, they also showed that there is a main factor, the psychophysical correlate of which has been called 'sharpness' by von Bismarck. A sound is sharper the more energy it has in higher regions of the critical band scale. Von Bismarck also found that the fine structure of the spectrum - complex tone or noise - had only a marginal effect on perceived sharpness.

A further experiment by Plomp et al. (1971) on the dissimilarity between tones that differ in fundamental frequency, in spectrum or in both dimensions suggests strongly that pitch and timbre are processed independently. From the structure of the judged (dis) similarities between each stimulus pair one can infer how the two dimensions are related to each other in the perceptual domain (for example: Garner, 1972). If the two dimensions for a genuine two-dimensional space, like a flat surface in physical space, the dissimilarity between two stimuli will be equal to the square root of the sum of squares of the dissimilarities along each dimension (so-called Euclidean metric). An example of this is provided by the dimensions brightness and saturation in vision. The observer probably does not notice that there are two dimensions involved. But if the two dimensions are obvious and compelling, so that it is very difficult for an observer to see what the relation is between the two dimensions, the dissimilarity between two stimuli is equal to the sum of the dissimilarity along each dimension (so-called city-block metric). The observer perceives these dimensions separately. The results of Plomp's experiment strongly suggest a city-block metric for the similarity space of pitch and sharpness.

These results make it reasonable to assume that the ear has different mechanisms for the analysis of the pitch of tones. There is no reason to suppose that pure tones are not subjected to an evaluation by these two analysers. Although pure tones seem in a sense to vary along a single dimension for a physicist, since frequency and spectrum are coupled in a one-to-one manner, for the ear they vary in two dimensions.

1.4 Pitch Scaling and Interval Transposition with Pure Tones

Psychophysicists have tried to determine experimentally the relation between the physical entity frequency and the subjective entity pitch, without defining 'pitch' further. Stevens and his co-workers were the pioneers in the field of pitch scaling (Stevens et al., 1937), using their fractionation method in which subjects adjust the frequency of a variable tone so that its unspecified pitch appeared half as great as that of a standard. The determination of the relation between pitch and frequency has also been replicated with different methods, by Stevens et al. (1940) - equisection method; Siegel (1965) - fractionation; Beck and Shaw 1961) - magnitude estimation; Carvellas and Schneider (1972), and Parker and Schneider (1974) - non metric techniques. The results of these experiments vary somewhat with the method used, but one can say that there is a consistent picture of the global relation between pitch and frequency in these kind of experiments, expressed in the 'mel-scale'.

The mel-scale, in line with its name, pretends to be the scale on which melodies are constructed, despite deviating markedly from the musical or logarithmic scale. Marks (1974) argued that the mel-scale is a scale for pure tones, while the musical scales are constructed with complex tones. However, it is quite obvious that pure tones can be used to construct melodies. Attneave and Olson (1971) found in a transposition experiment that melodic relations between pure tones behave according to a logarithmic scale and not according to the mel-scale, since over a wide range of frequencies equal melodic distance meant equal frequency ratio.

To explain the discrepancy between the mel-scale and the logarithmic scale, we assume that in the two kinds of experiments the observers react to different qualities of the tones. If we consider why some experiments produced the mel-scale and other experiments the logarithmic scale we can see that two factors play a role: (1) the musical experience of the observer; (2) the width of the intervals employed in the scaling experiment.

Concerning the first Stevens et al. (1937) and Attneave and Olson (1971) indicate that the musical experience of the observer influences the performance in the experience. In Stevens, the musical observer had trouble in understanding the task, while in Attneave's original paradigm the nonmusical observers had trouble in responding consistently. These results do not mean, however, that experiments with musical observers result in one scale and with nonmusical observers in the other scale. The difference in behaviour can be understood by assuming that the relative importance of the two qualities differ in the two observed groups. Musical observers pay attention primarily to the musically important (chroma) pitch aspect while nonmusical observers concentrate on the timbre aspect. This analysis is supported by Stevens' report that the musical observer learned to disregard octave and other musical interval relations in the course of the experiment, while Attneave could help his nonmusical observers by providing more musical context, in which case these observers also transposed on a logarithmic scale.

Concerning the second point, another complicating factor is the width of the interval used in the scaling experiment. As was said before, a pure tone that changes in frequency changes in pitch and in timbre. Probably, however, the subjective changes are not equally large in both dimensions. A small frequency change of a pure tone may give rise to a clear pitch step without a substantial change in timbre. It could be reasoned that the smallest pitch step is about a semitone and the smallest timbre step about a critical band width* (consider for instance, the width of the response histo-

---

*   The critical band has a width of approximately 3 semitones or 1/3 octave. The measurement of the intensitites of a steady state complex tone in successive 1/3 octave bands gives a good first order approximation for the physical correlate of timbre of that tone (Plomp, 1972).

gram of NAPs in an absolute identification experiment for tones varying in frequency). This is in line with Harris' (1960) finding that scaling experiments w'th intervals smaller than about 4 semitones result in a logarithmic scale, while scaling with intervals larger than a musical fifth resulted in the mel-scale.

1.5 Combining the Evidence for Two Pitch Qualities

The results of the three experimental fields of pitch perception can be summarised as folllows:

(1)   the experiments on absolute pitch show that a number of observers can identiy so many tones of different frequency and with such an error pattern, that it seems that they identify tones as varying in two dimensions.

(2)   The experiments on pitch and timbre of complex tones show that pitch and timbre (spectrum) are two clearly distinguishable perceptual qualities of a tone and that sharpness is a main factor in the perceptual timbre space.

(3)   The experiments on pitch scaling with pure tones indicate that two distinct scales are found depending upon details of experiment set-up, viz. the mel-scale and the logarithmic scale.

We can link the results of these experiments by the assumption that these results all relate to the same two basic dimensions of pitch, one characterized by tone height, sharpness and mel-scale, the other by chroma, low fundamental pitch and logarithmic scale.

Bachem (1950) and considered tone height a quality of pitch that increases in a monotonic way with frequency of a pure tone. He further stated that noises also have tone height. Von Bismarck (1974) ascribed the same characteristics to his concept sharpness and related it to the critical bandwidth. The close relation betwen the mel-scale and the critical bandwidth as a function of frequency has already been mentioned often in the literature. So it seems reasonable to suppose that the mel-scale measures that quality of the pure tone that results from the timbre analyser.

More attention has to be given to the relation between chroma and the quality of pitch as it arises from the experiments on pitch of complex tones and the scaling experiment of Attneave and Olson. As a consequence of the fact that the notion of chroma is often used in relation with the phenomenon of absolute pitch, chroma has a connotation of having an absolute relation with frequency. The expression: the C-ness of a tone, is not unusual in this context. This notion is perhaps relevant as far as the introspection of an observer with absolute pitch is concerned. It does not mean, however, that an observer without absolute pitch cannot make use of the chroma dimension. An argument that chroma plays a role in relative pitch, is the fact that the transposition behaviour of the observers in the experiment of Attneave and Olson (1971) breaks down very sharply at about 5 kHz. This is the same frequency where Bachem (1954) observed the fixation of chroma. The difference between observers with and without absolute pitch has to be found in tone memory. not in tone perception mechanism (Siegel, 1974). Recognition of the chroma of a tone (like its C-ness) is in fact the recognition of the relation of that tone to one or more other tones in terms of a musical interval. The recognition of this fact lays the bridge between chroma and low pitch. Houtsma and Goldstein (1972) have shown that musical intervals are recognized on basis of low pitch. The fact that in their experiments the harmonic number of the few consecutive components of the complex tones varied in a random fashion, makes it very improbable that the timbre or tone height of the tones played a role. Finally, it has to be explained why a logarithmic scale is connnected to this pitch quality. From a number of experiments on pitch of complex tones it is evident that observers often make octave errors (Ritsma, 1966; Patterson and Wightman, 1976). There has to be a close similarity between octaves. If the observer recognizes this and considers the octave as a unit of pitch distance, his pitch scale will be a logarithmic scale of frequency.

THE PHYSIOLOGICAL COUNTERPART

2.1 Two Physiological Channels for Tone Frequency

From physiological measurements (e.g. Whitfield, 1967) we know that, in the auditory nerve, spikes are ordered in place (in which nerve fibres) and time. This is a two-dimensional physiological code in which information about the stimulus is transmitted. How is the two dimensional pitch perception related to this two-dimensional physiological code? A priori, it need not be the case that the specified perceptual dimensions correspond in a straightforward way with the specified nerve code dimensions. It is possible that only a single physiological dimension is used, and that the perceptual system reconstructs a two dimensional subjective space. It has been suggested that only the place code plays a role. Sharpness then is determined by the centre of gravity of the excitation on the basilar membrane and chroma is related to the relation between the distinguishable maxima of the excitation pattern of the basilar membrane stimulated by a complex tone (Bachem. 1950; Terhardt, 1974: Wightman, 1973). This theory, however, gives no explanation for the cases in which chroma pitch can be perceived without the occurence of clear maxima in the neuronal excitation pattern (as is the case with complex tones of only high harmonics, with large amplitude (Moore, 1973), and with pitch of modulated noise). Since it is difficult to imagine how the time code alone could be used as a mediator for both pitch and timbre, we therefore argue for the hypothesis that both codes are used.

There is little disagreement between investigators of the auditory system over the fact that sharpness is mediated by place code. The argument is that the sharpness scale is congruent with the critical band scale, while the critical band scale can be mapped linearly onto the basilar membrane: critical band corresponds to a fixed distance along the membrane (Zwicker, 1967; Marks, 1974).

Other pitch phenomena suggest that time code must be a mediator for pitch perception. Very direct evidence has been brought forward recently by Kengo Oghushi (1978), who shows that the small discrepancy between the low pitch of a complex tone and a pure tone corresponding to the fundamental of the complex tone can be related to the small displacements of the peaks in the interspike interval distribution. His case can be made even stronger than he put It himself (Van Noorden, 1981). Further arguments are:

(1)   pitch of amplitude modulated noise (Houtsma et al. 1980) and the sweep-tone of mistuned consonances (Plomp, 1967a);

(2)   synchronization of nerve spikes to the phase of the pure tone waveform may be lost at the same frequency as chroma is lost (viz. at approximately 5kHZ): and

(3)   the remarkable constancy of a transposed interval in frequency ratio over the entire range up to 5 kHz, as is shown by Attneave and Olson (1971).

To explain this last result on the basis of the place code, one has to invoke a learning process that relates different distances on the basilar membrane for each melodic interval. This seems unlikely. On the other hand it is quite well possible to conceive of a mechanism that determines the ratio of time intervals independently of frequency region.

Although these considerations do not have the power of a proof, they suggest that it is worthwhile to study the possible role of time coding in pitch perception.

2.2   The Spike Interval Distribution

If we study the distribution of spike intervals we see that, up to 4 or 5 kHz, nerve spikes are synchronized to the stimulating wave-form at the point of the basilar membrane where the monitored nerve originates (Rose et al., 1967). However, this synchronization is not very precise. A spike does not exist (in a certain neuron) for every cycle of the periodic stimulus and the time of occurence of spikes is not coupled to a very narrow phase of the waveform. which means that each individual interval between two successive spikes does not tell us very much about the frequency or period of the stimulus. We must then consider the statistics of the spike interval distribution. Fig. 1 gives a schematic representation of a spike interval histogram (SIH) evoked by a pure tone as it has been measured in an animal (cf. Rose et al., 1967). Obvious characteristics of these histograms are:

(1)   There are peaks at nT, multiples of the period T of the tone.
(2)   The heights of the peaks decrease with increasing n.
(3)   There is an exception to rule 2 at the smallest time intervals. The SIH shows a short absolute refractory period in which no spikes are found and a relative refractory period in which the probability of firing recovers gradually.

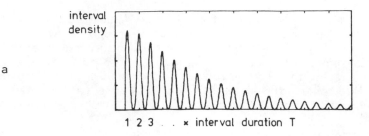

a

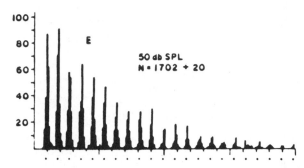

b

Fig. 1. (a)   The spike interval distribution in response to a pure tone of
1111 Hz in the auditory nerve of a squirrel monkey as measured by Rose et al. (1967) (by permission of the Journal of
Neurophysiology). (b) Schematic representation of the spike
interval distribution.

    The interval histogram registers the activity in a single nerve fibre.
Similar patterns of activity will be found in a large number of fibers. We
assume that at a certain level of perceptual processing the relevant information in the individual spike interval distributions are combined. The pitch
is associated to the peak pattern of the combined distribution as a whole.
However, this association even in the case of a pure tone is not always
unique. In situations with a very low signal to noise ratio and with the
attention of the observer directed at the relevant pitch range, the response
pattern is as if the listener reacts to the subharmonics of the pure tone
frequency (Houtgast, 1976). If one assumes that the auditory system
determines the relation between two pitches on basis of correspondence of
the peak pattern, it is easy to understand that there is a relatively large
correspondence between harmonically related tones, since in this case a
number of peaks will coincide.
    The occurrence of peaks at multiples of the stimulus period is a step in
the explanation of the origination of the low pitch of complex tones
(illustrated in Fig. 2). Say, the tone consists of the harmonics 3, 4 and 5.
These low harmonics will be resolved at the basilar membrane with separate
regions in which the pure tone components to a large extent determine the

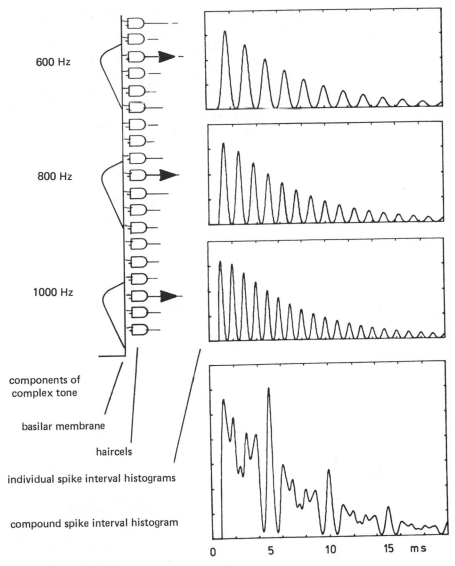

600 Hz

800 Hz

1000 Hz

components of
complex tone

basilar membrane

haircels

individual spike interval histograms

compound spike interval histogram

0   5   10   15   ms

Fig. 2.   Schematic representation of the origination of low pitch.

waveform. In this example the haircells produce an interval histogram of
the type shown in Fig. 1 and duplicated in the upper right corner of Fig. 2.
The pitch extractor combines the relevant feature of the interval histograms of a large number of neurons from different places along the basilar
membrane. A schematic representation of the resulting compound summed
histogram (CSIH) is shown in the lower right corner. The important feature
of this process is that the 3rd peak of the upper, the 4th peak of the middle
and the 5th peak of the lower histograms coincide. We therefore find a

relatively high peak at the shared subharmonic period and multiples thereof with a period corresponding to the low pitch of the complex tone.

It is clear that this description forms only a rough outline of a model. To be able to make quantitative predictions one should calculate the amplitude and waveform at each point along the basilar membrane and apply this to a haircell model in order to find the spike interval histogram in each nerve. At this stage of modeling however, it seems wise first to consider in the same qualitative way whether a number of the phenomena related to low pitch and other pitch phenomena do not contradict our ideas.

2.3 Existence Region of Low Pitch and Dominance of Components

To investigate whether there are indications that the distribution of spike intervals may play a role we have brought together some results of experiments concerning the pitch of complex tones (Fig. 3). These are:

(1) data on the range of complex tones that may give rise to low pitch (called the existence region of residue pitch, Ritsma, 1962);

(2) data on which harmonics of a complex tone are dominant in the determination of low pitch (Dominance region, cf. Plomp, 1976); and

(3) the existence region of chroma pitch.

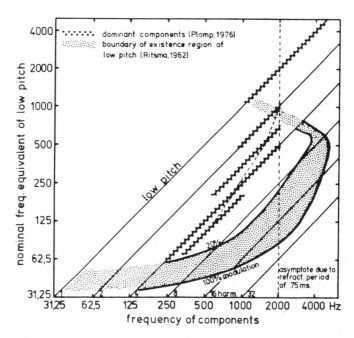

Fig. 3.   Some pitch phenomena in the range for which chroma exists.

Fig. 3 shows that low pitch from complex tones with 'missing fundamental' only exists for low pitches equivalent to frequencies below about 1000 Hz, while complex tones with fundamental frequency above this value have a tonal pitch (in the sense of Ritsma) only if the fundamental is present. This is in agreement with the data on the dominance in which the fundamental dominates at these high frequencies. For complex tones with frequencies below this 1000 Hz boundary the dominance region is situated around the 4th and 5th harmonic. In our opinion it is quite possible that this transition is related to the absolute and relative refractory periods found in the distribution of spike intervals. For the absolute refractory period values are found in the order of .75 ms, which means that the first peak in the spike interval histogram is completely occluded by the refractory period if the frequency is higher than 2 kHz (3/2 period = .75 ms). The fact that the dominance jumps from the first to the 4th or 5th harmonic indicates that the ear uses the highest peaks in the spike interval distribution, viz. those just beyond the refractory period. The fact that the dominance does not rise to higher harmonic values may be related to the pitch ambiguity that results from complex tones of only high harmonic number. This phenomenon is believed to determine the south east flank of the existence region together with the phenomenon of combination tones (Goldstein, 1973).

We are left with the question why tones with frequencies above about 2000 Hz to about 4500 Hz still have chroma pitch, although the first peak(s) fall within the refractory period. It is generally assumed that the spike interval distribution of these tones show a peak structure (sychronization). Since the first peaks are occluded by the refractory period and there will be several successive peaks about equally strong, the ear can only decide which chroma belongs to a tone if it gets some additional information, for instance from the place code. The fact that this additional information is obliterated in the case of the missing fundamental, may be the reason that a complex consisting of the frequencies 2000, 3000 and 4000 Hz does not have a tonal low pitch nominally equivalent to 1000 Hz.

It is difficult to estimate the weight of the contribution of a particular harmonic to the low pitch. It depends upon the number of interspike intervals the harmonic adds to the peaks in the CSIH corresponding to the low pitch. The level of the component, the harmonic number, the excitation pattern on the basilar membrane and the number of haircells among other factors have to be taken into account. It is clear that this estimation calls for a more precise model of the ear. We only want to make a suggestion concerning the role of the amplitude level of the component. If we study, for example, the measurements of Rose et al. (1967), we find that the stimulus level influences the form of the SIH. If the signal is just above the threshold of the nerve under consideration the height of the successive peaks decreases only very gradually. At higher levels the peaks fall off more rapidly. The mean firing rate increases by increasing the number of short interspike intervals at the cost of the number of long intervals. This means that the contribution of a weak component of a complex tone to the period of the fundamental frequency of the complex is relatively large. This mechanism may explain the fact that with stimuli for which it is difficult to perceive the low pitch, adjusting the level of the complex just above hearing thresholds helps to find the low pitch. (Terhardt 1976). It may explain also

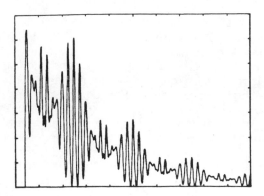

Fig. 4.   The compound spike interval histogram of harmonics 9, 10 and 11.

the fact that relatively weak combination tones contribute substantially to the determination of the low pitch (Ritsma 1970; Smoorenburg 1970).

2.4 Ambiguity of Pitch

The pitch of complex tones may be ambiguous. This means that two or more different pitches can be perceived depending upon the direction of attention of the observer. De Boer (1956) discovered the ambiguity in enharmonic complex tones, while Schouten et al. (1962) showed that the ambiguity is most prominent in complexes of only a few high components (for example: the 9th, 10th and 11th harmonic).

Fig. 4 indicates how the ambiguity can be understood on grounds of the CSIH. This histogram is constructed schematically on the naive assumption that the 9th. 10th and 11th component are resolved at the basilar membrane and contribute with equal weight. The diagram shows a multiplicity of peaks around 5, 10 and 15 ms. (In fact the group of five peaks around these values correspond to the five pitches that have been observed by Schouten et al., 1962, in this complex tone.) The fact that these components are not resolved at the basilar membrane does not change the CSIH dramatically, provided that the components have a certain phase relation. In this case the SIH of the individual nerve fibers will already show a peak structure similar to the CSIH of Fig. 4.

2.5 Some Small Pitch Shift Effects

There are number of small pitch shift effects that seem at first glance to contradict a time information model of pitch perception. How can, for instance, the pitch of a pure tone depend upon amplitude if pitch is based on time information? A possible place to look for an explanation for these effects is the absolute and relative refractory periods of the neurons. The refractory periods cause the peaks at the short side of the interval histogram not to be at an exact multiple of the stimulus period. A change in the amplitude of the tone may change the relative contribution of the various peaks to the pitch. The same mechanism could be responsible for octave enlargement (cf. Oghushi, 1978). Diplacusis may be explained by the assumption that the refractory period is not exactly the same for all neurons. The observed correlation between pitch shift and loudness fluctuations (Van den Brink 1970) and the predictbility of the diplacusis of the low pitch from the pitch of the components (van den Brink, 1975) would follow automatically.

2.6 Pitch of Amplitude Modulated Noise

There is considerable disagreement among investigators whether amplitude modulated white noise can elicit a pitch comparable with low pitch. Recently however, Burns and Viemeister (1976) showed that musical intervals between tones evoked by modulation of band limited or wide band noise can be recognized. The region of modulation frequencies where this is possible corresponds with the region of fundamental frequencies for which a low pitch can be determined. The recognition performance with AM noise, however, is lower than with pure tones (less salient).

This phenomenon can be understood on the assumption that this pitch is also determined by the CSIH. To understand how the histogram looks in the case of AM noise, one has to consider the period histogram of the spikes in the individual neurons first. The period histogram describes the firing probability as a function of the phase of the stimulus signal. The period histogram for a pure tone (sine wave) looks like a rectified sine wave because the firing probability is proportional to the momentary amplitude during one half period of the sine wave and is zero during the other half of the period. This long period of not firing is necessary in order to find, in the SIH, valleys between peaks that go down to zero (as in Fig. 1). If this period of not firing is shorter the valleys will be less deep. In the case of AM noise the period histogram is related to the modulating (envelope) waveform. The stochastic nature of the noise brings about that the firing probability is non zero everywhere the momentary envelope amplitude is non zero. For a 100% modulated white noise this occurs only for the short moment the envelope touches zero amplitude. The peak structure in the CSIH of AM noise will therefore be less salient.

The disagreement among the investigators about the question whether amplitude modulated white noise may elicit pitch may be due to the fundamental problem of how pitch sounds. It is easy to make the mistake of asking oneself, "can I hear a tone in AM white noise?" A perceived tone, however, is more than pitch alone. Even as a simple stimulus as a pure tones is a complex entity in perception, since there are elements such as loudness, roughness, direction, distance, volume, density, timbre and pitch of which the percept is built. We do not know whether or not an observer will perceive these elements separately. Since tone height is connected with the spectrum of the sound there is no reason to assume that AM white noise elicits this tonal element. If our assumption that chroma pitch is related to the time structure of the similus is right, it should be possible the AM white noise can mediate this pitch in a situation where chroma pitch can be perceived, such as in a musical context or in an experiment where musical intervals have to be identified. In the AM white noise case chroma pitch does not go together with the tone height quality.

2.7 Discussion

The pitch extracting mechanism of the auditory system can be con-ceived as a black box that transforms the input consisting of a complex of frequency components into the output, the frequency equivalent of the pitch of the complex. A mathematical model for this operation was described by Goldstein (1973). He assumed that the frequencies of the components are relayed to a decision mechanism through a noisy channel. The decision mechanism assumes that the frequency samples come from adjacent com-ponents of a harmonic complex and estimates in a theoretically optimal way the fundamental frequency for which the harmonics match the samples, after an estimation of the harmonic number has been made. Goldstein shows that a good agreement between theory and data can be achieved by assuming that the variance of the noise is a certain function of frequency. Taking Goldstein's theory as a framework, De Boer (1977) shows how the theories of pitch perception put forward by Wightman (1973a) and Terhardt (1974) can be considered as special cases of a generalized version of this theory, since their theories correspond with the cases for which the variance of the noise is large or small, respectively.

Our model is a suggestion how the ear performs the pitch extraction process and it does not contradict the above mentioned theories. It does, however, contradict the ideas of Wightman and Terhardt that the pitch extractor uses place code only and suggests an answer to the question Goldstein left open in his 1973 paper as to whether place or time code mediates the pitch extraction process. In a more recent paper, Goldstein and Srulovicz (1977) demonstrated that a model based on the spike interval histogram can explain the dependence of the just noticeable difference (jnd) of frequency on frequency and tone duration very well.

Our model and the latter finding lead back to earlier models of pitch perception (be it not all the way back) that assumed that the ear performs time analysis of the stimulus signal. On grounds of present knowledge of the peripheral ear, it cannot be assumed that all relevant information is present in a single neuron or a group of neighboring neurons (Wever volley principle; Ritsma 1962), since the dominant components are resolved at the basilar membrane and there is no particular preference of firing at intervals corre-sponding to the low pitch in individual neurons. The abundance of these intervals is found only in the CSIH.

The CSIH has some characteristics in common with the autocorrelation analysis of the signal as has been proposed by Licklider (1951, 1955) as a basis of pitch perception. It differs from the true autocorrelation function in the following ways:

(1)   If the signal is a pure sine wave the probability density function of the spike intervals is more like an autocorrelation function of the half wave rectified sine wave than of the sine wave itself (Duifhuis, 1971; Schroeder and Hall, 1974).

(2) The interval histogram is only an approximation of the autocorrelation function insofar as it is constructed in a limited time span. The stochastic process causes the longer intervals to be less numerous than the shorter ones (like a time window with an exponentially decaying weighting function).

(3) The influence of the refractory mechanism prevents the shortest intervals from occuring. This shapes the weighting function, on the short time interval side.

PITCH PHENOMENA IN THE LIGHT OF THE PHYSIOLOGICAL MODEL

To conclude the physiological considerations, we claim that it is quite possible for a tone presented to the ear to be analysed in (at least) two different ways. The characteristics of these channels can be brought into alignment with the two classes of perceptual pitch phenomena: tone height and chroma, as discussed in the first part of this paper. Tone height varies monotonically with frequency and is mediated by place code. Chroma shows characteristics that can be explained by the time code as the CSIH provides a mechanism that gives a special status to intervals like the octave, fifth, fourth, third and so on.

There is some similarity with the views held by Terhardt (1974) who assumes that in the perception of a pure tone a number of virtual pitches arise that are subharmonics of the tone under consideration. The peaks in the SIH correspond to these subharmonics. While Terhardt indicates how these subharmonics can explain the rules of harmony of music theory, and we agree with him in this respect, we do not agree with his explanation of how these virtual pitches arise in perception. Terhardt assumes that the auditory system has learned to recognize a set of components as a set of harmonics of a certain fundamental, because most natural sounds are harmonic complex tones. A pure tone component activates all pitches of which the stimulus could be a harmonic. If a number of stimulus tones all activate a certain pitch in common this will be the pitch of the complex. In our model, however, the subharmonics arise as a consequence of the probabilistic firing mechanism. In our opinion, it would have been possible for harmony to develop in a 'pure pure tone' world.

The two physiological codes provide a basis for understanding the phenomenon of absolute pitch, since absolute pitch observers may be able to use the time code dimension in addition to the place code dimension to make their identification of tones. The important question of why AP observers are able to do this and NAP are not, however, remains to be answered.

SUMMARY

The paper is a recapitulation of the findings in three areas of tone perception research, which have not often been confronted with each other in the past. These areas are: (1) absolute pitch; (2) pitch and timbre; and (3) pitch scaling, which teach us respectively that: (1) A number of observers can identify so many tones of different frequencies and with such an error pattern, that they must process tones along two channels; (2) Complex tones can vary in pitch and timbre quite independently; timbre is a multidimensional attribute of which sharpness is a main dimension; (3) Two pitch scales can be constructed depending on the observer's attention to the chroma or to the tone height dimension. This leads to the conclusion that a tone is analyzed along two basic pitch channels by the auditory system.

This two way perceptual analysis is brought in juxtaposition with what we know about the physiological analysis in the peripheral auditory system. A logical consistency appears if the tone height dimension is related to the tonotopical organization along the basilar membrane, and the chroma dimension to the temporal organization of spikes in the auditory nerves.

ACKNOWLEDGMENT

This paper is a further development of a series talks given at Bell Laboratories, Murray Hill, N.J.

REFERENCES

Attneave, F., 1959, "Application of information theory to psychology," Holt, New York.

Attneave, F., and Olson R.K., 1971, Pitch as a medium: A new approach to psychophysical scaling, Am. J. Psychol., 84:147-166.

Bachem, A., 1973, Various types of absolute pitch, J. Acoust. Soc. Am., 9:146-151.

Bachem, A., 1950, Tone Height and Tone Chroma as two differnt pitch qualities, Acta Psychologica, 7:80-80

Bachem, A., 1954, Time factors in relative and absolute pitch determination, J. Acoust. Soc. Am., 26:751-753.

Beck, J., and Shaw, W.A., 1961, The scaling of pitch, Am. J. Psychol., 74:242-251.

Bismarck, G. von, 1974, Sharpness as an attribute of the timbre of steady sounds, Acustica, 30:159-172.

Boer, E. de, 1956, "On the residue in hearing," Academic thesis, Amsterdam.

Boer, E. de, 1977, Pitch theories unified, in: "Psychophysics and Physiology of Hearing," E.F. Evans, and J.P. Wilson eds., Academic Press, London.

Brink, G. van den, 1970, Experiments on binaural diplacusis and tone perception, in: "Frequency analysis and periodicity detection in hearing," R. Plomp, and G.F. Smoorenburg, eds., Sythoff, Leiden.

Brink, G. van den, 1975, The relation between binaural diplacusis for pure tones and complex sounds under normal conditons and with induced monaural pitch shift, Acustica, 32:159-165.

Burns, E.M., and Viewmeister, N.F., 1976, Nonspectral pitch, J. Acoust. Soc. Am., 60:863-869.

Carroll, J.B., 1975, Speed and accuracy of absolute pitch judgments; some latter day results, Res. Bull., Educational Testing Service, Princeton.

Carvellas, J., and Schneider, B., 1972, Direct estimation of multi-dimensional tonal dissimilarity, J. Acoust. Soc. Am., 54:1839-48.

Drobisch, M.W., 1855, Abh. and Math. Phys, König. Sachs. Ges. Wiss. 4:1-120.

Duifhuis, H., 1972, "Perceptual Analysis of Sound," Thesis, University of Technology, Eindhoven.

Fulgosi, A. and Zaja, B., 1975, Information transmission of 3.1 bits in absolute identification of auditory pitch, Bull. Psychonomic Soc., 6:379-380.

Fullard, W., Snelbecker, G.F., and Wolk S., 1972, Absolute judgments as a function of stimulus uncertainty and temporal effects: Methodological note, Perc. and Motor Skills, 34:379-382.

Garner, W.R., 1962, "Uncertainty and Structure as Psychological Concepts," Wiley, New York.

Garner, W.R., 1972, "The Processing of Information and Structure," Wiley, New York.

Goldstein, J.L., 1973, An optinum processor theory for the central formation of the pitch of complex tones, J. Acoust. Soc. Am., 54:1496-1516.

Goldstein, J.L., and Kiang, N.Y.S., 1968, Neural correlates of the aural combination tone 2f1-f2, Proc. IEEE, 56:981-992.

Goldstein, J.L., and Srulovicz, P., 1977, Auditory nerve spike intervals as an adequate basis for aura frequency measurement, in: "Psychophysics and Physiology of Hearing," E.F. Evans, and J.P. Wilson, eds., Academic Press, London.

Harris, J.D., 1960, The scaling of pitch intervals, J. Acoust. Soc. Am. 32:1575-1581.

Houtgast, T., 1976, Subharmonic pitches of a pure tone at low S/N ratio, "J. Acoust. Soc. Am., 60:405-409.

Houtsma, A.J.M., and Goldstein, J.L., 1972, The central origin of the pitch of complex tones: Evidence from musical interval recognition, J. Acoust. Soc. Am., 41:520-529.

Houtsma, A.J.M., Wicke, R.W., and Ordubadi, A., 1980, Pitch of amplitude-modulated low-pass noise and predictions by temporal and spectral theories, J. Acoust. Soc. Am., 67:1312-1322.

Javel, E., 1972, "A Nurophysiological Investigation of Single Unit Responses to Some Periodic Complex Auditory Stimuli," Doctoral Thesis, University of Pittsburg.

Licklider, J.C.R., 1951, A Duplex theory of pitch perception, Experientia, 7:128-134.

Licklider, J.C.R., 1955, Auditory fequency analysis, in: "Proc. Third London Symposimum on Information Theory," C. Cherry, ed., Butterworth, London.

Marks, L.E., 1974, "Sensory Processes (The New Psychophysics), "Academic Press, New York.

Miller, G.A., 1956, The magical number seven, plus or minus two Psychol. Rev., 53:81-97.

Moore, B.C.J., 1973, Some experience relating to the perception of complex tones," Quart. J. Exp. Psychol., 25:451-475.

Moore, B.C.J., 1977, Effects of relative phase of the components on the pitch of three-component complex tones, in: "Psychophysics and Physiology of Hearing," E.F. Evans, and J.P. Wilson, eds., Academic Press, London.

Oghushi, K., 1978, On the role of spatial and temporal cues in the perception of the pitch of complex tones, J. Acoust. Soc. Am., 64:764-771.

Parker, S., and Schneider, B., 1974, Nonmetric scaling of loudness and pitch using similarity and difference estimates, Perc. and Psychophys., 15:238-242.

Patterson, R.D., and Wightman, F.L., 1976, Residue Pitch as a function of component spacing, J. Acoust. Soc. Am., 59:1450-1459.

Plomp, R., 1967a, Beats of mistuned consonants, J. Acoust. Soc. Am., 42:462-474.

Plomp, R., 1967b, Pitch of complex tones, J. Acoust. Soc. Am., 41:1526-1533.

Plomp, R., and Steeneken, H.J.M., 1971, Pitch versus timbre, Proc. 7th Int. Cong. Acoust., Budapest, 3:377-380.

Plomp, R., 1976, "Aspects of Tone Sensation," Academic Press, London.

Pollack, J., 1952, The information of elementary auditory displays, I, J. Acoust. Soc Am., 24:245-249.

Pollack, J., 1953, The information of elementary auditory displays, II, J. Acoust. Soc Am., 25:765-769.

Revesz, G., 1913, "Zur Grundlegung der Tonpsychologie," Veit and Company, Leipzig.

Ritsma, R.J., 1962, Existence region of the total residue I, J. Acoust. Soc Am., 34;1224-1229.

Ritsma, R.J., 1966, The 'Octave Deafness' of the human ear, IPO Annual Prog. Rep., 1:15-17.

Ritsma, R.J., 1967, Frequencies dominant in the perception of the pitch complex sounds, J. Acoust. Soc. Am., 48:191-198.

Ritsma, R.J., 1970, Periodicity detention, in: "Frequency and Periodicity Detection in Hearing," R. Plomp and G.F. Smoorenburg, eds., Sijthoss, Leiden.

Rose, J.E., Brugge, J.F., Anderson, D.J., and Hind, J.E., 1967, Phase-locked resonses to low-frequency tones in single auditory nerve fibers of the squirrel monkey, J. Neurophysiol., 29:769-793.

Schouten, J.F., 1938, The perception of subjective tones, Proc. Kon. Acad. Wetensch., 41:1086-1094.

Schouten, J.F., 1940a, The residue, a new component in subjective sound analysis, Proc. Kon. Acad. Wetensch., 43:356-365.

Schouten, J.F., 1940b, The residue and the mechanism of hearing, Proc. Kon. Acad. Wetensch., 43:991-999.

Schouten, J.F., Ritsma, R.J., and Cardozo, B.L., 1962, Pitch of the residue J.Acoust. Soc. Am., 34:1418-1424.

Schroeder, M.R., and Hall, J.L., 1974 Model for mechanical to neural transduction in the auditory receptor, J.Acoust. Soc. Am., 55:1055-1060.

Siegel, J.A. 1972, The nature of absolute pitch, in: "Studies in the Psychology of Music," Vol. 8, I.E. Gordon, ed., University of Iowa Press, Iowa City.

Siegel, J.A., 1974, Sensory and verbal coding strategies in subject with absolute pitch, J. Exp. Psychol., 103:37-44.

Siegel, R.J., 1965, A replication of the mel-scale of pitch, Am. J. Psych., 615-620.

Smoorenburg, G.F., 1970, Pitch perception of two frequency stimuli, J. Acoust. Soc. Am., 48:924-942.

Stanaway, R.G., Morley, T., and Anstis, S.M., 1970, Tinnitus not a reference
  signal in judgments of absolute pitch, Quart. J. Exp. Psych., 22:230-238.

Stevens, S.S., Volkmann, J., and Newman, E.B., 1937, A scale for the
  measurement of the psychological magnitude of pitch, J. Acoust. Soc.
  Am., 8:185-190.

Stevens, S.S., Volkmann, J., 1940, The relation of pitch to frequency: A
  revised scale, Am. J. Psych., 53:329-353.

Terhardt, E., 1974, Pitch, consonance and harmony, J. Acoust. Soc. Am.,
  55:1061-1069.

Terhardt, E., 1976, Ein Psychoakustisch begründetes Konzept der
  Musikalischen Konsonanz, Acustica, 36:121-137.

Ward, W D., 1953, Informaton and absolute pitch, J. Acoust. Soc. Am.,
  25:833.

Whitfield, I.C., 1967, "The Auditory Pathway," Monographs of the
  Physiological Soc., Arnold, London.

Wightman, F.L., 1973a, The pattern-transformation model or pitch, J.
  Acoust. Soc. Am., 54:407-416.

Wightman, F.L., 1973b, Pitch and stimulus fine structure. J. Acoust. Soc.
  Am., 53:417-426.

Zwicker, E., and Feldtkeller, R., 1967, "Das Ohr Als
  Nachrichtenempfänger," Hirzel, Stuttgart, 2nd ed.

Chapter XIV

SPECTRAL-PITCH PATTERN
A Concept Representing the Tonal Features of Sounds

Gerhard Stoll

Institute of Electroacoustics
Technical University, Munich
Munich, Federal Republic of Germany

INTRODUCTION

Recently the significance of tonal information for the sensation of timbre and pitch has been well recognized and emphasized. Accordingly a psychoacoustic concept was developed which enabled a quantitative description of that tonal information. This is the Spectral Pitch Pattern. Complex tones, as for example musical tones and voiced speech, possess not only fundamental pitch but, as is well known, also components such as harmonics, which can be 'heard out' as individual pure tones with corresponding pitches. This fact was extensively investigated and evaluated by Helmholtz (1863). The Spectral Pitch Pattern depicts these pitches and their relative salience.

The Spectral Pitch Pattern may be considered to contain the aurally relevant tonal information of any sound. It can be quantitatively described by ascertaining the sound pressure level excess LX, that is, the difference between the sound pressure level of one harmonic and that level which corresponds to the masking effect of all the other harmonics. A value LX<0 means that this component does not occur in the LX pattern and does not evoke an individual pitch sensation. The Spectral Pitch Pattern (SP pattern) consists of those components which possess a positive number of LX and evoke a spectral pitch. Subsequently the components are weighted depending on the spectral position and the number of LX.

PSYCHOACOUSTICAL SIGNIFICANCE OF THE SPECTRAL-PITCH PATTERN

The SP pattern has a fundamental significance for the perception of virtual pitch (or 'fundamental pitch'). A functional model of pitch perception of complex tones (Terhardt 1972a, 1972b) derived from the fact that virtual pitch is related to the spectral pitches of the partials. A numerical procedure for calculating the SP pattern and for a schematic and automatic extraction of virtual pitch from complex tonal sounds was proposed by Terhardt (1979a, 1979b). This procedure operates on the frequencies and amplitudes of the components of a complex tone. The extraction of virtual pitch is accomplished by the principle of subharmonic matching.

The LX pattern can also be applied to timbre. One part of a functional model for timbre differences of steady harmonic complex tones (Benedini, 1979) takes the tonal information into consideration; the calculation of timbre differences is based on those partials which can be resolved by the ear. The other part of the model uses the concept of sharpness (Bismarck, 1974), and describes the differences in timbre depending on different spectral envelopes of complex tones.

The LX pattern has another important role in ascertaining the pleasantness of sounds. The results of psychoacoustic experiments with common sounds, non-musical as well as musical (e.g. electric typewriter, electric coffee mill, church bell, musical chord, human voice), showed that the sensations of <u>tonalness</u>, <u>sharpness</u> and <u>roughness</u> had a significant influence on pleasantness (Terhardt and Stoll, 1980). (Tonalness characterizes the attribute of a sound to evoke more or less pitch strength). It was found that pleasantness was decreased by increasing sharpness and roughness, but increased with tonalness. For estimation of the quantitative value of the tonalness of a complex sound, the SP pattern is necessary.

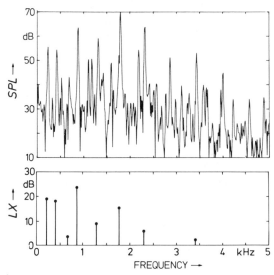

Fig. 1   Plot of the FFT spectrum (top) and the calculated LX pattern (bottom) of a church bell, manually excited with the original hammer and sound recorded in about 2m distance. The spectrum was calculated 40ms after the stroke. The peak SPL was set to 70 dB. The time interval of sampling was 80 ms. The LX pattern consists of 8 partials with the frequencies of 236 Hz, 426 Hz, 689 Hz, 883 Hz, 1314 Hz, 1798 Hz, 2321 Hz and 3437 Hz.

A quantitative evaluation of pitch salience based on the above described concept enables the determination of pitches of sounds which evoke more or less ambiguous pitch sensations. In the case of residue tones, musical chords, and other very complex sounds, one usually perceives several different pitches with different salience at once. For example, a residue tone evokes a virtual pitch corresponding to the fundamental frequency but in addition a pitch will be perceived with a salience corresponding to the lowest partial. Nonharmonic complex tones, such as bells and chimes, can contain many pitches, both spectral and virtual, of different salience. These effects can be considered with the aid of a recently developed computer program for quantitative evaluation of pitch (Terhardt et al., 1980). The essential part of this program is based on the amplitude spectrum. This new procedure predicts virtual as well as spectral pitches: thus a complete pitch analysis can be achieved by this program. The LX pattern is of fundamental significance, because the weights (salience) of the calculated pitches depend directly on the number, frequency, and quantitative value of LX of the resolved components. The example of a church bell demonstrates the results obtained by this computer program as well as the results of psychoacoustic measurements.

Fig. 1 shows the FFT spectrum of a church bell. Below, the calculated LX pattern is represented. Only 8 partials of this complex nonharmonic spectrum can be resolved by the ear. The components with the frequencies of 236 Hz. 426 Hz and 883 Hz can be perceived clearly, whereas the partials with the frequencies of 689 Hz and 3437 Hz for example can only be perceived faintly. In a psychoacoustic experiment the 'spontaneously' perceived pitches of this bell (as well as 16 others) was measured (Seewann and Terhardt, 1980). The sound of the bell was presented monaurally through earphones in random order with a loudness of 8 sones. After hearing the bell, the subjects had to match the frequency of a comparison tone (pure tone) with the pitch sensation of the test sound. The test sound and comparison tone pair were repeated until the subject was sure of his decision. Results of 18 subjects, some of whom were music students, are represented in Fig. 2, a pitch histogram containing 144 pitch matches. The results are described by the relative number of pitch matches (ordinate) within a frequency interval of 20% of the critical band, as a function of the center frequency of this interval. The pitch histogram shows 3 significant maxima: the centers of these maxima correspond to 215 pu, 435 pu, and 889 pu. The frequency of a pure tone with SPL of 60 dB (standard tone) is taken as a measure of the investigated pitch. So the value of the pitch units is identical with the frequency of this tone which evokes the same pitch as the investigated sound. Calculated pitches with the previously mentioned procedure and with a pitch weight ≥ 0.22 are also shown in this diagram. It is obvious that the 3 pitches with the highest pitch weights are practically identical with the answers of the subjects. These calculated pitches are 216 pu, 441 pu and 888 pu. It can be seen that the qualitative relationships between the three most prominent pitches obtained by the computer program and those obtained from the subjects are the same. Further it is obvious, by comparing Fig. 1 and Fig. 2 (note different axes!), that neither the most prominent predicted nor measured pitch correlates with the spectral pitch with the highest LX value, nor with the partial with the highest SPL of 70 dB.

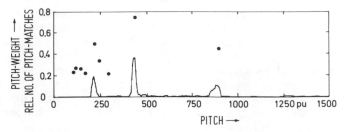

Fig. 2   Experimental pitch histogram of the church bell shown in Fig. 1 (relative number of pitch matches of 18 S's within an interval of 20% of the critical band), and the calculated pitch weights of virtual pitches (circles). Only those calculated pitches with a weight ≥0.22 are displayed.

VERIFICATION OF THE LX PATTERN BY PSYCHOACOUSTIC EXPERIMENTS

The first systematic experiments, after those of Helmholtz, on 'hearing out' the partials of complex tones were done by Plomp (1964) and Plomp and Mimpen (1968). They concluded from their results that only the first seven harmonics can be heard as individual pure tones.

The LX pattern of 4 different test sounds was experimentally invest-igated in the following way. The test sounds are: a complex tone with a low-pass filtered amplitude spectrum, and the vowels /a/, /ə/, and /i/. The vowels were generated by an electronic model of the vocal tract. The complex tone was produced by a pulse generator. All sounds had the same fundamental frequency of 200 Hz and they were low pass filtered at the twentieth harmonic. The higher harmonics of the complex tone were additionally attenuated with a special low pass filter to make sure that the acoustic intensity per critical band was constant. The sounds were presented monaurally through an electrodynamic earphone (Beyer DT 48) with a freefield equalizer and a sound pressure level of 60 dB.

The subjects had to detect the spectral pitch of the harmonics and were required to match a pure tone of variable frequency and sound pressure level to the individual pitches of the components of the test sound. The subject could vary the frequency of a pure tone by a voltage controlled oscillator (VCO) within a given interval which corresponded to the distance between two successive harmonics; that means that this range had the same value as the fundamental frequency. The starting point of the VCO was set so that the subject could match the pitch of only one harmonic. If the subject could match one harmonic, the frequency of the varied pure tone was registered with a frequency counter. If the subject was not able to hear one harmonic with the same pitch as the varied pure tone, a new starting point for matching another harmonic was given. The intervals were chosen randomly so that all the first 20 harmonics of the test sound could be matched in the same manner. The SPL of the comparison tone was adjusted to the level of the actually matched harmonic: thus the difference in loudness between the considered harmonic and the pure tone was reduced. Comparison tone and test sound were presented alternately, each for a duration of 1 sec with a short pause in between of 10 ms. After pause of 200 ms the pair was repeated until a match was accomplished, or 30 secs, the time maximally provided for each match, had elapsed. In one session all the first 20 harmonics could be matched twice. Three subjects with normal hearing took part in the experiments on 4 occasions on different days.

RESULTS

Fig. 3 shows the results in 4 sections, each comprising two diagrams. In the upper diagram of each section the physical spectra are represented by

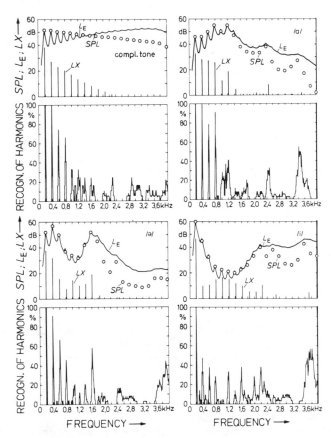

Fig. 3   Amplitude spectrum (circles), excitation level (drawn line), and calculated LX pattern (vertical lines) with pitch shifts of a complex tone and the vowels /a/, /ə/ and /i/, displayed in the upper diagrams (4 sections). The lower diagrams show the experimental pitch histograms obtained by 3 S's (relative number of pitch matches within an interval of 20% of the critical band).

circles. Also shown is a calculated representation of the excitation level L_E (Zwicker and Feldtkeller, 1967) with clear peaks at the lower harmonics and a broad maximum at the higher harmonics. In the present context only the LX pattern is relevant, since it is used to represent the relative pitch salience of every component. The positions of the vertical lines in the LX pattern on the abscissa indicate the spectral pitches. The pitches deviate numerically somewhat from the corresponding frequencies due to the effect of pitch shift by masking. With complex tones, the first harmonic usually decreases somewhat in pitch, while the higher harmonics increase in pitch. It is an advantage of our experimental method that these pitch shifts cannot produce artifactual results but are in fact taken into account. The numerical values of the pitch shifts vary somewhat from subject to subject. In the lower diagram of each section the experimental spectral pitch patterns are shown, that is, the relative number of probe tone matches to individual harmonics (ordinate), as a function of probe tone frequency (abscissa). The "relative number of probe tone matches" was obtained by summation of all the matches of the 3 subjects which fell in an interval of 20% of the critical band. A relative number of 100% means, for example, that the subjects matched successfully a particular harmonic within 30 seconds every time they were asked to do so.

For the complex tone, the calculated LX pattern shows a positive SPL excess of the first 11 harmonics. The first harmonic has the highest value - after this the SPL excess of the higher harmonics decreases. The pitch histogram shows that the first and second partials were recognized every time, and that the recognition rate for the higher harmonics decreased continuously. There is a high correlation with the calculated LX pattern: the correlation coefficient is 0.92.

For the vowel /a/, due to the formant structure the calculated SPL excesses for the first four harmonics are nearly identical. On the other hand, the 6th and 12th harmonics (which coincide with the 2nd and 3rd formants) can be easily recognized. In the experimental data the pitch shift of the 12th harmonic can also be seen. The center frequency of the distribution which belongs to this harmonic is clearly shifted somewhat towards higher frequencies. A remarkable number of pitch matches appear in the region around the 17th harmonic which coincides with the 4th formant. The correlation between experimental and calculated data is again high (0.93).

For the vowel /ə/ the first eight components evoke different saliences of the corresponding spectral pitches, in particular the 8th harmonic can be seen to have a relatively high SPL excess and a high experimental recognition rate. The experimental data show a broad maximum in the area of the 18th to the 21st harmonics which correlates very well with the 4th formant. The experimental results correlate with the predicted LX pattern with a correlation coefficient of 0.9.

For the vowel /i/ the SPL of the components lying between the first and second formants is rather low; thus there is much less masking in this frequency region. The corresponding spectral pitches are recognized relatively well, in spite of the low SPLs. The influence of the 4th formant on the experimental results is apparent in the region around the 18th harmonic, where a slight rise of the excitation level L_E takes place. The wide maximum in the experimental data reflects the fact that the pitch strength is not very well defined. The correlation between the calculated and experimentally measured pitch patterns is 0.7.

Our experimental results show that in the case of a complex tone with 200 Hz fundamental frequency, individual pitch recognition of the first 11 harmonics is possible. Significant differences between the vowels are to be seen, both with the calculated and with the experimentally measured spectral pitch patterns. Pitch matches above the 12th harmonic cannot be assigned to individual harmonics, but rather correspond to formants.

SUMMARY

The Spectral Pitch Pattern of a sound contains the relevant tonal information and consists of those components which can be heard as individual pure tones. First there is discussed the significance of the SP pattern for timbre and virtual pitch, and an example of the SP pattern of a church bell is given. In the second section psychoacoustic experiments to verify the SP pattern are described. The patterns of the vowels /a/, /ə/, /i/ and a complex tone were measured by subjects and the results compared with calculated data, obtained by a program which takes the relevant tonal information out of the physical amplitude spectrum.*

AKNOWLEDGMENT

Many thanks are expressed to M. Seewann and W Krafft for their assistance in working out the spectral analysis and psychoacoustic data. I am also grateful to E. Terhardt and S. Kemp for providing several valuable comments. This work was carried out at the Sonderforschungsbereich 50 Kybernetik, Munich, supported by the Deutsche Forschungsgemeinschaft.

REFERENCES

Benedini, K., 1979, Ein Funktionsschema zur Beschreibung von
    Klangfarbenunterschieden, Biol. Cybern. 34:111.
Bismarck, G. von, 1974, Sharpness as an attribute of the timbre of
    steady sounds, Acustica, 30:159.
Helmholtz, H. L. F. von, 1863, "Die Lehre von den Tonempfindungen
    als physiologische Grundlage für die Theorie der Musik," F. Vieweg &
    Sohn, Braunschweig.
Plomp, R., 1964, The ear as a frequency analyzer, I, J. Acoust. Soc. Am.,
    36:1628.
Plomp. R., and Mimpen, A.M., 1968, The ear as a frequency
    analyzer, II, J. Acoust. Soc. Am., 43:764.

---

* Sounds illustrating this chapter are presented in the recording included with this book. (See Appendix for details.)

Seewann, M., and Terhardt, E., 1980, Messungen der wahrgenommenen
        Tonhöhe von Glocken, in: "Fortschritte der Akustik" (DAGA '80),
        Munich, VDE-Verlag, Berlin.
Terhardt, E., 1972a, Zur Tonhöhenwahrnehmung von Klängen I.
        Psychoakustische Grundlagen, Acustica, 26:173.
Terhardt, E., 1972b, Zur Tonhöhenwahrnehmung von Klängen, II. Ein
        Funktionsschema, Acustica, 26:187.
Terhardt, E., 1979a, Calculating virtual pitch, Hearing Research,
        1:155.
Terhardt, E., 1979b, On the perception of spectral information in
        speech, in: "Hearing Mechanisms and Speech," Springer-Verlag,
        Heidelberg.
Terhardt, E., and Stoll, G., 1981, Skalierung des Wohlklangs von 17
        Umweltschallen und Untersuchung der beteiligten Hörparameter,
        Acustica, in press.
Terhardt, E., Stoll, G., and Seewann, M., 1981, Quantitative
        evaluation of pitch and pitch salience for complex tonal signals,
        submitted to J. Acoust. Soc. Am.
Zwicker, E., and Feldtkeller, R., 1967, "Das Ohr als
        Nachrichtenempfänger," Hirzel-Verlag, Stuttgart.

Chapter XV

SPECTRAL FUSION AND THE CREATION OF AUDITORY IMAGES

Stephen McAdams

Stanford University School of Medicine
and Center for Computer Research in Music and Acoustics
Department of Music, Stanford University
Stanford, California, USA

SUMMARY

The auditory system participates in the forming of images evoked by acoustic phenomena in the world around us. An important aspect of the imaging process is the distinguishing of different sound sources. Since the peripheral auditory system performs a spectral analysis on the incoming composite signal, mechanisms must exist to group spectral components according to their respective sources and to affect a kind of perceptual fusion of spectral components arising from the same source. There may be innate mechanisms and mechanisms acquired through experience in the world that have criteria for "deciding" whether a particular constellation of dynamic acoustic elements is likely to constititute a sound source. Of particular interest for music composition are the ways in which these mechanisms operate with respect to ambiguous acoustic information, the ways a listener can be beckoned beyond the boundaries of established patterns of perceiving. These have implications for the realms of "possible" perception.

INTRODUCTION

In order to be able to form images of sounds in the environment the auditory system must be able to decide which sound elements belong together, or come from the same source, and which elements come from different sources. I will address some of the issues involved both with the perceptual fusion of sound elements into a single source image and with the separation or distinguishing of different simultaneous images.

Asking the question "what cues are associated with perceptual fusion" is only asking a subset of the questions which ask what cues are associated with the formation of auditory images. Some images have unitary and unequivocal perceptual attributes regardless of the number of individual spectral components of which they are composed. These are strongly fused images. Others have dispersed or equivocal attributes, such as the constellation of pitches evoked by the sound of a church bell. But the pitches in this constellation still seem to belong together and can be perceived or conceived as a single image. Imaging proceeds as a kind of collecting of things that "belong together". The image emerges as a representation of this collection of the parts of a sounding body distributed across time and frequency.

'Belongingness' is a conceptual tool originally invoked by the Gestalt psychologists (Koffka, 1935; Kohler, 1947). I use it here to name a family of rules of relations that any given sensory/perceptual system uses to group things into functional units. However, these are not rigid rules which box the sensory world into non-mutable objects. The domain of the artist and composer is one which challenges the predominant sensory patterns and evokes (among other things) the conscious transformation of perception by directing or beckoning one's attentional focus to different levels of form and structure in the work. What may at one moment be an 'object' of focus for a listener may at another moment be an element collected into a composite image, wherein the object loses its identity but contributes to the quality of the more embracing image.

I.   FUSION

Nearly all of the sounds we encounter in the world can be analyzed into many frequency components which vary in frequency and amplitude over time. The auditory periphery performs such an analysis within certain limits of temporal and spectral resolution. However, we normally perceive such a complex sound as a whole rather than as many parts. We might say, then, that ordinary listening is SYNTHETIC rather than ANALYTIC, in the sense that it groups things together. This process by which simultaneous things are grouped into single entities may be called the process of PERCEPTUAL FUSION.

Why might it be useful for the auditory system to behave like this? Many types of sounds arise from objects we encounter repeatedly over the course of our lives. And these sounds usually behave in a fairly predictable fashion for each generating source. That is, the way the components of a source signal evolve individually and the way they maintain certain relationships remains reasonably constant from one occurrence to the next. We then categorize and recognize all of the constituent parts together, often even naming them as a group, such as an oboe tone, my father's voice, the word 'tone'. This kind of categorization results in a reduction of the amount of stored information that is necessary to represent the source in memory.

In addition, most of the biologically relevant sources of acoustic information we encounter are physical systems. These will behave under certain constraints which yield predictable patterns. For example, forced-vibration systems such as the voice and most musical instruments each have predictable resonances in their spectra and all have a series of partials that very closely approximate the harmonic series.

This consideration of the nature of the sources that are significant in our acoustic environment and of our relationship to them has led me to consider three kinds of cues that seem to contribute to the perceptual fusion of complex tones. These are:

1)   the harmonicity of the frequency content of a tone,

2)   the coordinated modulation of the spectral components, and

3)   the relative familiarity of the spectral envelope.

Certainly other cues are involved to some extent, but my research leads me to believe these are the most efficacious cues.

Harmonicity

There is a great deal of psychoacoustic and physiological research which indicates that the auditory system is biased toward the processing of harmonic, as opposed to non-harmonic, sounds. Psychoacoustic pitch research reveals that the most unitary and unequivocal pitch sensation results from harmonic complexes (de Boer, 1976). Various kinds of non-harmonic complexes have been found to yield multiple pitch sensations, often with three of more distinct pitches (de Boer, 1976; Cohen, 1980). As previously observed, many of the most relevant sources we deal with are harmonic, so it would not be surprising to find that the auditory system is biased toward interpreting harmonic signals as representing single sources and that non-harmonic signals might confound this interpretive mechanism in some predictable way. Two of the three pitch processing models currently in vogue (Goldstein, 1973; Terhardt, 1974;) invoke a hypothetical HARMONIC TEMPLATE-MATCHING MECHANISM assumed to operate somewhere in the central auditory nervous system. (Wightman's 1973 model is based on an autocorrelation mechanism which, nevertheless, gives very similar results in many cases.) The output corresponding to a given template would represent a given pitch and the magnitude of its output would correspond to the relative strength of the pitch sensation. The important property of such a template is that a harmonic signal best matches it and creates the least ambiguous pitch sensation. However, a non-harmonic signal might partially match to several templates, thereby creating multiple pitch sensations of various strengths depending on the degree to which each match was made. There is some physiological evidence for the existence of such harmonic signal identifiers (Katsuki, 1961; Keidel, 1974).

The harmonicity of a signal is a strong factor in the perceived fusion of a tone complex. Harmonic tones fuse more readily than non-harmonic tones under similar conditions and the degree to which non-harmonic tones do fuse is dependent upon their spectral content. In all of the studies on fusion to be discussed below, four types of spectral content were used:

(a)   harmonic series: $f_n = nF_o$

   where   n is the number of the partial, n = 1, 2, 3, . . . ;
            F_o is the fundamental frequency (n = 1);
            f_n is the frequency of partial n.

(b)   shifted harmonic series: $f_n = (n + k) F_o$

where k is the proportion of F_o by which each partial is shifted.

This may be written as $f_n = nF_o + kF_o$

A constant frequency is added to that of each harmonic partial. This stimulus has been used extensively to study the 'pitch shift' effect beginning with de Boer (1956).

(c)   stretched harmonic series: $f_n = n^s F_o$

where s is the stretch factor, s >1. This factor is most easily conceived of as s = log(b) / log(2), where b is the ratio to replace the standard octave ratio (2:1) of the harmonic series. For example, for b = 2.1, s + 1.07 and the partial ratios are 1, 2.1, 3.24, 4.41, etc.

(d)   compressed harmonic series: $f_n = n^s F_o$

where s is the compression factor, s 1. For example for b = 1.9, s = 0.93 and the partial ratios are 1, 1.9, 2.77, 3.61, etc. The series specified by

$$f_n = n^s F_o$$

has been used to study pitch perception, fusion and the perception of musical harmony (Slaymaker, 1970; Mathews and Pierce, 1980; Cohen, 1979).

The interest in these types of inharmonicity is that they represent a regular, predictable transformation of the harmonic spectral pattern and yet they do not exhibit the same property of having phase-locked partials as with harmonic partials. This points again to a certain uniqueness of the harmonic series and has implications for the parallel processing of spectral and temporal representations of the acoustic environment in the auditory nervous system. With harmonic signals, there would be a concurrence between a spectral pattern recognition mechanism and a temporal periodicity extraction mechanism. But with the non-harmonic signals described here, these two kinds of processing mechanisms would provide disparate results to a processor that tried to combine their respective outputs. This may be partly responsible for the equivocal response elicited by these sounds with respect to their perceived pitch and fusion.

As the sound is transformed to be less like the purely harmonic case, there is a decrease in the perceived fusion. To test this, four tone complexes with 16 partials, a fundamental frequency of 200 Hz, identical spectral envelopes and differing frequency contents, as described, were compared with respect to fusion. The harmonic tone was perceived as the most fused followed by stretched (s = 1.07), compressed (s = 0.93), and shifted (k = 0.5) tones, respectively. As there is a growing interest in the use of non-harmonic sounds in computer music composition, this area of research may help to map out some of the perceptual effects that are possible when these types of sounds are used in musical contexts.

Coordinated Frequency Modulation

The next major class of cues contributing to fusion that I will discuss includes three types of frequency modulation (small frequency perturbations) found in natural sources such as the voice and the wind and string instruments. The types I have studied include:

(a) periodic frequency modulation (vibrato),

(b) random frequency modulation (shimmer), and

(c) very slow frequency modulation as found in inflectional changes in the voice or expressive pitch changes in musical instruments (portamento).

Such perturbations are most likely to occur in physical forced-vibration systems wherein any perturbation of the driving force will result in perturbations of the spectral components that are proportional to their frequency. This has the effect of maintaining constant frequency ratios among the partials. It would not be surprising to find that the auditory system is adept at recognizing this kind of signal as a single entity. In fact, the importance of maintaining constant ratios for a fused percept has been shown by Bregman et al. (1978).

My interest in the temporal factors that mediate fusion was initiated by Michael McNabb and John Chowning at the Center for Computer Research in Music and Acoustics (C.C.R.M.A.). They demonstrated that a harmonic tone complex whose spectral power distribution conforms to that of a given vowel elicits a rather weak sensation of a voice (and exhibits a weak perceptual fusion) unless a small amount (0.5 - 2% of the component frequency) of vibrato and/or shimmer is superimposed on all of the spectral components simultaneously. The contrast between voice spectra with and without the modulation is very compelling. It seems that at least some modulation is required for strong fusion to occur. Without modulation, there can always be some analytic listening, or attending to individual spectral components.

This coordinated modulation is the strongest cue for the fusion of complex tones, particularly when combined with a familiar spectral envelope (see next section). In these studies, the four frequency content types (harmonic, shifted, stretched and compressed) were compared both with and without coordinated modulation, which took the form of either a combined vibrato and shimmer or a portamento function. Two spectral envelopes were used, the more familiar vowel (a), as in 'father', and the less familiar +6 dB/octave slope.

The frequency and amplitude of the vibrato and the center frequency, bandwidth and amplitude of the shimmer were adjusted to achieve a life-like singing vowel quality for the vowel spectral envelope. For these types of modulation the amplitude parameter controls the actual extent of modulation in frequency of the component upon which the function is being imposed. These values were then used with the less familiar envelope. As expected, the more familiar envelope fused better than the less familiar one. Also, the ordering of the frequency content types with respect to degree of fusion was the same as in the previous study. The increase in fusion with vibrato of all of the tones with the more familiar envelope was substantial, even for the non-harmonic tones. There was also an increase in fusion with vibrato for the less familiar envelope but the change was not nearly as dramatic as for the vowel envelope. This suggests that there is a strong interaction between the effects of the spectral shape and the coordinated modulation of the components. It may be that different values for the vibrato and shimmer parameters affect fusion differently for various spectral envelopes, and may also affect the relative degree of fusion for different types of inharmonicity. The perceived fusion was also strong with portamento, which seems to be even more effective in causing non-harmonic tones to fuse than the combined vibrato and shimmer.

The means by which these sounds have been generated should be noted at this point since it bears on the acoustic relation between the spectral envelope and the modulation functions. A computer synthesis 'instrument' was developed during the summer of 1980 at the Institut de Recherche et de Coordination Acoustique/Musicque (I.R.C.A.M.) in Paris by David Wessel and myself. This additive (Fourier) synthesis instrument allows for the specification of the spectral envelope entirely independent of the instantaneous frequency content. This means that as each frequency component is being modulated, in whatever fashion, its amplitude is being looked up on a sample-by-sample basis in a table that contains the spectral envelope (essentially a transfer function). If vibrato is being superimposed on a frequency component which lies on a steep slope of the spectral envelope, then a modulation in amplitude accompanies the frequency modulation. Also, if a long portamento is superimposed, the continually changing amplitudes of the partials 'trace out' the shape of the spectrum over the course of their modulation. This process is closely akin to the functioning of the voice (Lewis, 1936) and various musical instruments, and may serve as an important cue for the unequivocal identification of the spectral envelope. So any sort of frequency modulation of sufficient amplitude under these conditions could serve to accentuate the effect of the familiarity of the spectral envelope.

As mentioned previously, the fact that the components move in parallel, maintaining constant frequency ratios, is an important cue from the standpoint of the behavior of many natural sources. It is worth noting that the initial mapping of the frequency spectrum into the auditory system via the basilar membrane roughly corresponds to a logarithmic scale. This means that constant ratios maintain constant distances along the basilar membrane. Further, it has been shown repeatedly that this 'spatial' organization of the frequency domain in the auditory system is maintained (to some extent) as far as primary auditory cortex (see for example: Evans, 1975 - auditory nerve and cochlear nucleus; Guinan et al., 1972 - superior olivary complex; Roth et al., 1978 - inferior colliculus, Aitkin and Webster, 1971 - medial geniculate body; Merzenich et al., 1975 - auditory cortex). There is a marked regularity and richness of connections in the anatomical organization of many of the higher processing centers in the central auditory nervous system. It is easy to imagine that there are mechanisms which would respond to a regular and coordinated pattern of activity distributed over an array of cells and fibers in this system as the neural information proceeds from the periphery and branches out to many of these centers. It would not be possible, however, with present technology to make direct physiological measurements in hundreds or thousands of inter-connected cells and fibers simultaneously. Yet it is quite apparent that such a regularity in the sound has a substantial effect on the perception of sources.

Familiarity

Another major cue contributing to spectral fusion appears to be the familiarity of the spectral envelope. In other words, the fusion process seems to be especially sensitive to the shape and location in the frequency spectrum of resonance peaks characteristic of sounds we frequently encounter, such as formant bands in voice sounds and the broad resonances of various musical instruments (Strong and Clark, 1967). In fact, the auditory system is so sensitive to the frequency location of formant bands of the voice that the sensation of a given vowel is lost by merely transposing the spectral envelope up a major third (multiply every frequency by 1.25 and keep the relative amplitudes the same). Note that when a voice sings a major third higher, the formant frequencies change relatively little com-pared to the frequency components themselves. It would not be surprising, then, to find that the auditory nervous system can evaluate the shape of the spectral envelope of a source independently of its evaluation, at any given moment, of the presence of the frequency components whose amplitudes are shaped by that spectral envelope. This ability implies that the auditory system can 'recognize' (i.e. something in the system responds to the presence of) a particular overall pattern in the amplitudes of response of each more or less frequency-specific nerve fiber. This neural mechanism may be innate or it may be acquired through experience with the source.

Tones with more familiar spectral shapes, such as those from voices, seem to fuse more readily than more unfamiliar spectral shapes, such as a flat spectrum or a spectrum with a +6 dB/octave slope. If we assume that fusion implies the auditory system has decided that "this constitutes a reasonable source", then these results suggest that one of the criteria for fusion is that the spectral envelope be of a class of previously encountered spectral envelopes. It seems possible that the voice is a special case in this respect since the spectral shape is crucial to the identification of vowel sounds.

There are many other features aside from harmonicity and spectral envelope that contribute to familiarity, such as the relative rates of growth and decay of individual partials. Some of these have been addressed by Grey and Moorer (1977), and seem to be more important than the spectral enve-lope shape for the identification or recognition of many musical instrument sounds.

Conclusions Concerning Fusion

These results suggest that difficulties may arise in the creation of novel sources by computer music synthesis. If the sounds are too unfamiliar, they may not be perceived as single entities. However, with more systematic study, it may be possible to map out what kinds of transformations of familiar sounds will still yield unitary percepts. Then again, those areas of sound that do not allow easy fusion may also be pertinent to the composer with interests in playing the 'spectral field' as a whole rather than in playing specific 'instruments'. These issues will be discussed later.

None of these three classes of perceptual cues occurs in natural sources without the simultaneous presence of the others. I would expect that they interact with each other in complex ways to contribute to the total percept of a fused source. If familiarity or recognizability, in general, is a cue for the formation of auditory sources, then all of these factors may contribute to fusion by contributing to the predictability of the sound's behavior. This would imply that the combinations of these various factors that induce a fused image may be fairly restricted and specific. Further investigation is needed to test this notion. But as a general rule, it seems certain that fusion depends on the meeting of certain criteria by the sound as a whole. If it is 'decided' that enough criteria are met for the signal to constitute a reasonable source, fusion occurs. This 'decision' may be made by dynamic pattern recognition processes which use both innate and learned templates that model the spectral and temporal properties of relevant acoustic events in our environment and which would necessarily be such that a new inter-pretation of the nature of the source would result if new, conflicting information were obtained. This new interpretation would result in a new source image. I will present evidence in the next section that suggests that this is indeed the case.

II. PARSING

Let us now consider the processes by which we separate, or parse, two or more sources that are present simultaneously. In his seminal work on auditory psychophysiology, Helmholtz (1885) noted that

> ...when several sonorous bodies in the surrounding atmosphere simul-taneously excite different systems of waves of sound, the changes of density of the air, and the displacements and velocities of the particles of the air within the passages of the ear, are each equal to the alge-braical sum of the corresponding changes of density, displacement and velocities, which each system of waves would have separately produced, if it had acted independently. (p.28)

He suggested that the problem becomes one of determining the means possessed by our sense organs to analyze the composite whole into its original constituents. Take a typical example. You are listening to a mono-phonic recording of a symphony orchestra. There is a single pressure wave emanating from a single source of sound: the loudspeaker. And yet what do you hear? Although the distinction is not as good as it would be were you sitting in the concert hall, it is still easily possible to separately hear many of the instruments playing simultaneously. This occurs even though one of the strongest cues of source distinction is removed. Specifically, the instruments in an orchestra do not occupy the same physical location, so all of the localization cues which can normally be used to aid in forming separate source images are missing. Much research has investigated the nature of auditory grouping processes responsible for the parsing of rapid sequences of sounds into auditory 'streams' where a stream is the psychological representation of a source. This means that a stream could be an image of an actual or virtual source. (See McAdams and Bregman, 1979, for a review of research on auditory stream formation.)

I wish to discuss the cues that play a role in the separation of simultaneous sources. This is a phenomenon that is understood only incompletely. No man-made analysis system has succeeded in parsing more than three simple sources and yet the auditory system is remarkably sensitive and accurate in this respect. It does have its limits, however. Listen to the large sound masses played by the strings in Penderecki's "Threnody for the Victims of Hiroshima" and ask yourself how many individual instruments there are playing simultaneously in that section. Certainly you can identify that there are 'many', but 'how many' is difficult to determine because the sounds are all so closely related that they obscure one another and are not individually distinguishable. This is a perceptual manifestation of the dictum "1,2,3, infinity" !

I have identified several possible kinds of cues that may play a role in source parsing, or the formation of multiple, simultaneous source images. Three of these will be discussed here including:

(1)   tone onset asynchrony,

(2)   asynchrony of onset of coordinated modulation for different source spectra, and

(3)   the temporal correlation among the modulations belonging to separate sources.

Another area that will eventually need to be addressed is the frequency proximity of spectral components between separate sources.

Tone Onset Asynchrony

The onset of a given source and the distinction of its onset from those of other sources is an important cue for the fusion of components of that source and for the parsing of separate source images. As Helmholtz (1885) observed about fusion,

> When a compound tone commences to sound, all its partial tones commence with the same comparative strength; when it swells, all of them generally swell uniformly; when it ceases, all cease simultaneously. Hence no opportunity is generally given for hearing them separately and independently. (p. 60)

Modern research would modify this statement, but there are characteristic onset patterns for individual instruments that maintain certain relations among the growth and decay patterns of individual partials. Here again we have a kind of parallel action of several components being used as a criterion for their belonging together and possibly arising from the same source. It would seem that if such a criterion were used, the asynchronous onsets of subsets of components, which belong to separate sources, might provide sufficient information to parse them appropriately. Let us turn to Helmholtz again, who states that

> ...when one musical tone is heard for some time before being joined by the second, and then the second continues after the first has ceased, the separation in sound is facilitated by the succession of time. We have already heard the first musical tone by itself, and hence know immediately that we have to deduct from the compound effect for the effect of this first tone...(p. 59)

It has been verified experimentally that asynchrony of onset of the partials in two or three component steady-state tones decreases the degree to which they fuse into a single image. Bregman and Pinker (1978) presented a stimulus composed of a sine tone alternating with a two-component tone in which the synchrony of the components was varied. Asynchrony values of 0, 29 and 58 msec. were used. One result of the study was that an increase in the asynchrony of the components in the complex tone was accompanied by a decrease in the tendency for those components to fuse. Dannenbring and Bregman (1978) measured the tendency for asynchronous components in three-tone complexes to segregate. Asynchronies of 0, 35 and 69 msec. were used. Again, with greater asynchrony, more segregation and less fusion were perceived. Rasch (1978) measured masking thresholds of the higher component in asynchronous two-component tones and found less masking and greater ease in the perception of individual components with greater asynchrony. Asynchronies of 0, 10, 20 and 30 msec. were used. For synchronous tones, masking thresholds were in the range of 0 to -20 dB (relative to the intensity of the lower component). For an asynchrony of 30 msec., the threshold was as low as -60 dB. These low thresholds appeared to be independent of non-temporal features of the tones and were thus ascribed to asynchrony.

Grey and Moorer (1977) have found that there are small asynchronies in the onsets of different partials in musical instrument tones. This might seem to contradict the evidence above. However, these asynchronies are generally less than about 20 msec. and there is often a significant amount of onset noise that might mask any minor differences in relative time of onset. It seems that variation in the relative onset times of individual harmonics within this small time period affects the perceived quality of the attack characteristic as a whole while the tone remains fused. Tone onset asynchrony is a useful technique in musical practice for distinguishing certain 'voices', and it is obvious that this cue is used with great versatility by many jazz and classical soloists. Also, Rasch (1979) has described how asynchronization allows for increased perception of individualized 'voices' in performed ensemble music which also may be used in multi-voiced instruments such as the piano and guitar. Across these studies, asynchrony values in the range of 30-70 msec. have been found to be effective in source parsing. No studies of which I am aware have been reported which have tested the effect of asynchrony on separability of complex, time-varying sources.

Onset Asynchrony of Modulation

In the previous examples, the asynchrony of onset of a source image is a cue that contributes to the ability to separate it from other concurrent source images, even if these are merely sinusoidal source signals. As was implied in the discussion on fusion, a complex tone without modulation can, under certain conditions, be perceived as a composite of many sinusoidal 'sources'. When coordinated modulation is introduced (and certain other criteria for fusion are met), these components may then fuse and be perceived as one source, i.e. they all form a unitary image. If the modulation, for example, vibrato, is introduced gradually, there is a transformation from a percept of many simple sources to one complex source (at least in the case of harmonic complexes). This perceptual transformation occurs very quickly even though the physical transformation may take up to a second. This suggests that the processes that synthesize source images are continually comparing the 'current' image(s) with the new information from the environment and when enough information has been acquired to indicate that this interpretation is no longer valid, a new synthesis is effected and new source image(s) formed. In the above example, once the vibrato has reached a sufficient amplitude to inform the source image 'synthesizer', the 'synthesizer' reinterprets the information and forms a new image. It takes a while for this to occur, but when it does, it occurs rather quickly. (See also Bregman, 1978b, for a discussion of the cumulative nature of the formation of auditory streams.)

Now consider what this might tell us about the role of fusion in the distinction of many simultaneous sources. Sounds have been created in which all 16 harmonics of each of three different spectral subsets began simultaneously, but without any kind of modulation. Each subset had a spectral envelope of the vowel (a), and the fundamentals formed an augmented chord with the lowest fundamental at 200Hz (ca. A-flat below middle-C). This is perceived as a large tone mass with many different pitches, but with no apparent harmonic structure or vocal quality. Then, combined vibrato/shimmer functions (with amplitudes as before) were gradually imposed on each of the subsets in succession beginning with the subset with the lowest fundamental. The vibrato frequencies were 6 and 6.5 Hz and the random shimmer functions were independent. As each modulation function began, the associated group of partials fused into a singing male voice and was segregated from the rest of the background tone mass. This occurred with each subset in succession and the tone mass was no longer the dominant percept after the last voice fused. Also, there was a strong percept of a chord of three distinct pitches composed of a tonic tone, major third and augmented fifth. A similar sound was synthesized using stretched partials (s = 1.07) and stretching the fundamental relationships by the same factor as well. The perception of an evolution from tone mass to three distinct voices with three respective pitch/timbres was equally strong as for the harmonic stimulus. This suggests that even non-harmonic tones can be fused if an appropriate context is constructed.

Two notions are of interest here. The perceptual result of imposing the modulation on a subset of the tone implies that fusion plays a crucial role in the parsing of a sub-group of components from a larger group. Also, this moment of fusion can be considered as a kind of perceptual onset of a particular source image. The moment the components of a sub-group fuse, they are distinguishable from the rest as in independent image. If these three spectral subsets are imaged as sources at different moments, it may increase the ease with which they are segregated, making this situation similar in effect to an actual asynchrony of tone onsets.

A plenitude of musical possibilities is implied by this property of the source-image forming process. Some of the implications for music composition will be discussed later, but consider the possibilties for decomposing and recomposing a large number of spectral components into various source images with various kinds of modulation functions: a mass of partials that constitutes a puzzle with many different and interdependent parsing possibilities.

Temporal Correlation

The last parsing factor I will discuss, and one I believe to be particularly indicative of a class of cues that allows us to hear separate sources, is the temporal correlation between the modulating functions of separate source spectra. Most natural sources, whose signals are derived from forced-vibration systems, have some sort of modulation, and this has been shown to contribute to the perceived naturalness when such sounds are resynthesized by computer (Grey and Moorer, 1977). Complexes of rigidly unvarying sinusoidal signals only occur in laboratories. If the modulation functions for these spectra are independent, i.e. uncorrelated, it is likely that they derive from different sources. Conversely, if they are perfectly correlated, the most reasonable interpretation is that there is just one source. It is also logical that situations with intermediate correlation should yield ambiguous percepts. In the stimuli described in the previous section, the modulation functions were uncorrelated. This certainly was a key factor in preserving the segregation of sources initially signalled by their different times of modulation onset.

In an informal listening experiment the two extremes, perfect correlation and zero correlation, were investigated. In three different 16-component tones, the components were grouped into 8 even-numbered and 8 odd-numbered components and the correlation between their respective vibrato/shimmer functions was varied, i.e. the functions were either perfectly correlated (identical) or were uncorrelated (independent of one another). Three different types of frequency content were used: harmonic, shifted and stretched. A familiar spectral envelope, vowel (a̱), was used to enhance the fusion of each group of components. A stimulus was developed in which a gradual transition was made between perfectly correlated and uncorrelated modulation functions (combined vibrato and shimmer). Uncorrelated vibrato frequencies differed by 0.5 Hz and independent random waveforms were used for the shimmer components of the two modulation functions. The stimuli were 4 seconds long. For 1.5 seconds all 16 partials received modulation function A(f,t). Between 1.5 and 2.5 seconds, a gradual trading of modulation functions A(f,t) and B(f,t) was made for either the even or the odd partials, while the others continued to be modulated by A(f,t). Thus the separate functions modulating the two sets of components during this 1-second interval were partially correlated. At the 2-second point, halfway into the stimulus, the set of partials undergoing the transition had a modulation function composed of half of A(f,t) and half of B (f,t).

$$\text{Vib}_1(t) \;=\; A(f,t)$$

$$
\begin{aligned}
\text{Vib}_2(t) \;&=\; A(f,t), \quad\quad \text{for } 0 \le t \le 1.5, \\
&=\; (2.5 - t)\, A(f,t) + (t - 1.5)\, B(f,t), \quad \text{for } 1.5 \le t \le 2.5, \\
&=\; B(f,t), \quad\quad \text{for } 2.5 \le t \le 4,
\end{aligned}
$$

where

$$
\begin{aligned}
A(f,t) \;&=\; .015 f \sin(12\pi t) + .008 f \text{Ran}_1(t), \\
B(f,t) \;&=\; .015 f \sin(13\pi t) + .008 f \text{Ran}_2(t), \text{ and}
\end{aligned}
$$

Ran(t) is a uniform random waveform as described previously.

The perceptual result with harmonic stimuli is striking. The initial percept is one of a singing vowel with vibrato and a distinct pitch. At a point approximately halfway into the stimulus, a 'new' voice enters one octave above the original. This occurs regardless of whether the odd or even harmonics undergo the transition. This is an intriguing and seemingly paradoxical finding. In the case where the new modulation function is imposed on the even harmonics, a new source image is formed whose pitch and timbre derive from that spectral subset. However, the timbre of the odd subset is unaffected. It continues unperturbed while a new voice 'joins' it at the octave. Note that no new components have been added. The existing ones are merely parsed differently due to similar, yet independent, modulation functions superimposed on the spectral subsets. So while half of its harmonics are parsed into a separate source and assigned a pitch based on the spectral subset composed of the even harmonics, the contribution of those harmonics is not subtracted from the timbre of the original tone. This indicates either (1) that the even harmonics are still contributing to the original timbre, even after parsing, in which case they are contributing to two timbres, or (2) that the process that synthesizes timbre and then updates that interpretation when conflicting information is received, did not receive what it considered to be conflicting information and continued with the original interpretation. The case where the new modulation function is imposed on the odd harmonics is even more confusing. The same percept results as in the former case, i.e. a new voice is added at the octave and the original timbre is unchanged. Even though the modulation function on the odd harmonics changes, these appear to create a continuous, unperturbed tone; and while the modulation function on the even harmonics does not change, these appear to create a new voice when the odd harmonics are parsed into a different source. What is baffling in this case is the continuity of the original timbre. If there appeared to be some sort of break in the original tone and another tone of similar pitch and timbre appeared in concert with a new tone at the octave, it would be somewhat easier to explain.

(A similar kind of phenomenon was found by Rand (1974), who synthesized a stimulus such that part of the sound for the syllable da was sent to one ear and the rest sent to the other ear. The syllable was not perceived when either ear was presented alone. But when the sound parts were presented to both ears, one heard both a da and a sort of 'chirp' which resulted from the fragment of sound in one of the ears. The thing to note is that the 'chirp' sound was contributing to both the percept of the da and of the 'chirp'. This result would support the first hypothesis above. The implications for one sound contributing to more than one percept will be discussed in the next section.)

The effect of parsing the even and odd partials for non-harmonic tone complexes is very vague and unclear as compared with the harmonic partials. It may be possible to find appropriate parsings of the various kinds of non-harmonic complexes which will yield substantial changes in pitch. The fact that a reinterpretation of pitch can be mediated by source parsing, has interesting ramifications for modern pitch theories and for auditory perception in general.

III. THE BOUNDARIES OF 'ALLOWABLE' PERCEPTION

> Often I am permitted to return to a meadow
> as if it were a scene made-up by the mind,
> that is not mine, but is a made place
>
> that is mine, it is so near to the heart
> an eternal pasture folded in all thought
> so that there is a hall therein
>
> that is a made place, created by light
> wherefrom the shadows that are forms fall.
>
>   - Robert Duncan
>   from   "Often I am permitted
>   to return to a meadow"

I have suggested several factors that appear to contribute interactively to the perceptual fusion of a number of spectral components into a unitary image. These factors include the coordinated modulation of the spectrum, the harmonicity of the spectral content, and the familiarity of the spectral envelope. Learning and previous experience may play an important role in the fusion process, which is to say that perceptual grouping may be based on dynamic pattern recognition processes that have been acquired or modified by experience. This suggests that the fusion process serves to group those acoustic components together that constitute a 'reasonable' source. These pattern recognition processes may operate on at least the three dimensions indicated above, and certainly these dimensions interact with each other as far as recognizability and fusion are concerned.

Pattern recognition processes may be conceived of as 'templates' of classes of sources that are encountered in the environment. This kind of template does not represent a static 'object' with which it can be directly compared. Rather, it represents a class of rules of relations among and coordinated transformations of elements of a source characterizing a family of particular instances of a type of object. In this sense, what we deal with as a particular object in the environment really implies a process of relationship between the object and the perceiver of that object. The richness of these rules of source formation allows for the perception of invariance. A clarinet remains a clarinet regardless of its orientation in space, i.e. spatial orientation is one kind of transformation rule used in the visual system. And a clarinet tone remains a clarinet tone regardless of the register or the intensity being played, i.e. with experience, we learn the kinds of transformations in spectral relations within a clarinet tone that can accompany register changes, loudness changes, and so on.

But these rules also imply certain limits to our perception with respect to what we 'allow' ourselves to perceive. People have the tendency to confine their perception within the bounds of these learned rules rather than 'stretching' their perceptual abilities to meet with novel acoustic organization such as are found in 'new' music or 'old' music of other cultures. Listening to these musics requires an evolution of one's perceptual patterns.

Another implication of the fusion studies relates to the distinction made by Helmholtz (1885) between synthetic and analytic listening. When no modulation is superimposed on a complex tone, it is possible, within the limits of spectral resolution for steady tones, to 'hear out' individual spectral components, that is, it is possible to perceptually analyze the signal. When doing this kind of listening, one hears what Terhardt (1974, 1979) has termed the 'spectral' pitches of a tone complex. When attempting to listen to the tone as a whole, composite perceptual aspects such as the timbre and 'virtual' pitch(es) become apparent. This requires a certain kind of perceptual synthesis of elemental components in the signal. When we hear more dynamic sounds which have modulation, synthetic listening is much easier and more predominant and analytic listening becomes very difficult. In fact, with tones from wind and string instruments, it is virtually impossible to hear harmonics individually unless the instrumentalists play long steady tones and minimize any sort of modulation as much as possible (Erickson, 1975, Chap. 2). The emphasis on blending of individual instruments into larger timbral structures in the music of the late nineteenth and much of the twentieth century indicates the possibilities for using synthetic listening, though the tendency is for the auditory system to resist fusing these different sources.

With synthesized music we can now play with these two kinds of listening by composing the grouping or segregation of musical elements which may then present many simultaneous possibilities of organization for the listener. Some of the factors I have delineated as being important for the grouping of simultaneous sources are the asynchrony of onsets of source images (including actual tone onsets or the 'onset' moment of fusion of a newly formed source) and the temporal correlation among the modulation functions associated with different sources.

The ability to separate acoustic sources in the environment has obvious biological significance. The deer needs to separate the sounds of his munching on grass from those of an approaching predator. We need to separate the voice of a talking friend from the sounds of an oncoming truck. But these grouping processes do allow for some ambiguity which makes them rich as conceptual tools for source building and source transformation in music composition.

A notion that derives from the properties of source image formation is one proposed by Bregman and Pinker (1978): perceptual attributes, such as pitch and timbre, are assigned to sources. This implies that the source formation process first separates specific subsets of the spectrum that constitute different sources. Then pitch and timbre building processes (and perhaps loudness processes to some extent) operate on these parsed spectral subsets. It further implies that components grouped in one source cannot contribute to the perceptual attributes in another source (Bregman, 1978a). This is a nice notion but things are a bit more complicated than that. The principle seems to hold fairly well for the processing of the pitch of harmonic signals, but non-harmonic signals are not so easily dealt with in this way since they present a confusing picture to the pitch processor(s) in the first place. Also, with the stimulus discussed previously where the even and odd harmonics were gradually parsed into two sources with pitches an octave apart, some listeners observed that there was <u>not</u> a concomitant change in the timbre of the original source. There may be some mechanism in operation here whose criteria for reinterpretation of perceptual attributes of the source were not met.

> We are baby lives
> until we die
> -locked
> within some space-
> until
> some system wraps
> itself around
> our twisting, turning
> motion
> and tells us through
> the limitations
> that we are tied.
>
> BUT still we know
> that all conceptions

of boundaries

                                        are   -Michael McClure
                                        lies.   from "Antechamber"

Another area of richness for music that is implied by these grouping processes concerns the notion of the 'boundaries' of auditory objects. These boundaries may be considered in terms of the perceptual/cognitive structures underlying their perception (Miller and Carterette, 1975). The dimensional structures underlying the perception of timbre and pitch as determined by multidimensional scaling techniques have been described by Grey for timbre (1977; Grey and Gordon, 1978) and by Shepard and Krumhansl for pitch (Shepard, 1964, 1980; Krumhansl, 1979; Krumhansl and Shepard, 1979). For example, Grey has described a three-dimensional structure for timbre where each dimension is considered to represent an orthogonal perceptual dimension contributing to the perceived similarity of the timbres of different sounds. Grey used the tones of common Western musical instruments. Shepard claims that 'distance' in this geometrical representation of perceptual/cognitive 'space' represents the degree of dissimilarity such that identical sounds have the same location in the structure and very dissimilar sounds are far removed from one another. An instrument such as the clarinet, would be defined by a region occupied by the sounds of this instrument in a combined pitch/timbre space. This would represent all of the pitch/timbre possibilities of that instrument. No acoustic instrument could encompass the entire, possible space. Each instrument would have a bounded region, though there is certainly the possibilitiy that different instruments' regions would overlap. Those instruments with a wider pitch range and more timbral versatility would occupy larger or even multiple regions.

These instruments usually elicit unitary images, so these regions represent a range of possible pitch/timbre percepts for fused sources. Consider now the possibility of having elements of one pitch/timbre 'point' embedded in those of another. The resulting percept could be transformed by the context of a parsing process such that a gradual transition from one point in the space to two other points could be realised. This would correspond to a transformation from the combined image to the two individual images. This would represent a sort of non-linearity in the structure. The transformation is not perceptually continuous, but neither is it noticeably discontinuous. At some point after a pre-conscious transformation has taken place, one becomes aware of new presences in the music. This would imply the possibility of musically dissolving 'instrument' boundaries or 'voice' boundaries by means of sound synthesis. Perhaps with versatile and sensitive performers, some of these transitions could be made acoustically as well.

The possibilities for continual transformation of the spectrum in ways such as this present the opportunity to move away from the limited (bounded) conceptions of pitch and timbre. Changes in the grouping of a complex spectral field can result in very rich perceptual changes. Myriad fleeting images can continually be emerging from and submerging into one another. There can be a real subtlety of effect of a source image as in the light sources in the art of William Blake and Claude Monet. One is not struck by the identity or recognition of the source itself in these works. One is more drawn into the process of form-becoming of that which is illuminated by the source.

Awaking into song a discovery of a voice that we don't own, a voice coming through us. I give-up 'my' voice in order that the world may sing through me. To stand naked in the music is to let it enter our pores, to wash over pre-conceptions of what we think the music is. Listening taking place in-the-world (an actual world where there is music) to know where the music is, where 'we' are in the music, where the music is in 'us' is to come-to-our-senses, to find the music again.

Christopher Gaynor

In music, we move away from a concept of melody as a simple or complex succession of pitches and/or timbres. We move toward melody as a complex evolving organism given life by the active organizing of the time-varying spectrum by the listener. We may never have the ability to predict the experience of any listener since a lot of what is perceived by an actively attentive listener ultimately depends on what the listener brings to the music as well as what the music brings to the listener. The composer creates a universe within which the listener can create musical worlds and forms. The composer enfolds a universe, the listener unfolds a new music and is unfolded by a new music with each coming-into-being of the sounds of that universe.

Hearing is a dynamic process which engages a listener actively in interacting with the environment, not merely with the analysing and storing of acoustic information. We hear a world "as if it were a given property of the mind / that certain bounds hold against chaos." (Robert Dunco). We can limit our hearing of the world it is possible to hear, or we can allow ourselves to hear the possible in the world. "What is the realm of allowable perception?" is a question beyond the scope of this chapter, but one well worth contemplating. As William Blake has written in "The Marriage of Heaven and Hell:"

If the doors of perception were cleansed every thing would appear to man as it is, infinite.
For man has closed himself up, till he sees all things thro' narrow chinks of his cavern.

ACKNOWLEDGMENT

Much of the work reported here was done at the Institut de Recherche et de Coordination Acoustique/Musique (I.R.C.A.M), Centre Georges-Pompidou, Paris, France. I would like to thank David Wessel, Gabriel Weinreich, Andrew Gerszo, Marc Battier and the staff of I.R.C.A.M. for their valuable assistance in the development of the synthesis procedures and for helpful discussions and insights. I would also like to thank John Chowning, Christopher Gaynor, Earl Schubert and Rudolf Rasch for illuminating discussions of the concepts dealt with here and for characteristically thorough critiques of the manuscript. The author is supported by a National Science Foundation Graduate Fellowship. C.C.R.M.A. is supported in part by grants from the National Endowment for the Arts and the National Science Foundation.

This work is the subject of the author's doctoral dissertation research and represents (among other things) a preliminary report of work in progress.

REFERENCES

Aitkin, L.M., and Webster, W.R., 1971, Tonotopic organization in the medial geniculate body of the cat, Brain Res., 16:402-405.

Blake, W., ca. 1793, "The Marriage of Heaven and Hell," reproduction publ., 1975, Trianon, Paris.

Boer, E. de, 1956, Pitch of inharmonic signals, Nature, 178:535-536.

Boer, E. de, 1976, On the 'residue' and auditory pitch perception, in: "Handbook of Sensory Physiology", Vol. V/3, W.D. Keidel and W.D. Neff, eds., Springer-Verlag, Vienna.

Bregman, A.S. 1978a, Auditory streaming: Competition among alternative organizations, Perc. and Psychophys., 23:391-398

Bregman, A.S., 1978b, Auditory streaming is cumulative, J. Exp. Psychol./Human Perc. Perf., 4:380-387.

Bregman, A.S., McAdams, S., and Halpern L.D., 1978, Auditory segregation and timbre. Presented at the meeting of the Psychonomic Society, San Antonio, Texas.

Bregman, A.S., and Pinker, S., 1978, Auditory streaming and the building of timbre, Can. J. Psychol./Rev. Can. Psychol., 31:151-159.

Chowning, J.M., 1980, Computer synthesis of the singing voice, in: "Sound Generation in Winds Strings Computers," Royal Swedish Academy of Music Publication No 29, Kungl. Musikaliska Akademien, Stockholm.

Cohen, E., 1979, Fusion and consonance relations for tones with inharmonic partials, J. Acoust. Soc. Am., 65:S123(A).

Dannenbring, G.L., and Bregman, A.S., 1978, Streaming vs. fusion of sinusiodal components of complex tones, Perc. and Psychophys., 24:369-376.

Duncan, R., 1960, "The Opening of the Field," New Directions, New York.

Erickson, R., 1975, "Sound Structure in Music," University of California Press, Berkeley.

Evans, E.F., 1975, Cochlear nerve and cochlear nucleus, in: "Handbook of Sensory Physiology," Vol. V/2, W.D. Keidel, and W.D. Neff, eds., Springer-Verlag, Berlin.

Gaynor, C., 1980, Personal communication.

Goldstein, J.L., 1973, An optiumum processor theory for the central formation of the pitch of complex tones J. Acoust. Soc. Am., 54:1496-1516.

Grey, J.M., 1977, Multidimensional perceptual scaling of musical timbres, J. Acoust. Soc. Am., 61:1270-1277.

Grey, J.M., and Gordon, J.W., 1978, Perceptual effects of spectra modifications on musical timbres, J. Acoust. Soc. Am., 63:1493-1500.

Guinan, J.J., Norris, B.F., and Guinan, S.S., 1972, Single auditory units in the superior olivary complex. II: Locations of unit categories and tonotopic organization, Int. J. Neurosci., 4:147-166.

Helmholtz, H., 1885, "On the Sensations of Tone as a Physiological Basis for the Theory of Music," transl. by A.J. Ellis from the 1877 German edition, facs. ed., 1954, Dover, New York.

Katsuki, Y., 1961, Neural mechanisms of auditory sensation in cats, in: "Sensory Communication," W.A. Rosenblith, ed., Wiley, New York.

Keidel, W.D., 1974, Information processing in the higher parts of the auditory pathway, in: "Facts and Models in hearing," E. Zwicker, and E. Terhardt, eds., Springer-Verlag, Berlin.

Koffka, K., 1935, "Principles of Gestalt Psychology," Harcourt & Brace, New York.

Kohler, W., 1947, "Gestalt Psychology," Liveright, New York.

Krumhansl, C.L., 1979, The psychological representation of musical pitch in a tonal context, Cog. Psychol., 11:346-374.

Krumhansl, C.L., and Shepard, R.N., 1979, Quantification of the hierarchy of tonal functions within a diatonic context, J. Exp. Psychol./Human Perc. Perf.,5:579-594.

Lewis, D., 1936, Vocal resonance, J. Acoust. Soc. Am., 8:91-99.

Mathews, M.V., and Pierce, J.R., 1980, Harmony and nonharmonic partials, J. Acoust. Soc. Am., 68:1252-1257.

McAdams, S., and Bregman, A., 1979, Hearing musical streams, Comp. Mus. J., 3(4):26-43.

McClure, M., 1977, "Antechamber, and Other Poems," New Directions, New York.

Merzenich, M.M., Knight, P.A., and Roth, G.L., 1975, Representation of chochlea within primary auditory cortex in cat, J. Neurophys., 38:231-249.

Miller, J.R., and Carterette, E.C., 1975, Perceptual space for musical structures, J. Acoust. Soc. Am., 58:711-720.

Rand, T.C., 1974, Dichotic release from masking for speech J. Acoust. Soc. Am., 55:678-680.

Rasch, R., 1978, The perception of simultaneous notes such as in polyphonic music. Acustica, 40:21-38.

Rasch. R., 1979, Synchronization in performed ensemble music, Acustica, 43:121-131.

Roth, G.L., Aitkin, L.M., Anderson, R.A., and Merzenich, M.M., 1978, Some features of the spatial organization of the central nucleus of the inferior colliculus of the cat, J. Comp. Neurol., 182:661-680.

Shepard, R.N., 1964, Circularity in judgments of relative pitch, J. Acoust. Soc. Am., 36:2346-2353.

Shepard, R.N., 1980, Structural representations of musical pitch, in: "The Psychology of Music," D. Deutsch, ed., in press.

Slaymaker, F.H., 1970, Chords from tones having stretched partials, J. Acoust. Soc. Am., 47:1569-1571.

Strong, W., and Clark, M., 1967, Synthesis of wind-instrument tones, J. Acoust. Soc. Am., 41:39-52.

Terhardt, E., 1974, Pitch, consonance and harmony, J. Acoust. Soc. Am., 55:1061-1069.

Terhardt, E., 1979, Calculating virtual pitch, Hearing Res., 1:155-182.

Wightman, F.L., 1973, The pattern-transformation model of pitch, J. Acoust. Soc. Am., 54:407-416.

Chapter XVI

THE PERCEPTUAL ONSET OF MUSICAL TONES

Joos Vos[1] **and Rudolf Rasch**[2]

[1]*Institute of Perception*
 Soesterberg, Netherlands
[2]*Institute of Musicology, University of Utrecht*
Utrecht, Netherlands

INTRODUCTION

The perceptual onset of an acoustic stimulus such as a musical tone or a speech syllable can be defined as the moment in time at which the stimulus is first perceived. The physical onset, however, can be defined as the moment at which the generation of the stimulus has started. Generally the perceptual onset is delayed in relation to the physical onset. The time difference between physical and perceptual onset is caused, among other factors, by the fact that most music and speech stimuli are not immediately at their maximum level, but begin with a gradually increasing amplitude. At the very beginning of the physical stimulus its level is too low to attract the conscious attention of the listener. Only after the amplitude has increased to a certain level does the listener become aware of the presence of the stimulus. This first portion of an acoustic stimulus is called the rise portion. It is temporally defined either as a time interval between the physical onset and the moment that the maximum level is reached (this definition is used for percussive sounds) or as the time interval between the physical onset and the moment that a level of 3 dB below maximum level is reached (this definition is used for non-percussive sounds). The durations of rise portions are within the range of 5 to 100 msec in most cases and depend on the kind of instrument, on the frequency of the tone played, and on the way the player is starting the tone (Luce and Clark, 1965; Melka, 1970).

Adequate description of the perceptual onset is very useful in psycho-acoustical experiments designed to investigate the effects of temporal structure. Thus in dichotic listening experiments, at least a certain amount of variance can be eliminated if the manipulation of the temporal order of the stimuli is expressed in perceptual onset asynchrony instead of physical onset asynchrony (see Marcus, 1976). The same possibly holds for diotic and dichotic temporal order judgments. Again, in the performance of ensemble music, perfect (subjective) synchronization is only realized when the perceptual onsets of the simultaneous tones in different voices coincide (Rasch, 1979). Also in research on the production of isochronous rhythm patterns it should be taken into consideration that the musician isochronizes the perceptual onsets of the tones (Michon, 1967; Vos, 1973; Gabrielsson, 1974). The concept might also contribute to the understanding of prosody, an important factor in models of speech recognition. Finally, perceptual onset is probably a relevant parameter in the synthesis of music and speech by means of electronic devices.

During the last decade a number of investigations relevant to the question of the perceptual onset of an acoustic stimulus have yielded some models that describe perceptual onset as a function of stimulus parameters.

In Schuette's model (1977, 1978 a, b) perception is simulated by a first-order RC integrator circuit (leaky integrator), which is characterized by its time constant T. Inputs are tones with physical envelope functions and outputs are subjective envelopes. Schuette defined the perceptual onset of a tone as the moment at which the subjective envelope passed a certain percentage of its maximum value. It should be emphasized that in this model a variable threshold is used which depends on the physical envelope and tone duration.

Efron (1970a, 1970b, 1970c), however, in a coherent set of experiments on the relationship between the objective and subjective duration of a stimulus, found that perceptual onset was independent of stimulus duration.

In his 1970b experiments, Efron asked his subjects to report whether the onsets of two dichotically presented stimuli were simultaneous or not. The duration of the tone burst was fixed, the duration of the noise burst was varied and the level of the noise burst was adjusted to maintain equal loudness. From experiments using another method (Efron, 1970a), as well as from experiments using cross-model simultaneity judgments (Efron, 1970c) the same conclusion was drawn, ie. that stimulus duration is not relevant.

In the context of speech production and perception, the psychological moment of occurrence, termed the perceptual center (P-center) of syllables has been studied by Marcus (1976), Morton, Marcus and Frankish (1976), and Fowler (1979). Morton et al. (1976) assumed that P-centers are a property of the acoustic make-up of the stimulus, although they failed to uncover a relevant marker for it.

Fowler (1979) however, questions the significance of models that describe P-centers as a function of articulation-free acoustical parameters. According to Fowler (1979) a plausible hypothesis about P-center identity can be formulated in articulatory terms, that is, by differentiating between features like voicing, place of articulation (e.g. labial, velar, alveolar, palatal) and manner of articulation (e.g. plosives, fricatives, nasals). Marcus (1976) described the P-center in a two parameter finite-state model. This model involves an acoustic correlate of vowel onset (Peak Increment), together with stimulus onset and offset. Stimulus onset and offset are defined as the time at which the temporal envelope of the signal intersects a threshold of about 30 dB. Peak increment and its associated time of occurrence were defined as the largest increment in spectral energy between consecutive time slices in a frequency band from 400 Hz to 1500 Hz.

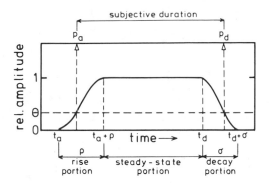

Fig. 1.   Temporal envelope of a musical tone, divided into three successive portions. The perceptual onset (p_a) of the tone is defined
as the moment at which the temporal envelope passes relative
threshold amplitude θ. The perceptual offset (p_d) of the tone,
although of minor importance in this study, can be defined in a
similar way.

A Simple Threshold Model Containing the Perceptual Onset of Musical Tones

The experiments to be described in this paper were designed to apply a
simple threshold model to the perceptual onset of musical tones. The
physical temporal envelope of a musical tone can roughly be divided into
three successive portions, the rise, the steady-state and the decay portions
(see Fig. 1). As a function of time the temporal envelope $E(t)$ can be
described as follows:

$$E(t) = R \left(\frac{t - t_a}{\rho}\right). \qquad t_a \leq t \leq t_a + \rho \qquad \text{rise portion}$$

$$E(t) = 1 \qquad\qquad t_a + \rho \leq t \leq t_d = t_a + \delta \qquad \text{steady-state portion (1)}$$

$$E(t) = D \left(\frac{t - t_d}{\sigma}\right). \qquad t_d \leq t \leq t_d + \sigma \qquad \text{decay portion}$$

in which $E(t)$ = temporal envelope

$\qquad\qquad$ $R(t)$ = relative rise function

$\qquad\qquad$ $D(t)$ = relative decay function

$\qquad\qquad$ t_a = physical onset (beginning of rise portion)

$\qquad\qquad$ t_d = physical offset (beginning of decay portion)

$\qquad\qquad$ ρ = rise time (duration of rise portion)

$\qquad\qquad$ σ = decay time (duration of decay portion)

$\qquad\qquad$ δ = tone duration (= $t_d - t_a$)

The relative rise function describes the evelope during the rise portion with the rise time ρ as time unit and the maximum amplitude as amplitude unit. This means that it is only defined for $0 \leq t' \leq 1$ (t' equals $(t - t_a)/\rho$). If the rise function $R(t) = v$ (v is relative amplitude) is monotonically increasing, then the inverse function $R^{-1}(v) = t$ is unambiguous. Throughout this paper, we will regard rise functions as monotonically increasing functions.

The relative decay function is defined in the same way as the relative rise function.

In our model, the perceptual onset of a tone p_a is the moment at which the temporal envelope during the rise portion passes a certain relative threshold amplitude θ:

$$R \left(\frac{P_a - t_a}{\rho} \right) = \theta \tag{2}$$

in which $\quad p_a \quad$ = perceptual onset
$\qquad\quad \theta \quad$ = relative threshold amplitude

If p_a is known, θ can be calculated with the held of equation (2). If θ is known, the perceptual onset can be calculated with the help of

$$R^{-1}(\theta) = (P_a - t_a) / \rho$$

or $\tag{3}$

$$P_a = R^{-1}(\theta) \cdot \rho + t_a.$$

In the same vein, the perceptual offset p_d is defined as the moment at which the decay portion of the temporal envelope crosses the relative threshold amplitude, which may or may not be the same as the threshold amplitude of the perceptual onset. The subjective duration of a tone is the time interval between the perceptual onset and offset of a tone.

The following paragraphs, describing an extension of our model will only deal with the perceptual onset.

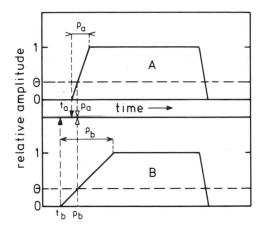

Fig. 2.   Temporal structure of a perceptually synchronous stimulus, containing tones A and B with physical onsets t_a and t_b, rise times ρ_a and ρ_b and maximum amplitude 1. The perceptual onsets p_a and p_b coincide in time and are by definition located at the moment at which the temporal envelopes pass threshold amplitude Θ.

The model can be extended to groups of tones, either simultaneous or successive ones. Two tones are called <u>perceptually synchronous</u>, when their perceptual onsets coincide in time. Thus, for two tones A and B that are perceptually synchronous, as is illustrated in Fig. 2 with physical onsets t_a and t_b, rise functions R_a and R_b, rise times ρ_a and ρ_b, and maximum amplitude 1, the perceptual onsets p_a and p_b coincide, so that

$$P_a = R_a^{-1}(\Theta) \cdot \rho_a + t_a = P_b = R_b^{-1}(\Theta) \cdot \rho_b + t_b$$

or   (4)

$$R_a^{-1}(\Theta) \cdot \rho_a - R_b^{-1}(\Theta) \cdot \rho_b = t_b - t_a.$$

This equation has only one unknown parameter, the relative threshold amplitude . The other terms are known in an experimental situation either as independent or as dependent variables. So it is possible to determine the relative threshold amplitude with the help of this equation. If the rise functions and rise time are identical ($R_a = R_b$, $\rho_a = \rho_b$), the perceptually synchronous condition results in $t_a = t_b$. In this case the envelopes of the rise portions of the tones will coincide entirely, and every amplitude between zero and one will be a solution of the above equation. The equation cannot then be used to determine the threshold amplitude.

This means that an experimental paradigm with simultaneous tones with different rise functions and/or rise times can be used to determine the threshold amplitude for the perceptual onset. If two tones have coinciding physical onsets ($t_a = t_b$), but different rise functions and/or rise times, the perceptual onsets will not as a rule coincide.

Tone sequences are defined as <u>perceptually isochronous</u> if the time intervals between successive perceptual onsets are all equal to each other:

$$P_{n+1} - P_n = T, \text{ for all values of n,}$$

in which T is the time interval between successive perceptual onsets. Fig. 3c shows the temporal envelopes of the tones A, B and A', which are perceptually isochronous. If we express p_a and p_b in the inverse rise functions R_a^{-1} and R_b^{-1}, as was done above for perceptually synchronous tones, the following equation results:

$$R_a^{-1}(\theta) \cdot p_a - R_b^{-1}(\theta) \cdot p_b = T - (t_b - t_b). \qquad (5)$$

From this equation, we can solve the relative threshold amplitude   under the same conditions as were necessary for solving equation (4). That means that an experimental paradigm with successive perceptually isochronous tones with different rise functions and/or times can also be used to determine the threshold amplitude for the perceptual onset.

If tones are physically isochronous, that is when the time intervals between successive physical onsets are all equal to each other, but have different rise times and/or functions, the perceptual onsets will not as a rule be isochronous.

In the model as described, there are only two stimulus variables, viz., rise time and rise function.

In our experiments, the effects of rise time and sensation level were investigated. These variables proved to have an effect on perceptual onset.

EXPERIMENT I

Method

Procedure - We used a paradigm in which a sequence of tones had to be adjusted in such a way that the onsets were perceived isochronously. Each trial started with a tone sequence that was decidedly non-isochronous. The starting sequence consisted of successive pairs of tones A and B with a different interval between the physical onsets of A and the following B, and between B and the following A (see Fig. 3a). The onset times of tones B, relative to those of A, could be adjusted by the subjects, by turning a knob. The experimental task was to adjust the onset times of tone B in such a way that the sequence ABABAB ..... was perceptually isochronous, i.e., that the perceived onsets of the tones followed each other with strictly the same time interval. This is illustrated in Fig. 3b. Because the tones A were repeated every 800 msec, the subjective repetition time T of the tones in the entirely isochronized sequence is 400 msec. Rise times were varied independently. The time interval $t_b - t_a$ was derived from the position

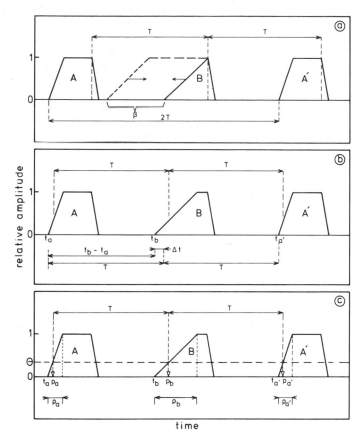

Fig. 3a.   Illustration of a perceptually non-isochronous starting sequence. The physical onsets of tones B could be adjusted by the subject within time interval β. At the start of a trial the physical onset of tone B was either at the beginning or at the end of β. The physical onsets of tones A, as well as the physical offset times of tones A and B were fixed.

Fig. 3b.   Temporal structure of a perceptually isochronous tone sequence in which the time intervals between successive perceptual onsets are all equal to each other. The physical onsets of tones A and B are t_a and t_b, respectively. The repetition time of tone A equals 2T, so that T is the perceptual repetition time. The dependent variable is denoted by the time interval $\Delta t = T - (t_b - t_a)$.

Fig. 3c.   Temporal structure of tones A, B and A' that are perceptually isochronous. The time interval between successive perceptual onsets is denoted by T. The perceptual onsets p_a, p_b and p_a' are defined as the moment at which the temporal envelopes pass relative threshold amplitude Θ.

of the turning knob at which the subject judged the tone sequence to be isochronous. Now all variables were known that are necessary for computing the threshold amplitude for the perceptual onset from equation (5).

In our tone sequences the physical offset times were kept isochronous, independent of the physical onset times. That means that tones B had different durations at the various stages of adjustment. However, since the perceptual offsets could also be considered perceptually isochronous, the subjective tone durations of tones A and B must have been equal in the final adjustments with isochronous perceptual onsets. Because of this relation between subjective onsets and durations, subjective duration could be (but not necessarily had to be) used as an extra cue for the isochronous adjustment.

An experimental series comprised 10 trials, which were all replications of the same condition. Four series were run consecutively. Each subject was tested individually. An experimental run lasted about half an hour. Between the runs there was a half-hour rest period, during which another subject was tested. The subjects were trained in the first runs. Knowledge of results was given to the subjects only with respect to the standard deviation of the 10 adjustments within a series. Standard deviations greater than 20 msec were exceptional. If they occurred, the series were repeated until results with standard deviations less than 20 msec were obtained.

The onset times of the tones B relative to those of tones A in case of a perceptually isochronous series was the dependent variable to be determined. The relative amplitude of the threshold for the perceptual onset was calculated as follows. In our experimental conditions, the rise functions of tones A and B were equal ($R_a = R_b$), so that we may say:

$$R_a^{-1}(\theta) = R_b^{-1}(\theta) = \alpha$$

We set $t_a = 0$ and $\Delta t = T - t_b$.

Then, equation (5) can be simplified to

$$\alpha \, (\rho_a - \rho_b) = \Delta t$$

or

$$\alpha = \Delta t \, / \, (\rho_a - \rho_b). \tag{6}$$

Since $\alpha = R^{-1}(\theta)$, $R(\alpha) = \theta$. Now, θ represents the relative threshold amplitude. In our experiments, we used the relative rise function

$$R(t') = 0.5 + 0.5 \sin [\, (t' - 0.5)\pi \,]$$

Thus,
$$\tag{7}$$

$$R(\alpha) = 0.5 + 0.5 \sin \left[\, (\frac{\Delta t}{\rho_a - \rho_b} - 0.5) \, \pi \right]$$

In this formula, Δt is the dependent experimental variable. It can be computed from the repetition time T (= 400 msec) and the adjusted physical onsets of tones B t_b.

The rise function and the rise times are features of the experimental conditions. If tones A and B have equal rise times ($\rho_a = \rho_b$), equation (6) cannot be solved. In this condition the envelopes should coincide in the case of a perceptually isochronous tone sequence, and Δt should be zero.

Stimuli

Waveforms were calculated with the formula

$$p(t) = \sum_{n=1}^{n=20} (1/n) \sin 2 \pi nft. \qquad (8)$$

This results in a waveform with a spectral envelope with a slope of -6 dB per octave. Fundamental frequencies of tones A and B were 400 Hz. The duration of tones A was always 150 msec, the duration of tones B depended on the adjusted onset of the moment. Rise times of tones A and B were independently varied. Decay times of A and B were held constant at 20 msec. The absolute rise function, as shaped by the analog gates, is described by

$$R(t) = 0.5 + 0.5 \sin [(\{t/\rho\} - 0.5) \pi]. \qquad (9)$$

In this formula, the physical onset is set at $t = 0$ and the maximum relative amplitude (1) is reached at $t = \rho$.

The decay function is described in a similar way:

$$R(t) = 0.5 - 0.5 \sin [(\{t/\sigma\} - 0.5) \pi]. \qquad (10)$$

Here, t equals 0 at the beginning of the decay portion. In this paper, rise and decay times are referred to as time interval ρ', which indicates the time interval necessary for the rise curve to increase from 10 to 90% of the maximum amplitude. For a rise or decay time ρ' as defined above, the time ρ between zero and maximum amplitude is given by:

$$\rho = \rho' (\arcsin 1/\arcsin 0.8) = 1.69 \rho'. \qquad (11)$$

The sound pressure level of the tones was 77 dB(A) in the highest level condition, measured as continuous signals. The other level conditions comprised tones of 57 and 37 dB(A).

Apparatus - A flow diagram of the apparatus is shown in Fig. 4. The experiments were run under the control of a PDP 11/10 computer. A continuous tone was generated in the following way. One period of the waveform was stored in 256 discrete samples (with 10 bit accuracy) in an external revolving memory (recirculator), which could be read out by a digital-to-analog converter. The sampling rate was given by a pulse train derived from a frequency generator. The tone was filtered by low-pass

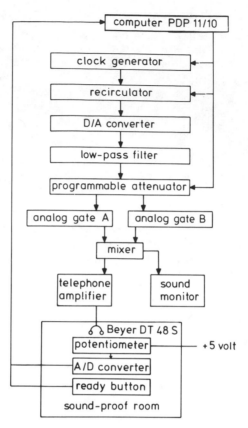

Fig. 4.   Flow diagram of the apparatus used. Tones A were established by
means of gate A, tones B by means of gate B.

filter with a cut-off frequency of 5 kHz. Sound pressure level was controlled by a programmable attenuator. Tone A was presented by passing it
through on/off gate A, tone B by passing it through on/off gate B. After
gating, the tones were mixed and fed to a headphone amplifier. The signals
were presented diotically (same signal to both ears) by means of headphones.
    Subjects were seated in a sound-proof room. The subjects had to find
out first in which area of the blinded knob the onsets of tones B could be
controlled. There were five such areas, which overlapped. Which area was
sensitive was determined by a random procedure. Two consecutive trials
could not have the same sensitive area. The voltage of the adjustment knob
was read out by an analog-to-digital converter, and was transformed into a
time measure of the onsets of tones B relative to the onsets of tones A.
Tests revealed that the accuracy of this measurement procedure, i.e.the
transformation of the voltage to the timing of t_b relative to t_a, was
within 1 msec. When the subject considered the tone sequence to be
isochronous, he pressed a ready-button.

Experimental design – The independent variables were:

(a)   rise time of tone A (5, 40, 80 msec);

(b)   rise time of tone B (5, 40, 80 msec); and

(c)   level of tones (37,57,77 dB(A)).

Within a sequence, tones A and B had the same level. The 27 different conditions were presented in 54 experimental series to four subjects. Each mean value is based on 80 trials.

Subjects – Four students at the University of Utrecht served as subjects and were paid for their services. They were musically trained.

Results

In the conditions in which tones A and B have equal rise times, Δt should be zero. Inspecting the mean Δt's in Table 1 for equal rise times, however a small but consistent tendency is found to place the onset of tone B too early. This adjustment effect, the subject's bias towards turning the knob consistently too far in one direction was also found by Marcus (1976), Schuette (1977) and Zwicker (1970). A similar effect, the occurrence of systematic time-order errors, was found when subjects are asked to produce a series of monosyllables in a rhythmical way (Fowler, 1978) and when auditory duration have to be compared or reproduced (Wundt, 1903; Woodrow 1934, 1935; Stott, 1935; Vos, 1979). The phenomenon seems to be independent of the task to be carried out.

Evidently mean Δt's are composed of a rise time effect (Δt_r) and an adjustment effect (Δt_a). It is assumed that Δt_a is not dependent on the rise times of tones A and B and that Δt is simply the sum of Δt_r and Δt . To test the assumption of the independence of the rise time effect and the adjustment effect, mean Δt's from the conditions in which $\rho_a < \rho_b$ have to be compared with the mean Δt's from the combinations in which $\rho_a > \rho_b$.

For the combinations in which ρ_a is shorter, or longer, than ρ_b, Δt is composed of Δt_r and Δt_a, while for the combinations in which ρ_a equals ρ_b, Δt equals Δt_a. If the rise time effect and the adjustment effect are mutually independent, the sum of the mean Δt's from the conditions in which $\rho_a < \rho_b$ and the mean Δt's from the conditions in which $\rho_a > \rho_b$ should equal twice the mean Δt of the conditions in which ρ_a equals ρ_b. (Note that Δt becomes negative when the physical onset of tone B is adjusted as t > T.)

Separate tests for the three levels of tones A and B showed that this was true within 3 msec or less. Given these small discrepancies, we concluded that the assumption of the independence of the rise time effect and the adjustment effect is tenable. Of course, since the rise times of tones A and B were varied orthogonally, the best estimate of the mean bias should be based on a whole set of Δt's at the same sound pressure level. The value of the adjustment effect was determined in such a way that the sum of the corrected Δt's within a set was zero. The adjustment effects for the 37, 57 and 77 dB conditions turned out to be 7.9, 8.1 and 7.2 msec respectively. In Table 1, the corrected mean Δt's are given for all

Table 1

Mean Δt's and corrected Δt's of all experimental combinations of rise times of tones A and B for the three presented levels of tones A and B, together with the corresponding relative thresholds. Thresholds cannot be derived for the conditions of equal rise times of tones A and B. The correction of Δt was -7.9, -8.1 and -7.2 msec in the 35, 57 and 77 dB conditions, respectively.

Rise time (msec)		37 dB(A)			57 dB(A)			77 dB(A)		
tone A	tone B	observed Δt(msec)	corrected Δt(msec)	threshold (dB)	observed Δt(msec)	corrected Δt(msec)	threshold (dB)	observed Δt(msec)	corrected Δt(msec)	threshold (dB)
5	5	4.4	- 3.5	-	4.0	- 4.1	-	5.0	- 2.2	-
5	40	32.0	24.1	-9.0	29.3	21.2	-10.9	24.5	17.3	-14.1
5	80	66.0	58.1	-7.2	54.2	46.1	-10.7	48.4	41.2	-12.4
40	5	-20.2	-28.1	-6.7	-11.4	-19.5	-12.2	-13.9	-21.1	-11.0
40	40	7.2	- 0.7	-	7.1	- 1.0	-	5.4	- 1.8	-
40	80	38.3	30.4	-7.5	30.9	22.8	-11.9	31.2	24.0	-11.1
80	5	-45.4	-53.3	-8.5	-34.4	-42.5	-11.9	-29.3	-36.5	-14.4
80	40	-19.6	-27.5	-9.0	-13.7	-21.8	-12.6	-11.6	-18.8	-14.9
80	80	8.8	0.9	-	6.7	-.1.4	-	5.0	- 2.2	-
		Mean level = -8.0			Mean level = -11.7			Mean level = -13.0		
		Stand. Dev. = 0.9			Stand. Dev. = 0.7			Stand. Dev. = 1.6		

Levels of tones A and B

experimental combinations of rise times of tones A and B for the three presented levels of tones A and B.

An analysis of variance was carried out on Δt. For this purpose a 4 (subjects) x 3 (rise times of tones A) x 3 (rise times of tones B) x 3 (tone levels) x 20 (replication) randomized block factorial design (Kirk, 1968) was used. The effects of the rise time of tone A (F(2,6) = 1258.1; p<.00005) and the rise time of tone B (F(2.6) = 612.8; p<.00005) were highly significant. The significant interaction effect between the level and the rise time of tone A (F(4,12) = 13.7; p<.0005) showed that with decreasing level, Δt increased when the rise time of tone A was short and decreased when the rise time of tone A was long. The interaction between level and the rise time of tone B revealed that with decreasing level, Δt increased significantly when the rise time of tone B was long and decreased when the rise time of tone B was short (F(4,12) = 20.1; p<.0005). For each sound pressure level there were 6 different conditions in which the threshold level for the perceptual onset could be computed. These different conditions comprised all combinations with unequal rise times. The relative threshold amplitudes were computed with the help of equation (7) and with the mean corrected Δt's as the dependent variable.

The relative levels were presented in Table 1. In the 37 dB condition the mean relative threshold was -8.0 dB and the standard deviation equalled 0.9 dB. In the 57 dB and 77 dB conditions the mean thresholds were -11.7 dB and 13.0 dB, the standard deviations 0.7 dB and 1.6dB, respectively.

Discussion

Inspecting the relative thresholds at each sound pressure level condition separately, an important conclusion can be drawn. Recall that the standard deviations of the different relative thresholds equalled 0.9, 0.7 and 1.6 dB in the 37, 57 and 77 dB conditions respectively. Considering this consistent result - i.e. that within each of the three intensity conditions, about the same relative threshold level was found in 6 physically different rise time combinations - we are justified in defining the perceptual onset moment of a tone as the time at which its envelope passes a certain threshold level.

Inspecting the mean relative thresholds between the different level conditions, it can be inferred

(a) that the relative threshold by which the perceptual onset is determined, shifts downwards with increasing level of the tones, and

(b) that the shift in threshold is small relative to the shift in stimulus level. Therefore, the threshold can be most conveniently described relative to the maximum level of the stimulus.

At our highest level condition a relative threshold of -13.0 dB was found. In a recent study on synchronization in performed ensemble music, Rasch (1979) defined the perceptual onset of a musical tone as the moment that its envelope exceeded a threshold of about 15 to 20 dB below the maximum levels of the signals. So Rasch's adopted level is fairly compatible with our data.

In the model of Schuette (1977) the perceptual onset of a tone was defined as the moment at which the subjective envelope passed a certain percentage of its maximum value. The subjective envelope equalled the output of a first-order RC integrator circuit, having the physical envelope functions of the tones as its input. Our results, however, show that the perceptual onset is located at the moment at which the physical envelope passed a certain percentage of its maximum value. A details comparison of our threshold model with Schuette's model was made by Vos and Rasch (1981). From this comparison it was concluded that the predictive power of the threshold model was much higher than that of Schuette's model.

Finally our results show that the perceptual onset is also dependent on the stimulus level. This may have important consequences for the performance and perception of music.

EXPERIMENT 2

It is a matter of everyday experience that the audibility of sounds like speech and music may be decreased in the presence of other sounds. Thus an orchestra may partially mask the sound of a soloist. In Experiment 1 it was shown that the relative threshold for the perceptual onset slightly increased with reduction of the levels of the tones. This lowering of the maximum levels of the tones corresponds to a reduction of the sensation level. The purpose of the second experiment is to investigate the effect on the relative threshold of altering the effective sensation level in more detail, through varying the signal to noise ratio.

Method

Procedure - The procedure was identical to that in Experiment 1. The s/n ratio, defined here as a level above masked threshold, is varied by changing the level of a continuous noise. Signal level is held constant. In addition, at the beginning of the first run the adequate levels of the continuous masker were determined individually for every subject, for three different s/n ratios of the tones. For a s/n ratio of 20 dB, for example, the level of the now isochronously presented tones was decreased by 20 dB and the level of the masker was adjusted until the tones could be detected in 50% of the cases.

Stimuli - The stimuli were the same as in Experiment 1. The sound pressure level of the tones measured as continuous signals was 77 dB(A). The continuous masker was pink noise with a spectral envelope of -3 dB per octave.

Apparatus - The apparatus was the same as in Experiment 1. In addition after appropriate attenuation, the output of the noise generator was fed to the headphone amplifier.

Design - The independent variables were:

(a)   rise time of tone A (5, 40, 80 msec);
(b)   rise time of tone B (5, 40, 80 msec);
(c)   level above masked threshold of the tones A and B (20, 30, 40 dB).

Within a sequence, tones A and B had the same level. The 27 different conditions were presented in 27 experimental series to four subjects.

Subjects - Two new students from the Institute of Musicology at Utrecht served as subjects and were paid for their services. One of the authors (JV) and a colleague also participated in the experiment. All subjects were musically trained.

Results - In Table 2, the corrected mean Δt's are given of all experimental combinations of rise times of tones A and B for each of the three levels above masked threshold. The adjustment effects were computed for the 20, 30 and 40 dB conditions separately, and turned out to be 8.5, 7.2 and 7.0 msec respectively. An analysis of variance was carried out on Δt_C, because the adjustment effect was to some extent dependent on the conditions. The effects of the rise time of tone A ($F(2,6) = 112.0$; p< .0001) and the rise time of tone B ($F(2,6) = 128.0$; p < .0001) were highly significant. The significant interaction effect between level above masked threshold and rise time of tone A ($F(4,12) = 3.8$; p <.03) showed that with decreasing level above masked threshold, Δt_C increased when the rise time of tone A was short and decreased when the rise time of tone A was long. The interaction between level above masked threshold and rise time of tone B revealed that with decreasing level, there was a trend for Δt_C to increase when the rise time of tone B was long and to decrease when the rise time of tone B was short ($F(4,12) = 2.3$; p<.12).

With the help of equation (7) the relative threshold amplitudes were computed with the Δt_C's for all combinations with unequal rise times. The relative levels are presented in Table II. In the 20 dB condition the mean relative threshold was -6.6 dB and the standard deviation equalled 0.9 dB. In the 30 dB and 40 dB conditions the mean thresholds were -7.1 dB and -9.2 dB the standard deviations 1.2 dB and 2.6 dB, respectively.

DISCUSSION

From the results of Experiment 2 it can be concluded that the relative threshold for the perceptual onset of musical tones decreases with increasing level above masked threshold. It should be noted that tones A and B were held at a constant level of 77 dB(A). The results of Experiment 2 can be related to those of Experiment 1, where a similar decrease of the relative threshold was found with increasing sensation level of the tones.

In Fig. 5, mean relative thresholds from Experiments 1 and 2 are plotted as a function of level above masked or absolute threshold. In experiment 1, the different tone levels of 37, 57 and 77 dB corresponded to sensation levels of 25, 45 and 65 dB, respectively. In Experiment 1, an increase of the sensation level of 40 dB resulted in a relative threshold decrement of 5 dB, while in Experiment 2, the increase of the level above masked threshold of 20 dB resulted in a relative threshold decrement of 2.6 dB. Moreover, the level of the relative threshold seems to be linearly dependent on the level above threshold. The relationship between level above threshold and relative threshold for perceptual onset can be roughly summarized by concluding that a 7 dB level above masked or absolute threshold increment results in a 1 dB relative threshold decrement. There

Table 2

Mean corrected Δt's of all experimental combinations of rise times of tones A and B for the three presented levels above masked threshold of tones A and B, together with the corresponding relative thresholds for the perceptual onsets. Thresholds cannot be derived for the conditions of equal rise times of tones A and B. The correction of Δt was -8.5, -7.2 and -7.0 msec in the 20, 30 and 40 dB conditions, respectively.

| Rise time (msec) | | Level above masked threshold of tones A and B | | | | | |
| | | 20 dB | | 30 dB | | 40 dB | |
tone A	tone B	Δt_c (msec)	Threshold (dB)	Δt_c (msec)	Threshold (dB)	Δt_c (msec)	Threshold (dB)
5	5	-3.8	–	-3.0	–	-1.3	–
5	40	26.7	-7.5	26.8	-7.4	25.3	-8.2
5	80	65.2	-5.6	62.8	-6.2	52.5	-8.7
40	5	-31.3	-5.3	-31.5	-5.2	-31.0	-5.4
40	40	-2.0	–	-0.7	–	-0.8	–
40	80	32.0	-6.8	29.5	-7.9	25.0	-10.4
80	5	-59.8	-6.8	-58.0	-7.3	-50.5	-9.3
80	40	-29.8	-7.8	-28.2	-8.6	-21.0	-13.2
80	80	2.7	–	2.3	–	1.5	–
		Mean Level =	-6.6	Mean Level =	-7.1	Mean Level =	-9.2
		Stand. Dev. =	0.9	Stand. Dev. =	1.2	Stand. Dev. =	2.6

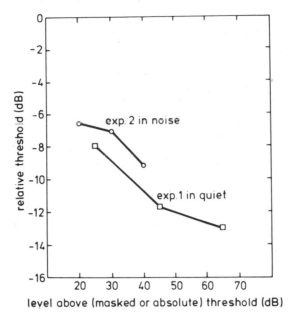

Fig. 5.   Mean relative threshold for the perceptual onset, plotted as a function of the sensation level of tones A and B. For reference purposes, also the mean relative thresholds from Experiment 1 are plotted.

remains a small difference between the levels of Experiments 1 and 2, for which no apparent explanation is available.

GENERAL DISCUSSION

From our experiments, we may conclude that the perceptual onsets of successively presented tones can be defined as the times at which the envelopes pass a relative threshold of about 6 to 15 dB below the maximum level of the tones. In a number of experiments, we have shown that the level of the relative threshold depends on the tone level above masked or absolute threshold. The data from the present experiments seem to suggest adaptation to a certain constant stimulus level. At the time the adaptation threshold is passed by the stimulus level presented, the onset of the stimulus is perceived. The experimental set-up, in which sequences of alternating tones A and B, having the same level were presented for a rather long time (one trial lasted about 30 to 120 seconds), may have evoked optimal conditions for adaptation.

The nature of our threshold model is at variance with theories of temporal summation in hearing.

Schuette's model (1978a) is based on temporal integration. A detailed comparison of the threshold model with Schuette's model is made by Vos and

Rasch (1981) who concluded that although Schuette's temporal integration model can explain the general trend of our data, it is much less powerful than our simple threshold model.

Perceptual Onset and Performed Music

In studies on the temporal structure of performed music, our threshold model can be applied to determine the perceptual onsets of musical tones. When music is performed on instruments with very short rise times, like the piano, harpsichord, and drums (Gabrielsson, 1974; Povel, 1977; Sundberg and Verrillo, 1977) the difference between the physical onset and the perceptual onset is very small. In these cases, level above threshold does also not have a great impact on this difference. However, when ensemble music is performed on instruments, producing tones with relatively long rise times (Rasch, 1979), such as bowed string instruments, the perceptual onset heavily depends on the relative threshold.

In such musical practice where dynamic differences are not very large, perceptual onset is only clearly affected by the rise times and rise functions of the different instruments. This, however, is a variable with which the respective musicians can cope by adjusting their physical onset times in order to establish the appropriate timing of the perceptual onsets of their tones.

Future research should be focussed on the perceptual onset of musical tones in synchronously perceived tone pairs. The sensation levels of simultaneously presented tones are especially dependent on the amount of auditory masking (Zwislocki, 1978). To apply our model to simultaneously produced tones, experimental results of binaural masking experiments with complex tones are needed. In addition, it would be interested to see if our model also works in cases of complex tones consisting of partials with unequal rise times and unequal physical onsets (Freedman, 1967; Grey and Moorer, 1977) and of tones with substantially differing amplitude envelopes (Strong and Clark, 1967).

CONCLUSION

From our experimental results we may conclude that:

(a)   the perceptual onsets of successively presented tones can be defined as the times at which the envelopes pass a relative threshold level;

(b)   within a range of 20 to 70 dB above masked or absolute threshold, the relative threshold for the perceptual onset lies about 6 to 15 dB below the maximum level of the tones;

(c)   a 7 dB level above masked or absolute threshold increment results in a 1 dB relative threshold decrement.

We propose as an explanation of the experimental results that adaptation of the hearing mechanism to a prevalent relative stimulus level is responsible for determining the level of perceptual onset.

SUMMARY

The perceptual onset of a musical tone can be defined as the moment in time at which the stimulus is first perceived. In the present experiments a simple threshold model for the perceptual onset was applied. A paradigm was used in which a sequence of tones had to be adjusted in such a way that the onsets were perceived at equally spaced moments in time. In Experiment 1 the threshold model was applied in a design in which the rise times of the tones were varied. In addition the maximum levels of the tones were varied from 37 to 77 dB(A). The results show that:

(a) the perceptual onsets of the tones can indeed be defined as the times at which the envelopes pass a <u>relative</u> threshold;

(b) that the relative threshold level decreases with increasing level of the tones; and

(c) that this shift in relative threshold level is small relative to the shift in the stimulus level.

In experiment 2 the effect of level above masked threshold on the perceptual onset was investigated in more detail by varying the level of a background noise. The results show that the relative threshold decreases with increasing level above masked threshold. The results from our experiments strongly suggest that the relative threshold is linearly dependent on the level above masked or absolute threshold and that a 7 dB increment of this level results in a 1 dB relative threshold decrement.

Our experimental results suggest that adaptation of the hearing mechanism to a certain relative stimulus level is responsible for perceptual onset. The applicability of our threshold model in various realistic musical situations is discussed.

ACKNOWLEDGMENT

This paper is an abridged version of "The perceptual onset of musical tones," to be published in <u>Perception & Psychophysics</u> (1981).

REFERENCES

Efron, R., 1970a, The relationship between the duration of a stimulus and the duration of a perception, Neuropsychologia, 8:37-55.

Efron, R., 1970b, The minimum duration of a perception, Neuropsychologia, 8:57-63.

Efron, R., 1970c, Effect of stimulus duration on perceptual onset and offset latencies, Perc. and Psychophys., 8(4):231-234.

Fowler, C.A., 1979, 'Perceptual centers' in speech production and perception, Perc. and Psychophys., 25(5):375-388.

Freedman, M.D., 1967, Analysis of musical instrument tones, J. Acoust. Soc. Am., 41(4):793-806.

Gabrielsson, A., 1974, Performance of rhythm patterns, Scand. J. Psychol., 15:63-72.

Grey, J.M., and Moorer, J.A., 1977, Perceptual evaluations of synthesized musical instrument tones, J. Acoust. Soc. Am., 62(2):454-462.

Kirk, R.E., 1968, "Experimental Design: Procedures for the Behavioral Sciences," Belmont, Calf.

Luce, D., and Clark, M., 1965, Durations of attack transients of non-percussive orchestral instruments, J. Audio Eng Soc., 13:194-199.

Marcus, S.M., 1976, "Perceptual centres," Unpubl. fellowship dissertation, King's College, Cambridge, Eng.

Melka, A., 1970, Messungen der Klangeinsatzdauer bei Musikinstrumenten, Acoustica, 23:108-117.

Michon, J.A., 1967, "Timing in temporal tracking," Diss., Inst. for Perception TNO, Soesterberg, Neth.

Morton, J., Marcus, S., and Frankish, C., 1976, Perceptual Centers, Psychol. Rev., 83(5):405-408.

Povel, D., 1977, Temporal structure of performed music, some preliminary observations, Acta Psychologica, 41:309-320.

Rasch, R.A., 1979, Synchronization in performed ensemble music, Acoustica, 43(2):121-131.

Schuette, H., 1977, "Bestimmung der subjektiven Ereigniszeitpunkte aufeinanderfolgender Schallimpulse durch Psychoakustische Messungen.,"Diss., Technical University, Munich.

Schuette, H., 1978a, Ein Funktionsschema für die Wahrnehmung eines gleichmässigen Rhythmus in Schallimpulsfolgen. Biol. Cybern. 29:49-55.

Schuette, H., 1978b, Subjektiv gleichmässiger Rhythmus: Ein Beitrag zur zeitlichen Wahrnehmung von Schallereignissen. Acoustica 41(3):197-206.

Stott, L.H., 1935, Time order errors in the discrimination of short tonal durations, J. Exp. Psychol. 18:741-766.

Strong, W., and Clark, M., 1967, Synthesis of wind-instrument tones, J. Acoust. Soc. Am. 41(1):39-52.

Sundberg, J., and Verrillo, V., 1977, On the anatomy of the retard, a study of timing in music. Speech Transmission Laboratory, Stockholm. Qart. Prog. and Status Rep. 2-3:44-57.

Vos, J., and Rasch, R.A., 1981, The perceptual onset of musical tones, Perc. and Psychophys. (in press).

Vos, P.G.M.M., 1973, "Waarneming van Metrische Toonreeksen," Thesis, University of Nijmegen, Neth.

Vos, P.G.M.M., 1979, "Critical duration ratios in tone sequences for the perception of rhythmic accent and grouping," Internal rep. 79 ON 10, University of Nijmegen, Neth.

Woodrow, H., 1934, The temporal indifference interval determined by the method of mean error, J. Exp. Psychol, 17:167-188.

Woodrow, H., 1935, The effect of practice upon time-order errors in the comparison of temporal intervals, Psychol. Rev. 42:127-152.

Wundt, W., 1903, "Grundzüge der physiologischen Psychologie," Vol. 3, (5th Ed.), W. Bertelmann, Leipzig.

Zwicker, E., 1970, Subjektive und objektive Dauer von Schallimpulsen und Schallpausen, Acoustica, 22:214-218.

Zwislocki, J.J., 1978, Masking: experimental and theoretical aspects of simultaneous, forward, backward and central masking, in: "Handbook of Perception," Vol. 4, E. Carterette and M. Friedman, eds., Academic Press, New York.

Chapter XVII

THE PITCH SET AS A LEVEL OF DESCRIPTION FOR STUDYING MUSICAL PITCH PERCEPTION

Gerald J. Balzano

Department of Music
University of California at San Diego
La Jolla, California, USA

INTRODUCTION

How shall we define the musical stimulus? Traditionally, music theorists interested in pitch phenomena have sought the definition in terms of ratios of whole numbers. Such ratios can provide a description of most, if not all, of the musical intervals in use today, and can be translated readily into ratios of physically realizable tone frequencies. Psychoacousticians, following the dictates of reductionism, have sought a finer grain of analysis than this, pointing out that the essential constituent of an interval is a tone, and that the study of music perception must ultimately refer to the perception of single tones and their frequency components. Accordingly, a great deal of scientific effort has gone into studying the perception of isolated tones.

In this paper I will argue that both of these levels of description are too fine-grained for representing music. I would propose instead the pitch set as a more realistic level of analysis appropriate to the study of music. Streams of pitches arrayed over time that do not generate a determinate pitch set, such as the intonation contours of normal human speech, do not generally elicit a state of the listener commonly associated with perceiving music. Given this observation, it is quite possible that properties of pitch sets, while not to be found at the level of single tones or ratios, are nonetheless directly operative in music perception. Without a description at this higher level, many of the most distinctively musical phenomena may be left out of account.

I will introduce a means of description different from those commonly received: I shall characterize pitch set structure in terms of the language of mathematical group theory. In music of the Western world today, the universal pitch set is the twelve-tone chromatic scale, and the group associated with it is C_{12}, a cyclic group of order 12. Felix Klein showed that certain groups of transformations described the fabric of projective,

Euclidean, affine, and topological spaces in geometry. I will use the structure of C_{12} to represent pitch space. Pitch sets will be viewed in terms of their 'shape'-like properties vis-a-vis three isomorphic spaces inherent in the structure of C_{12}.

In describing at the level of pitch set we do not necessarily forego lower levels of analysis. A two-tone interval is a pitch set, as is, for that matter, a single tone. Pitch sets with more than two members may be referred to as triads or chords, and pitch sets that are larger than this may be known as scales. Whenever the term 'scale' or 'triad' is used in this paper, I refer only to a pitch set, without further connotations such as simultaneity in time or frequent musical usage.

Any study of the 'musical stimulus' addressing the level of pitch sets must come to grips with the most historically enduring of all pitch sets, the major scale. When viewed from the level of single tones, there appears to be nothing special about this scale. When viewed from the level of ratios, however, the major scale does appear to possess a number of unusual properties (Helmholtz, 1885; Schenker, 1906; Benade, 1960), and this has been taken by some as a decisive advantage for the ratio-based approach. One startling, but satisfying conclusion we will come to from our pitch-set purview is that the major scale is not merely special, but unique, even in reference to a ratio-independent set of properties. And as we will see, the major scale is literally embedded in the structure of C_{12}.

The following is a sketch of an approach. Other facets of the approach may be found in Balzano (1978) and Balzano (in press).*

THE GROUP C_{12} AND ITS SUBGROUPS

The elements of C_{12} may be taken as the twelve basic pitch classes, represented by the integers 0, 1, 2, . . . ,11 modulo 12. Depending on the tuning system (e.g. Just Intonation, Pythagorean Intonation, Equal Temperament), differences among these integers translate either approximately or exactly into log frequency differences. The elements of the group are the twelve transformations - musical intervals - that generate the pitch classes. In situations where we assign a given pitch class to the 'origin' or zero-element of the group, the distinction between intervals and pitch classes becomes somewhat blurred. When we wish to emphasize the transformational nature of the group elements, the notation T_0, T_1, . . . , T_{11} will be employed. "I", for "identity", will be a synonym for "T_0". In

---

*   The following relevant references, in alphabetical order: Babbitt (1965), Boretz (1970), Budden (1972), Chalmers (1975), Fuller (1975), Gamer (1967), Lakner (1960), Lewin (1959, 1960, 1977), O'Connell (1962), Regener (1973), and Rothenberg (1978a, b), except Budden and Rothenberg are from music-theoretic sources. Babbit (1965) was an important stimulus for my own work, but otherwise the ideas presented in this chapter were developed largely independently of the sources cited above. For an excellent discussion of the intimate connections between group theory and perception, see also Cassirer (1944).

Table 1. Group Table For C_{12}

*	0	1	2	3	4	5	6	7	8	9	10	11
0	0	1	2	3	4	5	6	7	8	9	10	11
1	1	2	3	4	5	6	7	8	9	10	11	0
2	2	3	4	5	6	7	8	9	10	11	0	1
3	3	4	5	6	7	8	9	10	11	0	1	2
4	4	5	6	7	8	9	10	11	0	1	2	3
5	5	6	7	8	9	10	11	0	1	2	3	4
6	6	7	8	9	10	11	0	1	2	3	4	5
7	7	8	9	10	11	0	1	2	3	4	5	6
8	8	9	10	11	0	1	2	3	4	5	6	7
9	9	10	11	0	1	2	3	4	5	6	7	8
10	10	11	0	1	2	3	4	5	6	7	8	9
11	11	0	1	2	3	4	5	6	7	8	9	10

general, we will use the language of intervals-as-transformations when it is more natural to speak in active terms, and the language of pitch classes when we are describing group elements in terms of passive, spatialized places. Every statement we make may be formulated either way without affecting its truth value (Holland, 1972, pp.217-219).

A group consists of a <u>set</u> of elements and an <u>operation</u> defined over pairs of elements in the set. In order to constitute a group, the set must contain an <u>identity</u> element, one whose operation has no effect on any of the group elements. For each element of the set, there must be an <u>inverse</u> element also in the set, such that the combination of any element and its inverse yields the identity element. In addition to these constraints, a set of elements can constitute a group only if the set is <u>closed</u> under the operation; that is, the result of every combination of two group elements under the operation must yield an element that also belongs to the set.

It is easy to show that the set (0, 1, . . . , 11) constitutes a group under the operation of mod 12 addition. The identity element is evidently "0", and for each element g, its inverse g^{-1} is given by

$$g^{-1} = (12-g) \bmod 12 \qquad (1)$$

Thus 1 and 11 are inverses, as are 2 and 10, 6 and so forth. Finally, since the sum of two integers is always an integer, mod-12 reduction of the sum provides that it will belong to the set (0, 1, . . . , 11) and closure is thereby assured.

With respect to their effect on pitch class, the octave (p8) and unison (p1) are indistinguishable; both behave like an identity element in that they do not affect the pitch class they operate upon. In symbols, for any interval x,

$$p8 + x = x \qquad (2)$$

The effect on pitch class of any interval is the same as the combined effect of that interval plus the octave. The most natural mapping of the remaining 11 integers/intervals is to associate each interval with its integral number of semitones, so that m2$\longrightarrow$1, M2$\longrightarrow$2, . . . , M7$\longrightarrow$11. We adopt the convention of thinking of intervals as upward pitch transformations (though none of the results would be affected by assuming the opposite). Note the unusual congruence between mathematicians' and musicians' terminology: both call the relation between m2 and M7 by the same name, <u>inverse</u>.

Table 1 shows the complete group table. The "i" notation is used instead of the "T_i" notation for the sake of visibility, but it is helpful to conceive that the information in the table represents <u>combined effects of transformations</u>. The star (*) is used for the rule of combination instead of the plus sign of Equation 2. Thus 5 * 9 = 2 represents the fact that the combined effect of T_5 and T_9 on any pitch class is the same as the effect of T_2 alone. To express this relation as a function on pitch class places, we would write $T_5(9) = 2$:T_5 transforms pitch class 9 into pitch class 2. With the latter notation we can also express the effect of a transformation g (i.e. T_i) on an entire pitch set S, writing g(S). For example, $T_4(0, 3, 7) = (4, 7, 11)$, and in general for a set of size m, T_i $(S_0, S_1, . . . , S_{m-1}) = (S_0 + i, S_1 + i, . . . , S_{m-1} +i)$. Note that, while we use the * operator for combinations of transformations, we will often use the more intuitive plus sign for combining of pitch class places.

From the universal chromatic set of twelve pitch classes one can choose $2^{12} - 1 = 4095$ different pitch sets, including the full chromatic itself and the twelve trivial single-note pitch sets. Of the remaining sets, let us distinguish those that are transpositionally related to one another from those that are not Two pitch sets S and S' are transpositionally related if and only if S' = g(S) for some transformation g in C_{12}. We will call sets like S and S' members of the same <u>family</u>, for example, the F major scale and C major scale belong to the same family, and so do the two sets (0, 3, 7) and (4, 7, 11) treated above. If members of the same scale family are not distinguished, this results in a reduction to 351 distinct sets, 349 without the full chromatic and the single-note set.*

A number of subsets of the full chromatic are special in that they correspond to <u>subgroups</u> of C_{12}. For example, the set (0, 2, 4, 6, 8, 10) is closed under mod 12 addition, contains the identity, and contains the inverses of all of its elements. It is therefore a group contained within

---

* This number is different from that obtained by Forte (1964). In essence, Forte treats both transpositions and inversions as producing 'equivalent' scales. In so doing, he is implicitly using a larger group as a basis for invariance, namely D_{12}, the dihedral group of order 24. Using this group instead of C_{12} leads to a number of results that are questionable from the present point of view. For example, under D_{12}, the major triad (0, 4, 7) and the minor triad (0, 3, 7) are not distinguished.

C_{12}; a subgroup known as C_6, the cyclic group of order six. The corresponding pitch set is commonly known in music as the <u>whole-tone scale</u>, and its family consists of only two distinct members, $(0, 2, \overline{4, 6, 8, 10})$ and $\overline{(1, 3, 5, 7, 9, 11)}$. In a similar fashion, it can be shown that $(0, 3, 6, 9)$, $(0, 4, 8)$, and $(0, 6)$ are also subgroups of C_{12}, termed C_4, C_3 and C_2, respectively. Each of the corresponding pitch set families already has a name in standard musical terminology: the C_4 set corresponds to the diminished-7th chord, the C_3 to the augmented triad, and C_2 to the interval of a tritone. All subsets of C_{12} associated with subgroups have the property that their family is <u>incomplete</u>, consisting of fewer than 12 distinct sets. Thus there are only three distinct diminished-7th chords, four distinct augmented triads, and six distinct tritones.

With this background, we are ready to develop a number of basic properties of pitch sets more fully. The three main properties we will develop, together with information specific to the structure of C_{12} are more than enough to demonstrate the uniqueness of the major scale.

SOME DISTINGUISHING PROPERTIES OF PITCH SETS

We should be clear at the outset that our current level of description is more general than the term 'major scale' - it corresponds more closely to that of 'diatonic scale family', where by diatonic scale we mean nothing more than the pitch set $(0, 2, 4, 5, 7, 9, 11)$. The diatonic scale family is, as defined, the set of 12 group-generated transpositions of the set above. The <u>major mode</u> of the diatonic scale is represented by this same pitch set, but with the '0' element individuated as a reference or 'tonic' pitch. Note, however, that there is nothing in the theory of sets that provides for individuating a particular element of a set in this way, and we should like to see how far we can get without recourse to such a move. The fact that, of the seven possible tonics in this seven-note scale, fully six had seen extensive musical use until about the 17th century, recommends that we leave open the possibility that a tonic may be determined mainly be temporal-contextual factors, and not by intrinsic set-structural properties.

The 'Uniqueness' or 'Dynamic Quality' Property

We can consider what properties of a set might be conducive to the emergence of a 'tonic' element. It must be possible to <u>individuate</u> the elements of a set by virtue of their relations with one another. According to Zuckerkandl (1956), the chromatic scale possesses "no dynamic relations; every tone is as good as every other" (pp.38-39). Further, Zuckerkandl (1971) remarks about the dynamic qualities of pitches as members of pitch sets:

> The dynamic quality of a tone is part of the immediate
> sensation. We <u>hear</u> it just as we hear pitch or tone
> color but not under all circumstances. A tone must
> belong to a musical context in order to have dynamic
> quality. Within a musical context no tone will be

> without its proper dynamic quality. Outside the
> musical context, however - for instance, in the
> laboratory - tones have no dynamic qualities. Thus,
> the dynamic quality of a tone is its musical quality
> proper. It distinguishes the musical from the physical
> phenomenon (pp.19-20, original emphasis).

It is quite possible that these dynamic qualities reside in higher-level - but no less objectively specifiable - relations among members of a pitch set, each of whose elements has a unique set of relations with the others and therefore has the potentiality for a unique musical 'role' or 'dynamic quality'.

More formally, let a pitch set (scale) of cardinality (size) m be represented by $S = (s_0, s_1, \ldots, s_{m-1})$ with s_i a distinct element (pitch class) of C_{12}. In accordance with what we have said earlier, the initial element s_0 may be any member of the set, but it will be convenient if we stipulate that remaining set members will be written in 'ascending form', such that each s_1 is written in standard numerical order, mod 12. For example $(2, 4, 5, 7, 9, 11, 0)$ would be a perfectly acceptable way to write a diatonic scale. For each element of the set, define a vector of relations $V(s_i) = V_i = (v_{i0}, v_{i1}, \ldots, v_{i(m-1)})$ such that

$$v_{ij} = s_{i+j} - s_i \qquad (3)$$

where the subscript "i+j" is to be taken mod m. In the diatonic scale above, $V_2 = V(5) = (5-5, 7-5, 9-5, \ldots, 4-5) = (0, 2, 4, 6, 7, 9, 11)$. Now we can say that a set satisfies Uniqueness if and only if

$$V_i = V_{i'} \Longleftrightarrow i = i' \qquad (4)$$

That is, the vector of relations associated with each set element must be distinct.

The chromatic scale and the whole-tone scale - in fact, all of the sets associated with subgroups of C_{12} - fail to satisfy Uniqueness, since all the V_i are the same for every set element. A quick check will verify that V_i for every member of a whole tone scale is just $(0, 2, 4, 6, 8, 10)$. Other sets that fail Uniqueness in less drastic ways are $(0, 1, 4, 5, 8, 9)$, $(0, 1, 3, 4, 6, 7, 9, 10)$ and $(0, 2, 3, 5, 6, 8, 9, 11)$. In all cases it is the very symmetry and apparent elegance of the set that is its undoing with respect to Uniqueness. On the other hand, the uneven looking diatonic scale does satisfy Uniqueness. It is not difficult to show that the Uniqueness property entails and is entailed by completeness of a set's family.

I should like to claim that Uniqueness is not just an abstract property of a pitch set, but one with some perceptual content. By hypothesis, a melody based on a scale satisfying Uniqueness should be easier for a perceiver to deal with, because the notes of the melody are individuated not only by their particular frequency locations, but by their interrelations with one another. However, it turns out that many more sets satisfy Uniqueness than fail it, so more than this property is necessary to allow thorough differentiation among potential scales.

Scalestep-Semitone Coherence

All scales/sets partake of distance relationships based on the semitone unit of C_{12}. These semitone distances are in fact the constituents of the vector of relations V_i defined in the preceding subsection. Any set short of the full chromatic also gives rise to a new level of distance-reckoning, which we will call the scalestep. The number of semitones contained in a distance of one scalestep is given by the v_{i1} element of the v_i relations vector, and can be different at different points in the scale: a diatonic scale has some scalesteps that are 2 semitones wide, and others that are 1 semitone wide. More generally, v_{ij} describes the number of semitones contained in a distance of j scalesteps from the given scale member s_i. For example, in the diatonic set (2, 4, 5, 7, 9, 11, 0), $s_2 = 5$, $V_2 = (0, 2, 4, 6, 7, 9, 11)$, and we can read from the vector that a distance of (say) three scalesteps from scale element s_2 contains 6 semitones ($v_{23} = 6$).

In general, greater numbers of scalesteps correspond to greater numbers of semitones, but there is nothing that forces this to hold everywhere in the scale. For example, in the set (0, 2, 4, 9) a distance of two scalesteps from the element "0" corresonds to four semitones, and a distance of one scalestep from the element "4" corresponds to five semitones. Thus a larger number of scalesteps is associated here with a smaller number of semitones. We will say that, for scales like these, the relation between scalesteps and semitones is not coherent.

Symbolically, we can say that a set satisfies coherence if for any pair of scale elements s_i and $s_{i'}$

$$j < k \Rightarrow v_{ij} < v_{i'k} \qquad (5)$$

where j and k are scalestep-counting indices, and take on values from 0 to m-1 inclusive. Equation 5 states that larger numbers of scalesteps are always associated with larger numbers of semitones in a coherent scale. For sets satisfying this equation, scalesteps are a monotone increasing function of semitones. Notice that the entailment in Equation 5 applies in one direction only. The converse would require that all representatives of j scalesteps contain an identical number of semitones, and this, as we saw in the case of the whole-tone scale, would lead to a failure of Uniqueness.

I will not demonstrate it here, but it can be shown than any scale of odd cardinality containing a tritone will fail to satisfy Equation 5 strictly. The failure, however, will be localized to just the tritone interval ($v_{ij} = 6$) and can be remedied by relaxing the strict inequality on the right of Equation 5 for that interval:

$$j < k \Rightarrow v_{ij} < v_{i'k} \qquad \text{for } v_{ij} \neq 6$$

$$j < k \Rightarrow v_{ij} \leqslant v_{i'k} \qquad \text{for } v_{ij} = 6 \qquad (5a)$$

Perhaps the perceptual content of the Coherence property is obvious; if not, a few remarks are in order. Semitones are (approximately) a linear function of log frequency, and there is evidence, both (a) in the everyday fact of perceptual invariance of melodies under constant log frequency shifts, and (b) in the empirical literature (Attneave and Olson, 1971), that we do perceive musical pitch in terms of log frequency. Now, scalesteps cannot in turn be a linear function of semitones if the scale is to satisfy Uniqueness (recall the (0, 2, 4, . . . , 10) whole tone scale). But unless scalesteps are at least a monotone increasing function of semitones, perception mediated by log frequency will fail to yield consistent results in terms of scalesteps. As a consequence, perception would be 'stalled' at the semitone level. Indeed, just this sort of thing happens in the case of a tritone. When we hear an interval four semitones wide, in or out of context, we can safely identify that interval as a major 3rd, where its "thirdness" is a scalestep-level property. But when we hear an interval six semitones wide, we can often do no better than to identify it by the scale-neutral term 'tritone', since it may function either as an augmented 4th or a diminished 5th in a diatonic scale context. If all intervals were like the tritone, scalestep-level perception could never occur outside the specific context of a specific piece, and within this context only if the piece weren't changing keys too rapidly. Since learning to recognize intervals may require at least a temporary isolation of the interval from context, it is hard to see how learning to perceive scalestep-level qualities could occur unless scalestep-semitone coherence were satisfied.

Coherence may at first sight appear to be a rather superficial property of a scale. But it imposes powerful constraints on scales so that few sets conform to it. Of the 66 essentially different 5-note scales (i.e. scale families), only four satisfy Coherence, one of which is the familiar (0, 2, 4, 7, 9) pentatonic scale. Of the 80 essentially different 6-note scales, only two are coherent, one of which is the whole tone scale, and both of which fail Uniqueness. And of the 66 essentially different 7-note scales, only one, the diatonic scale, satisfies Coherence.

Simplicity of Scale Family

Our first two properties, Uniqueness and Coherence, were concerned with features of a scale determined by relational properties of its individual elements. Uniqueness is determined by relations of scale elements to one another, Coherence by relations of scale elements to the embedding system of semitone distances. Our third and most powerful property, which we will call Simplicity, concerns relations between members of a scale's family. Since all family members of a given set have the same cardinality and the same ensemble of V_{ij} relations, the only thing that distinguishes these transpositionally related sets is the pitch classes they contain. Let us therefore begin by defining the overlap of two members of a scale family as the cardinality of their intersection:

$$Ov(S, g(S)) = |S \cap g(S)| \qquad (6)$$

where $g(S) = g(s_0, s_1, \ldots, s_{m-1}) = (s_0 + g, s_1 + g, \ldots, s_{m-1} + g)$ in accordance with the definition of a scale family. Obviously Ov is a symmetric relation. Since S may be any member of the scale family without

Table 2. Matrix of Overlap Between Pairs of Pentatonic
Scale Family Members

Family Member	0	1	2	3	4	5	6	7	8	9	10	11
0	5	0	3	2	1	4	0	4	1	2	3	0
1	0	5	0	3	2	1	4	0	4	1	2	3
2	3	0	5	0	3	2	1	4	0	4	1	2
3	2	3	0	5	0	3	2	1	4	0	4	1
4	1	2	3	0	5	0	3	2	1	4	0	4
5	4	1	2	3	0	5	0	3	2	1	4	0
6	0	4	1	2	3	0	5	0	3	2	1	4
7	4	0	4	1	2	3	0	5	0	3	2	1
8	1	4	0	4	1	2	3	0	5	0	3	2
9	2	1	4	0	4	1	2	3	0	5	0	3
10	3	2	1	4	0	4	1	2	3	0	5	0
11	0	3	2	1	4	0	4	1	2	3	0	5

affecting overlap, we may write $Ov_S[g]$, the overlap associated with transformation g for scale S. And when it is clear what scale is being discussed, we will simplify the notation still further by dropping the "S" and writting $Ov[g]$. Since S is the same as $g^{-1}(g(S))$, it can easily be shown by substitution in Equation 6 and by the symmetry of Ov that $Ov[g] = Ov[g^{-1}]$ for all g. For example, any two diatonic scales a p5 apart ($g = T_7$) share six of seven notes, and so do any two diatonic scales a p4 apart ($g = T_5 = (T_7)^{-1}$).

The basic idea behind the Simplicity property is that spatial information can be deduced from patterns of overlap among scale family members. There are a number of alternative ways to proceed from this notion. One would be to treat values of $Ov[g]$ as similarity values between pairs of scale family members related by g. Given a matrix of pairwise similarity values such as that shown for the (0, 2, 4, 7, 9) pentatonic scale in Table 2, an implied spatial configuration of elements (scales) can be recovered by multidimensional scaling methods (e.g. Shepard 1962a, b; Kruskal, 1964a, b). Maximum Simplicity of scale family would correspond to minimum dimensionality of the space of scales. A different method, though one that leads to quite similar results, would be to define further predicates in terms of set operations, such as was done for Ov, and to develop the implied spatial relations directly. Goodman (1966) is a good example of this approach. It is the latter path that we shall take here.

A first attempt along these lines would be to observe that the closest possible relation among scale family members obtains when they share all elements but one. Let us call this relation adjacency and symbolize it "A". Formally,

$$A(R, S) \equiv Ov(R, S) = m-1 \qquad (7)$$

where m is, as usual, the number of elements in the scale under consideration.

The problem with "A" is that it is too strong a property to be of much use for most scales. Scales having any family members R, S satisfying A(R, S) are few and far between. For example, it can be shown either by exhaustive enumeration (Forte, 1964) or by formal proof that there are only three size-7 scales (out of 66) containing scale family members that satisfy "A": (0, 1, 2, 4, 6, 8, 10), (0, 1, 2, 3, 4, 5, 6), and (0, 2, 4, 5, 7, 9, 11).* The group elements (transformations) associated with adjacency in each case are $(T_2, T_4, T_6, T_8, T_{10})$, (T_1, T_{11}), (T_5, T_7), respectively. In the case of (0, 1, 2, 4, 6, 8, 10), the transformation $T_4(S)$ yields (4, 5, 6, 8, 10, 0, 2) = (0, 2, 4, 6, 8, 10), and Ov (S, T_4 (S)) = m-1. In general it can be seen that all of the transformations $(T_2, T_4, \ldots , T_{10})$ carry the subset (0, 2, 4, 6, 8, 10) into itself and the 'odd' element is the only nonoverlapping one. Similarly, inspection reveals that adding or subtracting 1 - transforming by T_1 or T_{11} respectively - for each element in (0, 1, 2, 3, 4, 5, 6), yields a set containing 6 notes in common with the original set. Neither of these first two scales is coherent, and neither has seen any musical usage in any culture, as far as I am aware. The third scale, (0, 2, 4, 5, 7, 9, 11), is of course the diatonic scale.

A more generally useful predicate can be defined over triples of scale family members. In the spirit of Goodman's (1966) 'betwixt' relation among manors of qualia, let us define a betweenness relationship among three scale family members, X, Y, Z as follows:

$$X/Y/Z \equiv [X \cap Z) \subset (X \cap Y)] \wedge [(X \cap Z) \subset (Y \cap Z)] \quad (8)$$

where "X/Y/Z" is to be read as "Y is between X and Z". The above definition is stated in a form closely analogous to Goodman's 'betwixtness'. From the definition, it follows that (a) no scale is between itself and any other scale ($\sim X/X/Y$), (b) betweenness is symmetrical with respect to its first and third arguments (if X/Y/Z, then Z/Y/X), and (c) other than the situation just described, betweenness is asymmetrical: for any three scales, at most one is between the other two (if X/Y/Z, then $\sim Y/X/Z$ and $\sim$ X/Z/Y).

The character of betweenness may be more intuitively appreciated from an immediate consequence of the above definition:

$$X/Y/Z \Rightarrow (X \cap Z) \subset Y \quad (8a)$$

In words, if Y is between X and Z, then all elements shared by X and Z are contained in Y. Figure 1 displays Venn diagrams of sets that do and do not satisfy the definition of betweenness. Loosely, only sets X, Y, Z satisfying X/Y/Z can be represented 'on a line' with Y represented 'between' X and Z.

---

*   The complete proof would take us too far afield here; interested readers should write to the author.

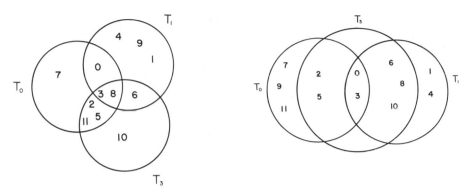

Fig. 1   Illustration of the betweenness relation. The triple of sets on the left does not satisfy betweenness, while the triple on the right satisfies $T_0/T_3/T_1$.

Most scale family members contain many triples in a betweenness relation. Considering the three sets just examined in the discussion of adjacency, we find the following:

(I)   In (0, 1, 2, 3, 4, 5, 6), it is easy to show that $T_0/T_1/T_2$. In addition, $T_0/T_1/T_3$, $T_0/T_1/T_4$, and in general $T_g/T_{g+i}/T_{g+j}$, so long as $i<j$ and $j<6$. (Addition of subscripts, remember, is modulo 12).

(II)   In (0, 2, 4, 5, 7, 9, 11), we have $T_0/T_7/T_2$, $T_0/T_7/T_4$, and in general $T_g/T_{g+7i}/T_{g+7j}$, so long as $i<j$ and $j<6$. We will discuss further the relation between this scale and (0, 1, 2, 3, 4, 5, 6) at a later point.

(III)   The set (0, 1, 2, 4, 6, 8, 10) exhibits no betweenness relations. If we relax Equation 8 to allow <u>improper</u> subsets to count for betweenness, we then get such relations as $T_0/T_2/T_4$, $T_0/T_2/T_6$, $T_0/T_2/T_8$, and $T_0/T_2/T_{10}$.

The next step, again following Goodman's lead, is to define <u>besideness</u> in terms of betweenness. In general, we will say that two scales are beside one another if they enter into at least one betweenness relation, and if no other scale is between them. Formally,

$$\text{Bsd}(X,Y) \equiv (\exists R: X/Y/R \lor Y/X/R) \land (\not\exists S: X/S/Y) \qquad (9)$$

Table 3. Besideness Relations for Family Members of
Harmonic Minor and Diatonic Scales

Family Member	Harmonic Minor	Diatonic
0	3,9	5,7
1	4,10	6,8
2	5,11	7,9
3	0,6	8,10
4	1,7	9,11
5	2,8	0,10
6	3,9	1,11
7	4,10	0,2
8	5,11	1,3
9	0,6	2,4
10	1,7	3,5
11	2,8	4,6

Pursuing the spatial analogy, it is proposed that the simplest scale families have a large number of betweenness relations and a small number of besideness relations.

The simplest kinds of besideness relations occur when each scale family member is beside exactly two others (as points on a line, for example). This situation can occur in two rather different ways, exemplified by the harmonic minor scale and the major scale in Table 3. In the former, T_0 is beside T_3, T_3 beside T_6, T_6 beside T_9, and T_9 beside T_0, but there are no besideness relations connecting these four scales with the other eight family members. Scales associated with (T_1, T_4, T_7, T_{10}) and (T_2, T_5, T_8, T_{11}) are similar; each set of four scales can be represented on the vertices of a square, but the relation between the three squares so obtained is indeterminate.

In the case of the diatonic scale each family member is again beside two others, but in this case the family is fully connected by the besideness relation: T_0 is beside T_7, T_7 beside $\overline{T_2}$, T_2 beside T_9, and so on up to the final link, Bsd (T_5, T_0). All other members of the scale family can thus be represented on the vertices of a dodecagon, as shown in Figure 2b. There is only one other size-7 scale that leads to a configuration as simple as this one, namely the previously cited $(0, 1, 2, 3, 4, 5, 6)$. For that scale, T_0 is beside T_1, T_1 beside T_2, and so on up to T_{11} beside T_0. The resulting space of scale relations is shown in Figure 2a.

For both of these scales besideness is essentially determined by a single parameter, either the group element T_7 (and its inverse) or the group element T_1 (and its inverse). While there are scales of different cardinalities that also have besideness determined by one or the other of these group elements, no scale of any cardinality gives rise to a space of scale relations determined by any other single group element. To see why this is so, we need to examine the concept of a group generator. Along the way we will develop the notion of a group isomorphism and present the three basic isomorphisms of C_{12} that are operative in music.

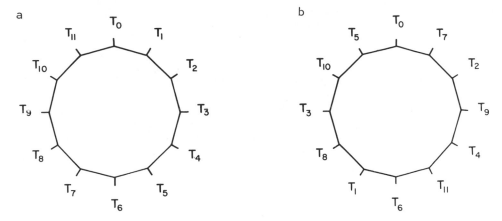

Fig. 2. Map of besideness relations for the scale (0, 1, 2, 3, 4, 5, 6). (b) Map of besideness relations for the diatonic scale. The figure also depicts isomorphic representations of the group C_{12} referred to in the text as "the cycle of semitones" (a) and "the cycle of fifths" (b).

GROUP GENERATORS AND THE ISOMORPHISMS OF C_{12}

Semitone Space and Fifths Space

The subgroups of C_{12} have been presented in an earlier section. The largest subgroup of C_{12} is C_6, which contains the elements (0, 2, 4, 6, 8, 10). Transformationally, the subgroup would be written $(T_0, T_2, T_4, T_6, T_8, T_{10}) = (I, T_2, T_4, T_6, T_8, T_{10})$. Note that every element in the subgroup is expressible as a power of T_2. Thus $T_2 * T_2 = (T_2)^2 = T_4$, $T_2 * T_2 * T_2 = (T_2)^3 = T_6$, and so forth. We say that the group element T_2 is of period six, since $(T_2)^6 = 1$, and that T_2 thereby generates the subgroup C_6. The same is true of T_{10}, the inverse of T_2, which generates the same six elements in reverse order.

Similarly, the subgroup C_4 consists of $(T_0, T_3, T_6, T_9) = (I, T_3, T^2_3, T^3_3) = (I, T^3_9, T^2_9, T_9)$. In this case we would say that T_3 and T_9 are of period four, and each generates C_4. In like fashion, $T_4(T_8)$ is of period three, generating the C_3 subgroup, and T_6 is of period two, generating C_2.

The only elements that do not appear in any of the subgroups of C_{12} are T_1 and T_7 (and their inverses). Both of these elements are in fact of period 12. and generate all of C_{12}. If a subgroup of C_{12} contained T_7, it would also have to contain all the powers of T_7 in order to satisfy the closure property for groups. Since the powers of T_7 exhaust C_{12}, no proper subgroup (analogous to 'proper subset') of C_{12} can contain T_7.

On the other hand, elements that <u>are</u> contained in proper subgroups of C_{12} cannot 'reach' all of the elements in C_{12}; only elements that generate all of C_{12} can do this. Thus, we cannot express the relation between every pair of group elements in terms of, say T_2 or T_3. In terms of T_2, the relation between group elements "4" (T_4) and "5" (T_5) is indeterminate. In essence, only T_1 and T_7 can serve as a complete basis for a space of scale relations as discussed in the previous section. Graphical representations of the structures generated by T_1 and T_7 - independently of any considerations of scales - are precisely those given in Figure 2. The said structures are both directly implied by C_{12}; indeed, they <u>are</u> C_{12}. We will call Figure 2a by the name "semitone space" or "the cycle of semitones", Figure 2b will be referred to as "fifths space" or "the cycle of fifths."

Unlike the versions of C_6 generated by T_2 and T_{10}, Figure 2a and 2b are not simply related by mirror reversal. But they are nonetheless fully <u>isomorphic</u> representations of C_{12}. What this means is that the mapping $A \longleftrightarrow B$: $i(\bmod \ 12) \longleftrightarrow 7i \ (\bmod \ 12)$ is one-to-one and structure-preserving. Any true statement about elements in system A is true of their images in system B. What is <u>different</u> about the two systems lies in the proximity relations among elements. In system A (Figure 2a), elements "2" and "3" are close together, "2" and "9" far apart, while the reverse is the case in System B (Figure 2b). But both of these isomorphisms are on an equal footing in the sense that neither is logically prior to the other.

It may be argued, however, that the two spaces in Figure 2 are not on an equal <u>perceptual</u> footing. With or without musical context, it might be said that the normative sense of 'closeness' of two pitches corresponds to that depicted in Figure 2a, not 2b. Additional constraints of some sort would be necessary to render the proximity structure of fifths space (Figure 2b) perceptually available information.

Furnishing such constraint would appear to be exactly the function served by a diatonic scale. The besideness and adjacency relations held by members of the diatonic scale line up precisely with the T_7-generated isomorphism of C_{12} called fifths space. If we examine the structure of a diatonic scale with respect to fifths space, we can see just how this is so. As Figure 3 shows, a diatonic scale corresponds to a connected region of fifths space. Transforming the scale by a perfect fifth corresponds to the minimal rotation of the region, such that m-1 elements are common to any two adjacent scales. We have shown how unusual this property is. The set (0, 1, 2, 3, 4, 5, 6) has similar properties, but with respect to the T_1-generated space.

From Figure 3, it can perhaps be appreciated that scales of any cardinality representable as regions in semitone space or fifths space, and only those scales, have besideness relations fully determined by T_1 or T_7, respectively. Thus the scales (0, 1, 2, 3, 4, 5), (0, 1, 2, 3, 4), (0, 2, 4, 5, 7, 9), and (0, 2, 4, 7, 9) are all similar in that respect. If we restrict our view to scales exhibiting Coherence, however, we are left with only two scales: (0, 2, 4, 5, 7, 9, 11), and (0, 2, 4, 7, 9). The former is the diatonic scale, and the latter is none other than the well-known and culturally

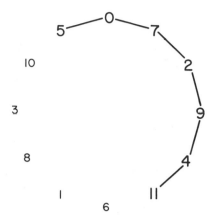

Fig. 3   The diatonic scale represented as a connection region of fifths
            space. Transforming the scale by T_2 or T_5 leads to a scale
            with six (out of seven) overlapping elements.

widespread pentatonic scale. Our inquiry into the structure of scales and of
the embedding group C_{12} has led us to the two most nearly universal
scales in the history of music. But our description of C_{12} is not complete
until we consider one more isomorphic representation.

Thirds Space

        Both of our previous isomorphisms of C_{12} have been 'one-dimensional'
in the sense that a single generator - like a basis vector in the theory of
vector spaces - spans all of the elements under consideration.
Higher-dimensional vector spaces can be realized by forming so-called
Cartesian products, and in an analogous fashion there exist product groups,
where each element is an n-tuple, each component of which is a member of
some group.   For example, the product group C_2 x C_3 consists of
2-tuples of the form (x,y,) where x is an element of C_2 and y is an
element of C_3.   We use the integers mod n as a model for C_n.
Combination of 2-tuples proceeds componentwise, so in C_2 x C_3

$$(x_1, y_1)*(x_2, y_2) = (x_1 + x_2 \text{ mod } 2, y_1 + y_2 \text{ mod } 3) \quad (10)$$

It is easy to verify that there are six such elements and that the
requirements for a group are satisfied.
        In some cases direct product groups can be isomorphic to simpler groups
whose elements are 1-tuples. It turns out that C_{12} is isomorphic to the
direct product of two of its subgroups, $C_3 x C_4$.   Elements of $C_3 x C_4$
are 2-tuples consisting of an element of the set (0, 1, 2) followed by an
element of the set (0, 1, 2, 3). The rule of combination for such (x, y) pairs
is analogous to $C_2 x C_3$. Thus $C_3 x C_4$,

$$(x_1, y_1)*(x_2, y_2) = (x_1 + x_2 \text{ mod } 3, y_1 + y_2 \text{ mod } 4) \quad (11)$$

It is not hard to see that there are 12 elements in this group, but to demonstrate an isomorphism with the group C_{12} we must show a one-one structure-preserving mapping of the twelve 2-tuples to the elements in the set $(0, 1, \ldots, 11)$. Here it is:

$C_3 \times C_4$	C_{12}
(0,0)	0
(0,1)	3
(0,2)	6
(0,3)	9
(1,0)	4
(1,1)	7
(1,2)	10
(1,3)	1
(2,0)	8
(2,1)	11
(2,2)	2
(2,3)	5

In general $(a,b) \longrightarrow [4a + 3b]_{12}$ (where the subscript "12" merely indicates that the right side is to be taken mod 12). The reader may readily verify that the 2-tuples on the left play analogous structural roles to their C_{12} images. For example, (1,1) is a generator of $C_3 \times C_4$; $(1,1)*(1,1)*(1,1)$ = (0,3), $7*7*7 = 9$ and 9 is the image of (0,3) (see above).

Graphically, $C_3 \times C_4$ would require two orthogonal axes, one generated by major thirds (C_3: (0, 4, 8) $\longrightarrow$ [(0,0), (1,0), (0,2)]) and the other minor thirds (C_4: (0, 3, 6, 9) $\longrightarrow$ [(0,0), (1,0), (0,2), (0,3)]). A doubly cyclic structure such as this one is representable on the surface of a torus in three dimensions. In Figure 4 we cut and unroll the torus and lay several torii next to one another to provide a more readable planar equivalent of the representation. To facilitate comparison with the other isomorphisms, the points of $C_3 \times C_4$ have been labelled with their C_{12} images rather than the 2-tuples. The points are labelled with "i" rather than "T", mainly eliminate to redundancy, but also to remind that the figure depicts a structure both of places and of transformations between places. We will call this final isomorphism "thirds space."

In fifths space, the simplest, maximally compact 'shapes' were intervals of the fifth itself and pitch sets consisting of chains of fifths. In thirds space, the situation is similar with regard to chains of major and minor thirds. But because thirds space is two-dimensional, there are also simple, compact shapes to be found that are not merely chains. The simplest of these is a unit right triangle with a major third and a minor third constituting the two perpendicular sides. If both sides are traced out in a positive-going direction, there are two possible kinds of triangles, representable as (0, 4, 7) and (0, 3, 7). These two pitch sets are musically well-known as the major triad and the minor triad, respectively.

From here we can ask about the effect of 'chaining' together these higher-order structures, just as we did for the lower-order generating intervals. The result can be seen outlined in Figure 4. When we sweep out a

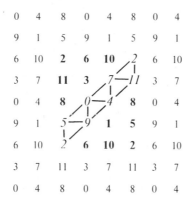

Fig. 4   Thirds space represented on a plane. The horizontal axis is in major-3rd (4 mod 12) units, the vertical axis in minor-3rd (3 mod 12) units. This space is isomorphic to semitone and fifths space. The parallelogram represents the region of a diatonic scale. The triangular constituents of the parallelogram correspond to the regions of major and minor triads. The boldface numbers contain the basic module of thirds space; adjoining modules are duplications.

region of thirds space by adjoining positive-going triangles together, we reach the point from which we began after obtaining six triangles interconnecting seven pitch places. And the pattern of those seven pitch places, forming a convex, space-filling region of thirds space, is the pattern of a diatonic scale.*

Other scales do not fare so well in attaining a simple structure vis-a-vis thirds space. The pentatonic scale, on an equal footing with the diatonic in fifths space, is not a compact region in thirds space. It contains five notes, but only two triads. Other fifth-generated chains suffer similar defects in thirds space. Our semitone-space diatonic analog (0, 1, 2, 3, 4, 5, 6), can be found in thirds space if we alter the 'handedness' of the space and construct triangles with one positive- and one negative-going side: adjoining six such triangles in the manner of our former diatonic scale construction yields (0, 1, 2, . . . , 6) or a member of its family. The constituent triangles themselves are sets of the form (0, 1, 4) and (0, 3, 4). Like the parent scale, these pitch sets have seen virtually no musical use.

With the addition of thirds space we exhaust the structure of C_{12}: the cycle of semitones and the cycle of fifths are the only single-generator spaces possible, and our $C_3 \times C_4$ thirds space is the only product group

---

*   The reader who wonders where the seventh triad had gone may find it in the 'seam' formed by joining the (11, 2) side of the uppermost triangle with the (2, 5) side of the lowermost triangle. This triad, the "vii$_0$" in major, is itself neither a major nor a minor triad, but a diminished triad belonging to the family (0, 3, 6) - a size-3 chain along the minor-3rds axis.

isomorphic to C_{12}. In particular, $C_2 \times C_6$, a group with twelve elements, is not isomorphic to C_{12}. For one thing, there are no elements in this group having period twelve, and therefore there are no group elements to correspond to semitones or fifths. In addition, there are three $C_2 \times C_6$ elements of period two, so there are too many elements that potentially correspond to a tritone. Higher-order product groups such as $C_2 \times C_2 \times C_3$ also fail to be isomorphic to C_{12}.

The reader is invited to consider the isomorphic semitone, thirds and fifths spaces as bases for melodic, harmonic, and key relations in music, respectively. We shall have more to say about this apparent correspondence in the closing section of the chapter. For now, note that the structural properties of C_{12} and of its scales have all been developed without recourse to the concept of a frequency ratio. Indeed, all the properties of our pitch system that have been the subject of the last two sections are logically independent of ratio concerns, including the special nature of the diatonic scale, the major and minor triads, and the cycle of fifths.

The present theoretical framework provides a role for several kinds of experiments in musical perception, many of which have yet to be performed. In the next section I will review the results of several experiments that are congenial to the present framework, in an attempt to sketch out the kind of experimental tradition that is in the spirit developed here.

EMPIRICAL RESEARCH

From the psychophysical and ratio-based traditions of pitch perception research, we have inherited studies on the perception of such things as beats, harmonics and combination tones. On the whole, it must be concluded that human perceptual sensitivity to these phenomena is rather low. Consider: (a) Many theoretically possible combination tones cannot be heard at all, and those that can are audible only under restricted frequency-amplitude conditions (Plomp, 1976). (b) It has long been known that detecting harmonics requires a mode of listening anathemic to the perception of a running musical context (Helmholtz, 1885), and even under the best conditions humans seem to possess no significant sensitivity to harmonics beyond the sixth or seventh (Plomp, 1964). (c) The presence of beats, besides being difficult to distinguish from vibrato, is apparently not even functionally related to the perception of 'in-tuneness', contrary to many commonly held beliefs (Corso, 1954).

By way of contrast, musicians and nonmusicians alike show ample evidence of perceptual sensitivity to pitch set structure. The many studies that show some kind of advantage - or any kind of differential performance - under 'tonal' versus 'atonal' pitch contexts all exemplify this basic finding.* For example, the ability to detect a changed note in a melodic sequence is greater when that sequence is tonal than when it is atonal

---

*   In the cases to be reported, the 'tonal' contexts corresponded to pitch sets representable as regions in fifths space, usually the size-7 region

(Frances, 1958). In general, memory for the pitch of a given tone is better when the latter is embedded in a tonal context (Dewar, Cuddy & Mewhort, 1977; Dewar, 1977; Krumhansl, 1979). These findings appear to hold up equally well regardless of the degree of musicality of the listener. In some cases, it is actually the less musically inclined listener that shows the larger effects (Dewar et al., 1977).

The important but often-missed implication of these findings and observations is not that they show tonal music to be 'better' or even 'more familiar', but that they imply a direct sensitivity on the part of the perceiver to differences in the structure of pitch sets. To attempt to explain away such findings in terms of "familiarity" begs the whole question of what the determinants of perceived familiarity might be. So when Lundin (1953) says, "these responses are part of our cultural attitudes, and even though one does not have specific musical training, this does not mean he has not acquired the typically cultural reactions", (p.146) he does not appear to realize that his "typical cultural reactions" presuppose an ability to perform a perceptual discrimination. The common property most likely to serve as a basis for this discrimination is the structure of the pitch set.

Perception of Dynamic Qualities

In this section we will consider experiments on the 'dynamic qualities' (Zuckerkandl, 1956) of the degress (notes) of diatonic scales.

The use of a diatonic scale in a musical context usually involves the selection of a tonic or tonal center, which then acts as a point of reference or perceptual origin for other degrees of the scale. If the pitch "0" is selected as a tonic for the set (0, 2, 4, 5, 7, 9, 11), we have the major mode of the diatonic scale. We symbolize the corresponding scale degrees by elements of the set ($\hat{1}$, $\hat{2}$, $\hat{3}$, $\hat{4}$, $\hat{5}$, $\hat{6}$, $\hat{7}$).

Given the apparent importance of establishing a tonic in a musical context, the first question one might ask about the dynamic qualities of scale degrees is: how are they perceptually related to the tonic degree? Under a strict psychophysical view, we would expect the answer to be that perceptual relatedness is determined by differences in tone height, perhaps as measured by log frequency. Taking the notion of octave equivalence into account might lead one to predict that differences in tone chroma (see Revesz, 1954; Bachem, 1950; Shepard, 1964) would control perceptual relatedness. By this scheme, pitch classes "5" (degree 4) and "7" (degree 5) might be equally related to "0" (degree 1) since the pitch class difference or chroma difference is the same in these two cases.

It turns out that neither of the above notions is sufficient to account for the structure of affinities displayed between the tonic and other pitches. Krumhansl and Shepard (1979) put the question to empirical test by

---

known as the diatonic scale. 'Atonal' contexts did not necessarily consist of larger pitch sets, but pitch sets more thinly spread over fifths space.

playing the first seven notes of an ascending or descending major scale, followed by a variable eighth tone. The latter could be any one of 13 pitches contained in the octave spanned by the first tone and the tone an octave above (for ascending scales) or below (for descending scales). The task for subjects was to judge how well the final note completed the sequence in each case.

Of the 24 subjects in the experiment, only the six subjects with the smallest amount of musical experience showed anything like an effect of tone height. Every subject gave the highest ratings to the tonic and its octave neighbor. For all subjects, tones belonging to the scale received significantly higher ratings than tones outside the scale. And, for the more musical subjects anyway, the pattern of responses could be nicely modeled by a combination of distances on the cycle of semitones and the cycle of fifths. That is, the farther away a given final note was from the tonic, as measured by distance in semitone space and fifths space, the less well it was judged to complete the scale and thus substitute for the tonic (see also Shepard, in press). There are also a hint in the data that third-relatedness played a significant role in determining judgments, but the authors did not specifically examine the data from this point of view.

In a related study, Krumhansl (1979) looked at judgments of perceived similarity among all possible pairs of pitch classes. Before each pair of pitches to be judged, subjects heard the same diatonic context-inducing scale or triad (the triad used was the tonic triad, $\hat{1}$-$\hat{3}$-$\hat{5}$-$\hat{8}$). The results for pitch pairs containing the tonic as a member looked very similar to the Krumhansl and Shepard (1979) study. The overall matrix of rated similarities was subjected to multidimensional scaling, with a resulting conical configuration resembling that given in Figure 5. Points in the figure are labeled with pitch class numbers using "0" as the tonic ("12" is the pitch an octave above "0"). This configuration shows a clear role for third- and fifth-relatedness in determining perceived similarity. The pitch classes most closely related to one another are the members of the tonic triad, (0, 4, 7), scale degrees, $\hat{1}$, $\hat{3}$ and $\hat{5}$. At the next level in the configuration are the remaining diatonic tones - 2($\hat{2}$), 5($\hat{4}$), 9($\hat{6}$) and 11($\hat{7}$) - that, together with the member of the tonic triad, constitute the diatonic region of fifths and thirds space. The five chromatic tones outside the scale are displaced to another level of the configuration. Within each level of the configuration, the ordering of tones is apparently determined by semitone-space relations. Whether the diatonic context was induced by the full scale or the tonic triad did not affect these findings.

While such studies constitute strong evidence for the importance of abstract group-theoretic pitch relations, it might be argued that subjects' judgments were somewhat removed from direct perceptual experience. Perhaps, the argument would go, the contribution of abstract pitch relations in these experiments is a cognitive effect occuring during the process of forming a judgment, and not a true perceptual effect. I will now present some new data that address this issue.

The subjects in the study to be described were all college students in a large introductory course in music theory and 'ear training' designed for non-music majors. Many of these students had had little or nothing in the way of formal musical training.

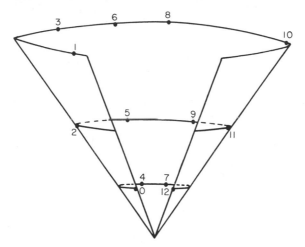

Fig. 5   Multidimensional scaling configuration depicting judged similarity of pitch pairs in a diatonic context. "0" is the tonic of the implied context. The configuration is somewhat idealized (after Krumhansl, 1979).

The experimental task, <u>degree discrimination</u>, was not unlike a standard pitch discrimination task, except that notes that were octave-related had to be treated as equivalent. Prior to the first trial of the study, and <u>ad lib</u> thereafter, listeners heard two octaves of an ascending major scale, to set the context for the trials to follow. Each trial involved the presentation of a tone belonging to a particular subset of the full scale. The subsets of present concern are ($\hat{1}$, $\hat{5}$) and $\hat{1}$, $\hat{7}$). The total ensemble of tones for these subsets are shown in Figure 6. The listener's task was to discriminate the tonic degree from the other scale degree in the subset (either $\hat{5}$ or $\hat{7}$), and to depress one of two buttons as soon as the decision had been made. Both correctness and latency of response were recorded on each trial. All stimuli were delivered by a PET-2001 microcomputer; tone spectra resembled that of a square wave. The actual frequencies used varied from subject to subject, but in each case approximated equal-tempered tuning within the frequency resolution of the computer.

On the whole the subjects were rather good at the task. Mean response latency over 49 subjects was 1260 milliseconds (msec), and mean percent correct was 87.4%. No subject performed at less than 74% accuracy, and even the longest mean response latency was barely over 3 seconds. The $\hat{1}$-$\hat{7}$ discrimination was performed 170 msec faster than the $\hat{1}$-$\hat{5}$ discrimination (1175 vs 1345 msec, respectively), and 4.6% more accurately (89.7% vs 85.1%). Both of these differences were highly significant statistically, $F(1, 48) = 8.71$, $p < .005$ for latencies, and $F(1, 48) = 36.55$, $p < .001$ for percent correct. Besides being reliable over the 49 subjects, the $\hat{1}$-$\hat{7}$ advantage also generalized over the five tones in the ensembles, $F(1, 4) = 20.30$, $p < .001$ for latencies and $F(1, 4) = 9.237$, $p < .05$ for percent correct.

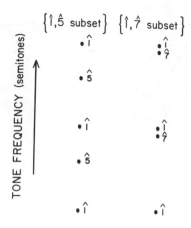

Fig. 6   Tone ensembles used in degree experiments.

Thus we see that, even on a speeded discrimination task, perceived similarity of scale degrees is mediated not be frequency separation, but by fifth-relatedness. In terms of our group isomorphisms, we would say that perceptual closeness in this task appears to be determined by distance in fifths space, and not distance in semitone space.

Table 4. Results of Degree Discrimination Studies

Pitch Subset	First Study		Three Months Later	
	Latency (msec)	% Correct	Latency (msec)	% Correct
$\hat{1}$ - $\hat{5}$	1345	85.1	885	90.4
$\hat{1}$ - $\hat{7}$	1175	89.7	840	93.1

These data were collected right near the beginning of the course, before students could have arguably become 'indoctrinated' to music-theoretic beliefs. To the extent that such beliefs or knowledge could affect one's perception, as is sometimes claimed, we would expect evidence of enhanced perceptual similarity of 1 and 5 to be even stronger for students who were thus indoctrinated. But follow-up measurements did not confirm this idea. Data collected on essentially the same group of students three months later (the course lasts an entire school year) revealed a general improvement of about 400 msec in latencies, down to a mean of 863 msec, and an improvement of about 4% in correct responses, up to 91.8%. But the size of the $(\hat{1}, \hat{7})$ - $(\hat{1}, \hat{5})$ difference was greatly <u>reduced</u>, such that the $(\hat{1}, \hat{7})$

advantage was only 45 msec (as opposed to 170 msec) and 2.7% (as opposed to 4.6%). These differences were still statistically reliable over subjects, but just barely so for the latencies, $F(1, 52) = 3.98$, $p < .05$ for latencies, and $F(1, 52) = 17.39$, $p < .001$ for percent correct. Being increasingly indoctrinated to the idea of 1 and 5 being similar apparently did not make 1 and 5 more perceptually confusable. The two sets of data values are shown in Table 4.

It might be argued that confusability of pitches related by fifths, as found here, was somehow due to the spectral composition of the tones. I have collected some pilot data with pure tones that suggest such is not the case. Also it should be noted, first, that no classical pitch discrimination experiment using complex tones has found any hint of the pattern of results reported here; pitch discrimination, we are told, is mediated by the frequency separation of the fundamentals. Secondly, we should recognize that tones of greater spectral complexity are more representative of what is actually found in music, so any result that occurred only with pure tones would be of limited generality or interest in any case. There is really no paradox here, as long as it is conceded that discrimination of pitched dynamic qualities is not the same thing as, nor is necessarily reducible to, pitch discrimination.

As a final informal result on the notions of Uniqueness and dynamic quality, consider the task of deciding what kind of scale a given melody is based on. On an examination, students in my ear-training class were given four melodies to listen to, and asked to decide for each melody whether it was based on a pentatonic scale, a major scale, a harmonic minor scale, a whole tone scale, or a chromatic scale. The pentatonic, major, and harmonic minor scales consist of 5, 7 and 7 notes, respectively, and all satisfy Uniqueness. The whole tone and chromatic scales consist of 6 and 12 notes respectively, and both fail Uniqueness. Of the four melodies played on the examination, one was based on the pentatonic, one on harmonic minor, one on the whole tone, and one on the chromatic scale. Tabulation of the 42 identification errors that occurred showed the following breakdown: fully 23 errors involved whole-tone/chromatic confusions, and 15 errors involved confusions within the pentatonic/major/minor class. Only 4 out of 42 errors were between-class errors; in general, scales satisfying Uniqueness were hardly ever confused with scales failing to satisfy Uniqueness. While the result is only suggestive, it supports the idea that abstract properties of pitch collections are indeed perceptible.

Scalestep-level Perception

When a scale is coherent, the scalestep-level distances it induces on its intervals are both a determinate function of semitones and a consistent (i.e. monotonic) function of semitone distances. It was argued earlier that only coherent scales are conducive to the perceptual learning of scalestep-level properties of intervals. The question to be treated here is whether such perceptual learning does in fact occur: are higher-level scalestep properties of intervals perceptible? Data from several experiments appear to suggest that the answer is <u>yes</u>.

The global cultural context of diatonic scales has determined the names of the twelve intervals from m2 to p8 inclusive: what makes a minor 3rd and a major 3rd both <u>thirds</u> is predicated on nothing more or less than their function in a diatonic scale. But it is another thing entirely to suggest that this global context in which intervals are heard and learned actually determines the way they <u>sound</u> to listeners. Yet that seems to be a reasonable description of what actually occurs in the course of learning to identify the twelve intervals, as we shall see.

Plomp, Wagenaar, and Mimpen (1973) tested the recognition of simultaneous intervals by musicians. To induce errors, these investigators played the intervals at very short durations, the longest of which was 120 msec. What they found was that most of the confusion errors involved intervals separated by a semitone, but of these, an overwhelming majority of the errors were to intervals that shared the same scalestep value. I will refer to such intervals as <u>scalestep-equivalent</u>. Thus a major 2nd is a semitone away from both a minor 2nd and a major 3rd, but it is scalestep-equivalent to only the minor 2nd (since they are both <u>seconds</u>). What the data of Plomp et al. reveal is that scalestep equivalence is a powerful determinant of perceptual confusability, even when separation in semitones is held constant.

Killam, Lorton and Schubert (1975) replicated and extended this finding to situations involving

(a) longer durations,

(b) sequential (melodic) as well as simultaneous (harmonic) intervals, and

(c) a non-expert subject population, namely a class of students involved with <u>learning</u> to recognize intervals.

As in the case of Plomp et al., scalestep-equivalent intervals were the locus of many more identification errors than could be accounted for by closeness in semitones.

The result was further replicated and extended by Balzano (1977a, 1977b), who measured latencies as well as errors in a slightly different experimental paradigm. Briefly, a trial in these experiments consisted of a visually presented <u>probe</u>, which was the name of one of the twelve basic intervals (m2-p8), followed by <u>stimulus</u>, a harmonic or melodic interval that either did or did not match the interval named by the probe. Subjects, all skilled interval recognizers, responded by pressing one of two keys, labelled SAME and DIFFERENT, as soon as they thought they knew the answer. On DIFFERENT trials, the stimulus could be any one of the eleven intervals not named by the probe. The data showed that, even with semitone distance between probe and stimulus held constant, latencies were significantly longer and errors significantly more frequent when the probe and stimulus intervals were scalestep equivalent. The latency difference, in particular, was as high as 258 msec for harmonic intervals, one of the largest response latency differences I have seen in binary choice experiments of this general kind.

In a related experiment, Balzano (1977a) found evidence that intervals may be recognized at the scalestep level <u>directly</u>, without meditation through the semitone level. By this I mean that subjects appeared to recognize, say, a major 3rd, as a "3rd" directly, rather than by a two-stage process of the form "major 3rd, therefore 3rd." The test was designed as follows: In addition to the semitone-level probes in the other experiments, a number of scalestep-level probes were used as well. An example of the latter would be the visual probe "3rd", indicating that the subject should respond SAME if the stimulus is either a minor 3rd or a major 3rd, and DIFFERENT otherwise. Now there is considerable evidence that it is more difficult to look (Sternberg, 1967; Cavanaugh, 1972) or listen (Clifton & Cruse, 1977) for two things than for just one, but that is not what happened here. Rather, the scalestep-level probes led to responses that were significantly <u>faster</u> and more accurate than semitone-level probes. Stated slightly differently: for a given interval, say a major 3rd, it was easier and faster for subjects to verify this interval as an instance of the higher-level category "3rd" than the lower-level category "major 3rd". It would seem , therefore, that the "3rdness" of an interval is perceptually available prior to its 'minor-3rdness'.

It has often been suggested (e.g. Trotter, 1967) that, even for naive listeners, scalestep-level properties are more perceptually salient than semitone-level properties. Thus the sense in which adjacent moves of an ascending major scale are the 'same' seems to be more evident than the sense in which they differ. In a more rigorous context, Dowling (1978) has demonstrated a variant of this phenomenon. He played a standard melody followed by a comparison melody and asked subjects whether the two melodies were the same or not. Melodies were based on diatonic scales, and 'same' comparison melodies were exact transpositions of the standard, i.e. melodies based on the same scale degrees of a different member of the standard melody's scale family. On a number of trials, the comparison melody was not an exact transposition of the standard to another scale, but a scalestep-preserving movement of the melody to a different point in the same scale. Results indicated that musical and non-musical subjects alike had considerable difficulty in distinguishing the scalestep-equivalent nontranspositions from true transpositions. So even - if not especially - the listener who is not musically trained appears to perceive melodies in terms of scalestep-level, and not merely semitone-level, relations. If it weren't for the scalestep-semitone coherence of diatonic scales, this could not occur, of course, but it is nonetheless surprising just how potently scalestep-level properties enter into the perceptual process.

Scale Families, Pitch Set Overlap and Key Relatedness

In the subsection on dynamic qualities we saw some evidence for the perceptual reality of fifths-space distance relations. Here we address a similar issue, this time regarding the behavior of pitch sets under transposition, i.e. scale families. Since we generally listen, not to scales per se, but to melodies based on scales, the most natural way to approach this question is through studies of melody recognition. Given that a melody retains its identity under transposition, is there any difference in the extent to which this is true as a function of key relateness? Does a melody originally heard in C major somehow retain more of its perceptible identity when transposed to the adjacent key of G major than the distant (in fifths space) key of F# major?

The evidence of this question is mixed but generally positive. Cuddy, Cohen and Miller (1979) used a forced-choice melody recognition task, where a standard melody was followed by two comparison melodies, one target and one foil. Both targets and foils were transposed versions of the standard; foils had a single note altered by a semitone. Transpositions were sometimes by a fifth, i.e. to an adjacent key on the cycle of fifths and sometimes by a tritone, the largest possible distance in fifths space. The results showed a small but reasonably consistent advantage (about 4% overall) for the fifth transpositions.

Bartlett and Dowling (1980) performed a similar study, with two differences:

(a)   The task was yes-no rather than forced-choice; subjects heard only one comparison melody on a trial, and decided it was the 'same' as the standard or not.

(b)   The construction of foils was different; in particular, many of the foils were melodies that had been both transposed to a new key and translated along the scale to a new scale degree.

These foils, like those in Dowling (1978), preserved scalestep-level relations but violated semitone-level relations. The results showed a reliable key-distance effect, not on the targets, but on the foils. When a foil was transposed to a distant key, it was easier to distinguish from a correct transposition (i.e. recognize as a foil) than when the foil was transposed to a near key. Both adults and grammar school children show this effect. It is not simply due to a response bias for saying "no" to far-key transpositions; if it were, targets would have showed the same effect. But for our present concerns, it would not be diastrous if response bias were involved anyway, for even a response bias that is sensitive to key distance is evidence of a perceptual ability to respond to that variable.

To what extent are results like these a function of pitch overlap? Diatonically-based melodies, as we have seen, will have more pitch overlap with transpositions to near than to far keys, so the only way to examine this question is to use non-tonal melodies - more specifically, melodies whose pitch content is thinly spread through all of fifths space. Cohen (1977; Cohen, Cuddy & Mewhort, 1977) performed several experiments using melodies based on both diatonic pitch sets and pitch sets satisfying the above description. The task was basically the same as Cuddy et al (1979), and as there, the p5 (near) and tt (far) transpositions were used. What Cohen found was an interaction between the factors of pitch set and transposition. Diatonic melodies showed an advantage for the p5 transpositions, while atonal melodies showed a tritone advantage. The atonal pitch sets employed by Cohen were (0, 1, 2, 6, 7, 10) and the whole scale, both of which exhibit greater pitch class overlap under T_6 (tt) than T_7 (p5). So, for these experiments anyway, the ability to detect a correct transposition of a melody appeared to be a direct function of overlap (Ov) as previously defined.

The final set of experiments to be described in this subsection, those of Balzano (1977a), are quite different from those we have just discussed, in that melody recoginition was not studied, but interval recognition by skilled musicians. These experiments nonetheless fit into the present context because they document a perceptual sensitivity to key-relatedness as reckoned by distance in fifths space, moreover one that cannot have been mediated by pitch class overlap per se. In these interval recognition experiments, the base tone (i.e. the tone lower in frequency) of the intervals tested was restricted to a very small set of pitches. In three of the experiments, the base tone was always an E, an A, or a C♯ (pitch set (0, 4, 7)), each one on one-third of the trials; in two other experiments, the base tone was either a G or a C♯ (pitch set (0, 6)), each on one-half of the trials. The reasoning ran as follows (see Balzano, 1977a, for a fuller discussion): With the former base-tone set, 2/3 of the intervals presented in an experimental session were based on E or A, adjacent keys on the cycle of fifths. The other 1/3 of the intervals were based on a pitch more remote from the first two in fifths space. It was expected that the overall effect of this manipulation would place the subject in a perceptual mode similar to that for the key of A major, and therefore that recognition would be significantly worse to intervals based on the tone (C♯) that was more remote from A in fifths space. The G-C♯ base tone set, on the other hand, exhibits a purely symmetrical structure on the cycle of fifths, so neither tone should show any perceptual advantage over the other; in particular, the disadvantage for C♯ should no longer occur.

The results confirmed these ideas. While only one of the three experiments using the E-A-C♯ base-tone set showed a significant advantage for intervals based on A over intervals based on E, in all three experiments, intervals based on A and E were responded to more accurately and rapidly than those based on C♯. In the two experiments using the G-C♯ ensemble there were essentially no base-tone effects; if anything it was C♯ that led to faster and more accurate responding. Pitch overlap cannot account for these results, since all of the basic intervals were tested on each base tone; that is to say, the upper tone of the intervals was free to vary, and was not restricted, for example, to intervals from the base tone's major scale.

Summing up the results of this subsection, we can tentatively say that perceptual distance between transposed melodies is a function of pitch set overlap. For the case of diatonic melodies, this directly implicates the cycle of fifths as a basis for perceptual distance, but not necessarily in the case of atonal melodies. In the absence of pitch set constraints, overlap becomes nonfunctional, and here fifth-space distance appears to act as a perceptual default. It is evident that much more research remains to be done to clarify these matters.

CONCLUDING REMARKS

Experiments were performed long before the notion of a psychoacoustical theory ever arose, and they continued to be performed throughout history, not by scientists but by persons mainly attempting to discover the types of experiences pitch had to offer. What they hit upon, independently and all over the ancient worlds, was that different <u>pitch collections</u>. sets of pitches known as scales, each presented a potentially unique medium for embedding pitch sequences called melodies. Just as the desired movement of a melody over time shaped the character of these pitch set materials, so it was found that the character of the pitch set in turn shaped the perceptible quality of its melodies; different pitch sets thus became associated with different meanings. That this could occur constituted a very important discovery about pitch perception.

An account of the distinctive properties of pitch sets and their elements has not been forthcoming from state-of-the-art auditory theory. I have attempted to provide the beginnings of such an account in this chapter by using the language of set and group theory to develop a number of basic properties of pitch sets. The group C_{12} has been treated as a 'ground' for the musical 'figures' that are pitch sets, and three isomorphic representations of C_{12} have been presented as alternative 'grounds' for pitch sets and events.

The properties of pitch arrays that have been the subject of this chapter are not found at the level of tone sensations. But 100 years after Helmholtz, it is still far from clear that the sensations of tone truly are a basis, physiological or other, for the theory of music. It may or may not be true that "music stands in a much closer connection with pure sensation than any of the other arts" (Helmholtz, 1885), but the present theory is founded on the idea that it is the perception of patterns and relations the tones enter into and not the sensations of tone themselves that accounts for our ability to appreciate music. Given that such patterns and relations are made available in music through the medium of pitch sets, a theory outlining properties of pitch sets would appear indispensable to an effort to understand music perception in context. To the extent that the properties of the embedding pitch system (C_{12}) both constrain and interpret properties of it subsets, a theory of the pitch system would also seem a necessity. I have tried to provide a foundation for these basic necessities, but more important than the specific details presented here is the fact that a logically coherent, empirically supportable alternative to Helmholtz and the psychophysical tradition is indeed possible. We have seen in this chapter that a pitch-set level of description grants easy access to an order of phenomena that are both eminently musical in nature and at the same time difficult to provide a theoretical rendering of in lower-level terms. Perhaps even more importantly, human musical behavior itself yields readily to an analysis in the higher-level language proposed here. From a pitch-set perceptive, we may well be led to ask different kinds of questions and to search for new kinds of phenomena. It may even turn out that the most fascinating properties of human pitch perception still remain to be discovered.

SUMMARY

Properties of single pitches and properties of pitch sets belong to two different grains of analysis of the musical pitch stimulus. It is suggested that musically important properties of pitch are more directly a function of predicates defined at the latter grain. Starting from the observation that the global pitch system in Western music exhibits the structure of the mathematical group C_{12}, a number of systematic properties of pitch sets – subsets of C_{12} – are formally developed. At the same time, three isomorphic spatial representations of the inner structure of C_{12} are presented, and the familiar diatonic scale is revealed to have unique properties both with regard to the abstract description of pitch sets and with regard to the spatial character of C_{12}. Empirical evidence is reviewed and presented in support of the perceptual reality of these formally developed properties, and the general claim is made that listeners are directly sensitive to such pitch set properties. The sensations of tone may well be a function of frequency and frequency ratios, but the perception of music need not be, and indeed appears instead to be a function of higher-order properties of pitch sets that are independent of ratios.

REFERENCES

Attneave, F., and Olson, R.K., 1971, Pitch as a medium: A new approach to psychophysical scaling, Am. J. Psychol., 84:147-166.

Babbitt, M., 1972, The structure and function of musical theory, in "Perspectives on Contemporary Music Theory," B. Boretz and E.T. Cone, eds., Norton, New York. (Reprinted from College Music Symposium, 1965(5).)

Bachem, A., 1950, Tone height and tone chroma as two different pitch qualities, Acta Psychologica, 7:80-88.

Balzano, G.J., 1977a, "Chronometric Studies of the Musical Interval Sense," Doctoral diss., "Dissertation Abstracts International", Stanford University, 38, 2898B (Univ. Microfilms, No. 77-25, 643).

Balzano, G.J., 1977b, On the bases of similarity of musical intervals, J. Acoust. Soc. Am., 61-S51(Abs.)

Balzano, G.J., 1978, The structural uniqueness of the diatonic order, in "Cognitive Structure of Musical Pitch," R.N. Shepard (Chair), Symposium presented at the meeting of the Western Psychological Association, San Francisco, April 1978.

Balzano, G.J., in press, The group-theoretic description of twelve-fold and microtonal pitch systems, Comp. Mus. J.

Bartlett, J.C., and Dowling, W.J., 1980, Recognition of transposed melodies: A key-distance effect in developmental perspective, J. Exp. Psychol./Human Perc. Perf. 6:501-515.

Benade, A.H., 1960, "Horns, Strings and Harmony," Doubleday, New York.

Boretz, B., 1970, The construction of musical syntax. I, Persp. New Mus., 9(1):23-42.

Boynton, R., 1975, The visual system: Environmental information, in "Handbook of Perception" Vol. 3, E.C. Carterette and M.P. Friedman, eds., Academic Press, New York.

Budden, F.J., 1972, "The Fascination of Groups," Cambridge University
    Press, London.
Cassirer, E., 1944, The concept of group and the theory of perception,
    Philos. Phenomenolog. Res., 5:1-36.
Cavanaugh, J.P., 1972, Relation between the immediate memory span and
    the memory search rate, Psychol. Rev., 79:525-530.
Chalmers, J.H., Jr, 1975, Cyclic scales, Xenharmonikon, 4:66-74.
Clifton, C., Jr, and Cruse, D., 1977, Time to recognize tones: Memory
    scanning or memory strength? Quart. J. Exp. Psychol., 29:709-726.
Cohen, A.J., 1975, "Perception of Tone Sequences from the
    Western-European Chromatic Scale: Tonality, Transposition and the
    Pitch Set," Doct. diss. Queen's University at Kingston (Canada),
    "Dissertation Abstracts International," 1977, 37:4179B.
Cohen, A.J., Cuddy, L.L., and Mewhort, D.J.K., 1977, Recognition of
    transposed tone sequences, J. Acoust. Soc. Am., 61:S87-S88 (Abs.)
Corso, J.F., 1954, Unison tuning of musical instruments, J. Acoust. Soc.
    Am., 26:746-750.
Cuddy, L.L., Cohen, A.J., and Miller, J., 1979, Melody recognition: The
    experimental application of musical rules, Canad. J. Psychol.,
    33:148-157.
Dewar, K.M., 1977, Cues used in recognition memory for tones, J. Acoust.
    Soc. Am., 61:S49(Abs).
Dowling, W.J., 1978, Scale and contour: Two components of a theory of
    memory for melodies, Psychol. Rev., 85:341-354.
Forte, A., 1964, A theory of set-complexes for music, J. Mus. Theory,
    8:136-183.
Frances, R., 1958, "La Perception de la Musique," J. Vrin, Paris.
Fuller, R., 1975, A structuralist approach to the diatonic scale, J. Mus.
    Theory, 19:182-210.
Gamer, C., 1967, Some combinational resources of equal-tempered systems,
    J. Mus. Theory, 11:32-59.
Goodman, N., 1966, "The Structure of Appearance," (2nd ed.), Bobbs-Merill,
    Indianapolis.
Helmholtz. H. von, 1885, "On the Sensations of Tone as as Physiological
    Basis for the Theory of Music, "A.J. Ellis, ed. and trans., 1954, Dover,
    New York.
Holland, J. 1972, "Studies in Structure," Macmillan, London.
Killam, R.N., Lorton, P.V., and Schubert, E.D., 1975, Interval recognition:
    Identification of harmonic and melodic intervals, J. Mus. Theory,
    19:212-233.
Kohler, W., 1938, Physical Gestalten, in "A Source Book of Gestalt
    Psychology," W.D. Ellis, ed., Routledge & Kegan Paul, London.
Krumhansl, C.L., 1979, The psychological representation of musical pitch in
    a tonal context, Cog. Psych., 11:346-374.
Krumhansl, C.L., and Shepard, R.N., 1979, Quantification of the hierarchy
    of tonal functions within a diatonic context, J. Exp. Psychol./Human
    Perc. Perf., 5:579-594.
Kruskal, J.B., 1964a, Multidimensional scaling by optimizing goodness of fit
    to a nonmetric hypothesis, Psychometrika, 29:1-27.
Kruskal, J.B., 1964b, Nonmetric multidimensional scaling: A numerical
    method, Psychometrika, 29:115-129.

Lakner, Y., 1960, A new method of representing tonal relations, J. Mus. Theory, 4:194-209.

Lewin, D., 1959, Intervallic relations between two collections of notes, J. Mus. Theory, 3:298-301.

Lewin, D., 1960, The intervallic content of a collection of notes, J. Mus. Theory, 4:98-101.

Lewin, D., 1977, Forte's interval vector, my interval function, and Regener's common-note function, J. Mus. Theory 21:194-237.

Lundin, R.W., 1953, "An Objective Psychology of Music," Ronald Press, New York.

O'Connell, W., 1962, Tone spaces, Die Reihe, 8:34-67.

Plomp, R., 1964, The ear as a frequency analyzer, J. Acoust. Soc. Am., 36:1628-1636.

Plomp, R., 1976, "Aspects of Tone Sensation," Academic Press, New York.

Plomp, R., Wagenaar, W.A., and Mimpen, A.M., 1973, Musical interval recognition with simultaneous tones, Acustica, 29:101-109.

Regener, E., 1973, "Pitch Notation and Equal Temperament: A Formal Study," University of California Press, Berkeley.

Revesz, G., 1954, "Introduction to the Psychology of Music," University of Oklahoma Press, Norman, Oklahoma.

Rothenberg, D., 1978a, A model for pattern perception with musical applications. I, Pitch structures as order-preserving maps, Math. Systems Theory, 11:199-234.

Rothenberg, D., 1978b, A model for pattern perception with musical applications. II, The information content of pitch structures, Math. Systems Theory, 11:353-372.

Schenker, H., 1906, "Harmony", republ. 1973, O. Jonas, ed., E.M. Borgese, trans., MIT Press, Cambridge.

Shepard, R.N., 1962a, The analysis of proximities: Multidimensional scaling with an unknown distance function, I, Psychometrika, 27:125-139.

Shepard, R.N., 1962b, The analysis of proximities: multidimensional scaling with an unknown distance function, II, Psychometrika, 27:219-246.

Shepard, R.N., 1964, Circularity in judgements of relative pitch, J. Acoust. Soc. Am., 36:2346-2353.

Shepard, R.N., in press, Structural representations of musical pitch, in "Psychology of Music," D. Deutsch, ed., Academic Press, New York.

Sternberg, S., 1967, Two operations in character recognition: Some evidence from reaction-time measurements, Perc. & Psychophys., 2:45-53.

Trotter, J.R. 1967, The psychophysics of melodic interval: Definitions, techniques, theory and problems, Aust. J. Psychol., 19:13-25.

Zuckerkandl, V., 1956, "Sound and Symbol," Princeton University Press, Princeton.

Zuckerkandl, V., 1971, "The Sense of Music," Princeton University Press, Princeton, rev. ed.

Chapter XVIII

IMPACT OF COMPUTERS ON MUSIC
An Outline

Ernst Terhardt

Institute of Electroacoustics
Technical University, Munich
Munich, Federal Republic of Germany

INTRODUCTION

Since the early days of programmable computers, i.e. for at least 30 years, it has been said that the computer provides a means to overcome the technical and acoustic limitations of conventional musical instruments, to explore and occupy new musical worlds, and thus to heavily affect our musical life and experience. Nowadays, computers are everywhere present and we have become accustomed to use their data and signal processing power in many areas of human life. However, the computer's role in music actually as yet is very limited. The music we normally hear from the radio, from records, and in concert, is largely independent of computers. If new musical worlds have been discovered, they do not appear to be specific of computers. It might seem thus that the euphoria of the early computer pioneers has led them to over-estimate the real significance of computers for music. Yet this conclusion would probably be a grave mistake. There are several indications that the forthcoming decade will bring an enhanced and almost explosive infiltration by computers of all life domains, and the musical domain will no longer be an exception. History readily shows that everything technologically realizable actually is realized if it is commercially promising, no matter whether a comprehensive scientific and conceptual basis exists, or not. Cheap, yet powerful programmable pocket calculators, computer-controlled TV games, chess computers that can be beaten only by expert chess players, language translators, speech-understanding and talking computers, and digital music synthesizers are now on the market. It is highly probable that in a few years there will be offered electronic (computer-controlled) successors of the eighteenth and nineteenth century mechanical music boxes, capable of (re)producing any kind of music under the control of a human 'conductor' (and listener); computers which automatically 'compose' and realize music (perhaps vast amounts of trivial music for commercial purposes); computers which 'listen' to the performance of one or more human players and immediately respond by producing musical sounds in a partly deterministic, partly random way; software for home computers providing support to music education and practicing.

These and several other applications of computers to music represent a striking challenge to those scientific disciplines which are to provide the essential conceptual and methodological means for realization - psycho-physics and musical theory. The real value and long-term success of those computer applications will to a considerable extent depend on our understanding of the psychophysics of music. This aspect especially induced the present consideration of the impact of computers on music.

On approaching this topic it is adequate to begin by taking notice of the manifold, partly controversial facets of today's musical reality: music is the result of ingenious inspiration on one hand, and an industrial product on the other (for example, in many releases of popular and film music); a science, and a subject of pseudo-scientific speculation; a medicine to body and soul, and sometimes also a poison; a pleasing experience, and an annoying factor; a means of therapy, and sometimes a danger for health; an object of fruitful endeavor, and a means for wasting time; a socially integrating medium, and a vehicle to isolation from society. On considering the use of computers in music, one should be aware that not only the positive aspects may be enhanced and developed by the computer's signal processing power, but also the negative ones.

Systematically, the medium 'music' may be subdivided into four significant domains of endeavor and activity: Research, Learning/Teaching, Realization and Music Therapy. Table 1 shows a condensed survey of what can be done with the support of computers in these domains. In the first part of the present paper the basic preconditions and implications of this approach will be examined and illustrated by considering the particular problem of music realization by computers. In order to find out what the computer-specific problems and impacts are, it is useful to begin by considering the conventional process of music realization in a cybernetic approach. In the second part, the impact of computers on music will be

Table 1. Domains of computer applications in music

Research	Learning/Teaching	Realization	Music/Therapy
acoustical analysis;	foundations of hearing music theory:	composition;	interactive realization of music as a therapy
auditory analysis;	analysis of musical sounds;	interactive music creation;	
music theory;	practising;	new tonal systems;	
music therapy	foundations of electronic realization	sound modification	

further illustrated by considering some recent results of our own research on the psychoacoustic foundations of music theory. It will be shown with some examples, that this type of research is of basic significance for computer applications in music.

PSYCHOPHYSICS OF MUSIC REALIZATION

The term 'music realization' indicates a concept according to which music exists in different manifestations - something to be 'realized' in one domain of manifestation logically must already exist in another domain. In fact, there exist three basically different domains of musical reality whch may be described as symbolic, acoustic, and auditory representation of music (Table 2). These three domains of musical reality correspond perfectly to the basic philosophical concept of Popper (1972) and Eccles (1973, pp 189), asserting that everything that is existent in human experience can be assigned to three basically different 'worlds'. According to Eccles, world 1 comprises the acoustic representation of music (the sound pressure oscillations and movements of air particles, specified by physical parameters, as in Table 2). World 2 is characterized by the 'states of consciousness', i.e. subjective knowledge and sensory, mental and emotional experiences. Obviously, world 2 comprises the sensory experience of music, i.e. its auditory representation. Auditory sensations usually are described by parameters as pitch, loudness, timbre, etc., as described in Table 2. Finally, there is world 3, comprising 'knowledge in the objective sense', i.e. "records of intellectual efforts..., theoretical systems". This world is specific of everything which usually is labelled 'cultural'. Hence it comprises music in its essential, i.e. symbolic form. The non-material, symbolic contents of a musical score, eventually comprising symbolic specifications of the tones to be played, the musical intervals, harmonies etc. (see Table 2), are typical examples of this specific domain of musical reality.

Table 2. The three basic representations of music

Symbolic Representation (Score)	Acoustic Representation (Sound Parameters)	Auditory Representation (Sensory Parameters)
tones	frequencies	pitch, chroma
intervals	amplitudes	tonal affinity
harmonies	phases	virtual bass notes
timbre	modulation-parameters	sensory consonance
rhythm		timbre, loudness
	noise parameters	
dynamics		rhythm

This conceptual approach is, of course, not self evident a priori. Rather, it is a theoretical concept with the purpose to better understand the entity of human experience. The three worlds concept itself is a cultural product, and as such pertinent to world 3. It is justified to the extent that it is actually helpful in understanding complex human experiences, as, for example, the realization of music. In fact, for understanding the psycho-physics of music realization this concept is extremely useful - even indispensable. Many misconceptions and false conclusions could have been avoided by taking advantage of that concept properly.

As an example, consider the term 'musical tone'. This term does by no means exactly specify what is actually meant, because the term 'tone' is usually also used with respect to the symbolic, acoustic, and auditory representations of tones. Even the "American National Standard Psycho-acoustical Terminology (1973)" is ambiguous on this point. Two different definitions of tone are given: (1) "A tone is a sound wave capable of exciting an auditory sensation having pitch", and (2) "A tone is a sound sensation having pitch". Likewise, the term 'pitch' is in many cases used quite carelessly, meaning 'perceived tone height' in one case, 'tone frequency' in another, and 'tone category' (for example, A, B-flat, etc.) in the third. The ANS Psychoacoustical Terminology specifies that "Pitch is that attribute of auditory sensation in terms of which sounds may be ordered on a scale extending from low to high ...". Thereby the term 'pitch' is strictly assigned to world 2, i.e. the world of (auditory) sensations. For the sake of conceptual clarity, this unambiguity and simplicity of definition must be highly appreciated. It may be useful to note here that the wide-spread concept which asserts that pitch is a bimodal entity, composed of 'tone height' and 'tone chroma' is a superfluous conceptual complication, apparently born from confusion of the terms 'tone' and 'pitch'. While a tone actually may be characterized by several sensory attributes (i.e. pitch and chroma, among others), this is not true for pitch. Pitch on its own part is an attribute. In fact, psychophysical and musical evidence strongly suggests that the one-dimensional definition of pitch provides the most adequate conceptual approach to understanding musical tone perception (Terhardt, 1979).

As another example, consider the problem of tone scales, their intonation and perception. On the basis of the present concept it becomes clear that a tone scale is just a series of tone symbols which represent corresponding tone categories (for example, C, D, E, F, etc.); thus a tone scale is an entity existing in world 3. Quite another thing is the scale's intonation. As a matter of definition, one may either consider 'frequency intonation', thus describing a certain physical aspect of the tones, or 'pitch intonation', describing the (musically most relevant) perceptual aspect. In the first case, a certain relationship to world 1 (physical objects) is realized, in the second to world 2 (sensory experience). It may become clear now that a tone scale as such, as well as its intonation, cannot be really understood or even adequately discussed without considering the complex inter-relationships between pitch perception (i.e. 'frequency-to-pitch transforma-tion') and categorization of musical tones. All the presently existing 'theoretical' scale intonations such as, for example, the 'just', 'Pythagorean', and 'equally tempered' intonation are constructed on an ad hoc basis and

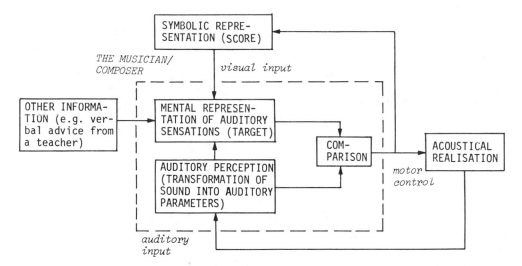

Fig. 1.   Cybernetic model of music realization.

thus must be considered as preliminary approaches to an appropriate theory of intonation which as yet does not exist. The enharmonic distinctions (for example, that between E-flat and D-sharp) may have some merits for certain music theoretical approaches, provided that they are strictly confined to the symbolic domain. No ad hoc theory can, however, tell us anything useful about corresponding intonation distinctions.

Once the conceptual distinction between the three domains of musical reality has been understood and accepted, the process of music realization can be described schematically as in Fig. 1. The essential information flow between the three domains is shown. The schematic illustrates that music realization is not a straightforward process but a complex mutual interaction of categorical (symbolic, or verbal), auditory, and acoustic representations of music. It is obvious that the process comprises, among others, the following psychophysical items:

- the technique of symbolic representation;
- visual and other non-auditory perception;
- auditory perception;
- learning and memorizing;
- evolution and application of theoretical concepts;
- motor control of the musical instrument;
- the physics of the musical instrument;
- the room acoustics involved in auditory feedback.

Although each of these psychophysical items on its own part stands for a number of complex problems which are by no means sufficiently understood as yet, the whole realization process i.e. composition and performance of music, obviously works quite well. This is due to the strong coupling between the three domains through feedback loops provided by the human sensory and motor organs. It is particularly this system of feedback loops which, on one hand, guarantees proper functioning of the whole system if used in its natural way, on the other hand makes scientific understanding of the process so difficult. From communication- and system-theory it is well known that almost nothing can be said about the functioning of a system composed of subsystems containing feedback loops, if the functional parameters of only one or the other subsystem are known. Rather, quite confusing conclusions about the function of the whole system may be drawn from such a limited knowledge. This probably is the ultimate reason why many (most?) musicians unconsciously prefer largely to ignore the psychophysics of what they are actually doing, rather than to attempt to operate on the basis of incomprehensive knowledge. They can hardly be blamed for that.

This cybernetic consideration of the realization process may also throw some light on the problem of finding the objective parameters which characterize the musical quality of a musical instrument. In Fig. 1, the instrument is represented by the box 'acoustical realization'. Since it is just one part of a complex system containing several feedback loops, almost nothing can be said about the instrument's musical value unless its physical parameters are considered in combination with all the other system parameters. However, while the physical parameters of a musical instrument can be determined quite precisely, several other parts of the whole system have been explored only to a limited extent as yet. A lot of experimental and theoretical research remains to be done. Fortunately, as already mentioned, the whole process, i.e. the conventional way of composing and performing music, works quite well, in spite of considerable gaps in our psychophysical insight. This is no longer true, however, when the use of computers in music realization is considered.

MUSIC REALIZATION BY COMPUTER

The simplest function which can be taken over by a computer would seem to be that of a musical instrument (acoustical realization in Fig. 1). In fact by such a technique sounds may be realizable which cannot be obtained from conventional musical instruments, thus expanding the sound material available to the composer and musician. This applies in particular to systematically non-harmonic sound spectra. Yet this type of application is not quite typical of computers. In principle, new sounds may be (and actually are) created by other techniques as well, for example, analog electronic synthesizers, and special non-electronic devices. Moreover, having a computer simulate a musical instrument does not basically change the described features and problems of the realization process. The typical, challenging, and promising impact of computers is their ability to take over larger parts of the realization process, eventually even all of it. In this case we arrive at a procedure which can be described as in Fig. 2. The music to be realized is entered into the computer system in one or the other symbolic form, thus specifying certain musical parameters as, for example, tone category, harmony, etc. Those parameters may be concerned with details (for example, pitch, loudness, and timbre of individual notes) or more with

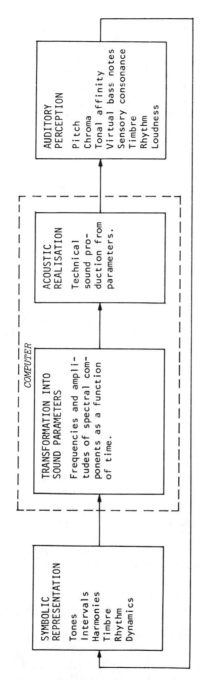

Fig. 2. Schematic illustration of music realization by computer.

global, holistic features (for example, harmony, consonance/dissonance, tonality/atonality) depending on the degree of sophistication of the system. The realization by computer of that music into audible sound takes place essentially in two steps: transformation into sound parameters, and acoustic realization. From the foregoing consideration of the psychophysics of music realization it is clear that the first of these two steps is by far the more significant, complex and difficult, since it implies that almost the whole psychophysics of music realization has to be taken into consideration and its essential principles implemented in algorithmic form.

This requires comprehensive insight into the psychophysics of music realization so that large gaps in that insight can no longer be tolerated, as in conventional realization. For example, in order to determine automatically the precise fundamental frequency, part tone spectrum, and sound pressure level of one single tone of which the desired perceptual parameters (pitch, timbre, loudness, etc.) are symbolically specified, several complex psycho-acoustic phenomena as, for example, the principles of pitch and loudness perception, pitch shifts, masking (simultaneous, backward, forward), etc. need to be implemented by approriate computer algorithms. This requires the availability of sufficiently reliable psychoacoustic models. Consider for example the two most elementary auditory sensations - loudness and pitch. While a comprehensive theory of loudness has existed for some decades (Fletcher and Munson, 1933; Zwicker, 1958), adequate models of pitch have been available only recently (Terhardt, 1972; 1974; Goldstein, 1973). Other, musically highly relevant psychoacoustic parameters as, for example, timbre. roughness, consonance, harmony, and rhythm, can be modelled algorithmically now, at least approximately (for a survey see Terhardt, 1978). Much psychophysical research remains to be carried out in order to adequately solve this problem. Here it becomes obvious that the use of computers in music produces strong demands and challenges, but also valuable suggestions to psychophysical research. At present, according to the knowledge of the author, only very simple, partially heuristic, models of musical psychophysics have been implemented to carry out the trans-formation of symbolic representation into sound parameters by computer programs (see Buxton, 1977). Thus the efficacy of music realization by computer can be considerably enhanced by developing that transformation further on a psychophysical basis.

The second main task of the computer, i.e. acoustic sound realization, is a matter of digital sound synthesis and/or control, i.e. a purely technical problem which can be considered and solved apart from psychophysics and music theory. Many appropriate and useful solutions to this problem have been developed and are still evolving (Moorer, 1976).

The fourth box in Fig. 2 (auditory perception) and the feedback to the first box complement the typical computer realization system, illustrating that the composer/performer may modify his musical score depending on what he hears.

These considerations of several basic aspects of musical realization (by computer) may suffice to suggest that the computer will significantly contribute to music, and in what respect. It is hoped that the analysis of the problem will help to recognize the potential advantages of this technique, and the specific problems arising in connection with it.

   The psychophysical and theoretical basis essential for getting full advantage of the computer's abilities is quite underdeveloped as yet. A new type of music theory needs to be developed which is more than just an analytic reduction of existing music to certain general principles (as is conventional music theory). Rather, that theory should be universal, not only giving space for new musical idioms, but even providing conceptual aids for them. In spite of its generality, that theory must be strictly algorithmic to be implementable on computers. These requirements are quite ambitious. But by the systematic exploration of the psychophysical fundamentals of music, in particular auditory psychophysics, this goal can be approached.

   This particular aspect will be further illustrated in the following sections by some examples which are chosen from the author's own research work.

EXAMPLE I: PSYCHOACOUSTICS, MUSICAL CONSONANCE, AND NEW TONAL SYSTEMS

   For thousands of years it has been felt by musicians and musical scientists that there seem to exist certain basic percetual criteria governing the production and perception of music. The most prominent and significant approach to verify this feeling is that of Helmholtz (1863). It is also the present author's conviction that the structure of music is governed by basic psychophysical criteria to a much larger extent than, for example, human speech. As pointed out above, the use of computers in music requires much more insight into psychophysics than does conventional music realization. Fortunately, the computer itself provides a powerful tool for obtaining that insight. This is crucial, since most of the psychophysical relationships are so complex that their practical consequences can be tested and used only by help of the computer.

   The basic principles which usually are considered as governing music one way or another are consonance and harmony. Large discrepancies exist among musicologists concerning their opinion about the origin and universal relevance of these principles. It is frequently said, that these phenomena cannot be considered as psychoacoustically based and thus universal criteria of music. because "the evaluation of consonance and dissonance is dependent on musical culture and has changed through cultural development". This assertion, however, is in conflict with obvious facts. While it may be true, that historically the major third was only accepted with some delay as a consonant interval (in addition to the octave, fifth, and fourth), there is no evidence that the meaning of the consonance/dissonance label has significantly changed beyond that. Although, for example, the major seventh and the tritone interval may play quite another role in nineteenth and twentieth century than they did before, and may also be perceptually more gladly accepted by the listener today than in earlier centuries, these intervals are still called 'dissonant' if it comes to the point. This is quite remarkable because the meaning assigned to the terms consonance and harmony probably would have been more or less deliberately changed if perceptual reality had demanded that. Instead, no significant change took place, indicating that there actually exist certain basic perceptual criteria which

can be readily associated (and almost independently of cultural development) with the labels 'consonant/dissonant', and 'harmonic/inharmonic'.
Another strong argument is the relative weight which is assigned in
contemporary musical life to harmonic/tonal vs. 'atonal' music. It is quite
evident that a large majority of people distinctly prefer the harmonic/tonal
music either represented by music from the seventeenth to nineteenth
century, or contemporary popular music. It appears quite safe to the author
to conclude from this evidence that there exist strong perceptual criteria on
a comparatively basic level which determine the distinction between
'consonant/harmonic' and 'dissonant/inharmonic', apart from cultural development.

   Although it is almost trivial it seems appropriate to notice that not only
conventional harmonic/tonal music, but also twentieth century music and
the above mentioned sociological behavior can be understood much better by
accepting and studying evident psychophysical constraints, than by denying
their existence. It should be noted that the existence of psychoacoustically
based consonance/harmony criteria by no means implies that music is
forever condemned to be strictly harmonic/tonal. Rather, by studying the
consonance/harmony phenomenon and learning from its psychoacoustic
principles one may find out conceptual approaches toward new, extended
musical languages.

   Our approach comprises three parts: (1) systematic description and
definition of musical consonance; (2) exploration of its psychoacoustic
foundations; and (3) drawing consequences from the discovered principles.

(1) The definition of musical consonance (Terhardt, 1976) is based on
traditional musical experience which shows that there are two main
components, called 'sensory consonance', and 'harmony' (i.e. musical
consonance = sensory consonance + harmony). Sensory consonance represents the universal aspect of 'pleasantness' or 'non-annoyance' (i.e. the
perceptual dimension 'unpleasant - pleasant'), which is a feature of any
sound, i.e. not specific to music. Harmony represents the music-specific
phenomena: 'tonal affinity' (octave-, fifth-, fourth-affinity); 'compatibility'
(of simultaneous and/or successive tones); 'fundamental-note-relation' (root);
'tonality' (existence of tonic). Thus harmony represents and governs the
essential functional features of tonal music, while sensory consonance
essentially stands for a sort of superficial 'cosmetic' aspect of music. It
should be noted that this conceptual approach was in principle already
realized and followed by Helmholtz. The aspect of sensory consonance was
by him labelled 'Konsonanz', the aspect of harmony 'Klangverwandtschaft'.

(2) The psychophysical foundations of musical consonance, according to our
approach, are the following: Sensory consonance is essentially dependent on
the sensations roughness, sharpness and tonalness (Terhardt and Stoll, 1981).
In the particular case of musical chords, roughness is the most determinant
factor, at least with regard to intonation. This is in full agreement with
Helmholtz's results and conclusions.

   Harmony (in the sense specified by Terhardt, 1976) is based on a
learning process pertaining to speech perception. In that process, virtual
pitch (i.e. the pitch assigned to a complex of part-tones as an entity) is

established, taking advantage of the auditory experience that the part-tones of voiced speech elements are harmonically related (octave, fifth, fourth, etc.). The fundamental notes (roots) which are assigned by the auditory system to musical chords are of the same nature as the well-known psychoacoustic percept of virtual pitch ('residue pitch', 'low pitch').

(3) Several consequences can be drawn from this theory of musical consonance, for example, concerning the intonation of tone scales, and tonal analysis of music. One particular consequence is that the traditional diatonic scales are largely predetermined by the harmonic part-tone structure of musical tones and the human voice, since those harmonics establish a series of basic tonal categories. While the categories (and thus the tone scales) are functionally significant (pertaining to 'harmony'), their intonation is a secondary aspect (pertaining to 'sensory consonance'). Thus the relationship between the part-tone structure and the tone scale in case of the natural i.e. traditional tonal system can be illustrated as in the left part of Fig. 3. The intervals are specified in terms of semitones (ST). The straight lines depict for any given note (abscissa) the height of the corresponding harmonics (ordinate; six harmonics are taken into account; 12 ST correspond to the frequency ratio 2:1; 19 ST to 3:1; 24ST to 4:1; 28ST to 5:1; and 31 ST to 6:1). The singularity of musical intervals within the scale (abscissa; octave 12 ST; fifth 7 ST; fourth 5 ST) is caused by the principles of harmony (tonal affinity, etc.), as suggested by arrows.

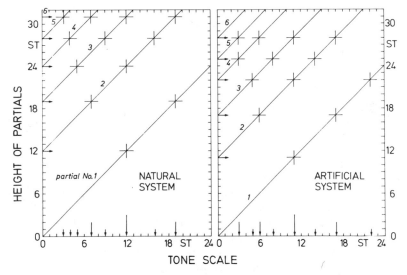

Fig. 3.   Illustration of the relationships between part-tone structure and tone scale with preferred (singular) intervals, for the natural tonal system (left part) and an arbitrary artificial system (right part). All intervals are expressed, in a categorical sense, in semitones, ST. Arrows indicate how, through a principle of compatibility and coincidence, the singular scale intervals are predetermined by the part-tone structure.

The right part of Fig. 3 illustrates, as an example, how these principles may be used to construct a new, artificial tonal system. A certain non-harmonic, yet systematic part-tone structure of musical tones is arbitrarily assumed, in which the second part-tone is 11 ST higher than the first, the third part-tone 17 ST, the fourth 22 ST, the fifth 25 ST, and the sixth 28 ST above the first part-tone. (For the sake of easy realization, the part-tones were selected from the equally-tempered semitone scale). By the same formalism as in the natural system, new singular scale intervals (abscissa) are obtained, comprising 11 ST, 6 ST and 3 ST, respectively (arrows). In this system, the most consonant interval (in terms of harmony as well as sensory consonance) is 11 ST wide, thus being identical with the conventional major seventh. Of course, this and the other artificial singular intervals will not readily be perceived as harmonic, in contrast to the natural octave, fifth, etc. Rather, a learning process is required which may take place through repeated listening to musical sounds of that system.

The crucial point of this approach is that full compatibility of part-tone structure and tone-scale structure is maintained, so that the same principles of musical consonance that are found in the natural system apply to the artificial system. The development and optimization of such artificial tonal systems, as well as their realization even using an interactive learning process are typical and promising computer applications in music.

EXAMPLE II : TONAL ANALYSIS

It has only recently been recognized that pitch is a perceptual quality with quite manifold implications. In music, on one hand, the pitch of musical tones plays a quite elementary role, and in psychoacoustics the pitch of pure tones in fact is considered as an elementary sensory attribute. Psychoacoustics, on the other hand, has discovered that the pitch of musical tones (i.e. complex tones) is a type of Gestalt attribute which is established through a complex perceptual process (virtual pitch; Terhardt, 1972). The theory of pitch perception, as mentioned already, also readily provides the explanation and formal deduction of the fundamental notes (roots) of musical chords. Thus the theory of pitch may be used to carry out 'pitch analysis' of musical sounds in a rather wide sense; we therefore prefer to call this type of musical analysis 'tonal analysis'.

We recently developed a computer program for tonal analysis (Terhardt et al., 1981), whose essential functional parts are depicted in Fig. 4. The goal approached by this program is to obtain, from any tonal sound signal, the various pitch qualities which may be evoked; and a quantitative estimate of the relative salience of the various pitches is provided. Spectral, as well as virtual pitches are taken into account.

Fig. 5 illustrates the tonal analysis of a major triad ($C\sharp_5$, E_5, A_5) played on a piano. (It was played mf, with about equal intensities of tones, without pedals.) A graphical representation of the amplitude spectrum as obtained in the first step of the procedure is shown, and from the series of extracted pitches the five most prominent ones are specified together with corresponding salience estimates ('weight'). It is apparent that the complex structure of the Fourier spectrum is reduced to a few

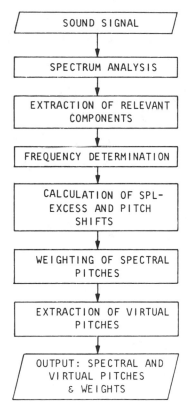

Fig. 4.   Flow chart of a computer-realized system for tonal analysis, entirely based on psychoacoustic data and models.

essential tonal qualities, as is actually the case in auditory perception. In this particular case, the most prominent pitch is that of the highest chord note (A5), while in second place a pitch corresponding to A3 occurs, which represents the chord's fundamental note. The procedure thus solves a problem on a psychoacoustic basis which traditionally has been assigned to music theory: finding the root(s) of a given musical chord. The fundamental notes (roots) of various chords obtained by the procedure are largely consistent with traditional music theory. However, in many cases the procedure provides unexpected new information on the perceptual tonal features of sounds. It is found, for example, that the root is never unambiguous. Musical chords differ only gradedly in the relative salience of competing roots, rather than being divided into chords having a root and chords lacking it. The major triad is singular in so far as its root ambiguity is smallest. Thus one can say that there is no musical chord possessing an absolutely unique root, but neither is any chord completely lacking a root.

The main advantages of the tonal analysis procedure are thus the following:

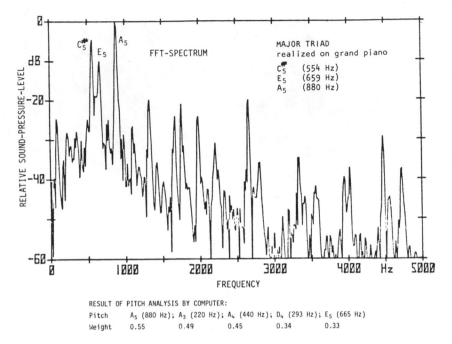

Fig. 5.   Tonal analysis of a major triad. Top, amplitude spectrum. (The spectral analysis was made 40ms after the onset of tones.) Bottom, pitch and salience estimates. Time window of FFT: 80 msec. Sampling frequency: 12.8 kHz.

Analysis is carried out automatically.
Analysis takes into account analytic tonal features (spectral pitches) as well as holistic ones (virtual pitch; roots).
Analysis takes into account the actual physical sound rather than just a musical score (thus effects of instrumentation, intonation, etc. are included).

Tonal analysis by computer may thus with considerable benefit be applied in practically each domain of musical activity: realization, learning/teaching, therapy and research.

As another illustration, let us finally consider a famous problem of music theory: the so-called Tristan chord (Fig. 6). There exist several different musicological analyses of that chord which have in common that they are all concerned with the whole musical phrase in which the chord is embedded rather than the isolated chord. Of course, the real musical and functional role of a chord cannot be fully understood without taking its musical context into consideration. However, the pronounced speculative component which is apparent in the case of the Tristan chord may be considerably reduced by knowing as much as possible about the perceptual tonal features of the isolated chord. We have therefore analyzed the Tristan chord, played on a piano. The resulting seven most salient pitches

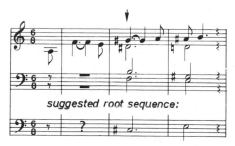

suggested root sequence:

Fig. 6.   The first few measures of introduction to 1st act of "Tristan und
            Isolde" by R. Wagner: the Tristan chord (arrow).

and weights are shown in Table 3. It should be noticed that this distribution
of pitches and weights is an example rather than a general validity. As
mentioned already, the particular result will to a considerable extent depend
on the acoustical parameters of realization. As in the foregoing example,
the highest chord note $(G^{\#}_4)$ has the highest weight. (Note that this
is consistent with the dominance of the soprano voice usually observed in
music.) In the second place, $D^{\#}_5$ occurs, which may be evaluated as
just an octave replication of the chord note $D^{\#}_4$. The $G^{\#}_3$
represents a pitch which is present neither in the chord nor in its
harmonics. Thus it is a candidate for a root; one can observe that a
$G^{\#}_3$ which is really played in addition to the other chord notes
readily melts into the whole sound, hardly changing anything (thus being
fully 'compatible'). However, it is probably not adequate to consider the
$G^{\#}_3$ as a significant root because its position is right within the tonal
region covered by the chord notes. The next three notes in the table
$(G^{\#}_5, D^{\#}_4$ and $F_3)$ are again merely chord notes, or their
octave replications. One might be inclined on first sight to assign to F_3
the role of a real bass note identical with the chord's root. However, the
interval between the F_3 and the higher notes is too small to support the
view that F_3 functions as a root.

Thus on considering the six most salient pitches in Table 3, a
pronounced perceptual dominance of the chord notes becomes apparent, in
contrast, for example, to the major triad considered before where the root

Table 3. Result of tonal analysis of the Tristan chord
$(F_3, B_3, D^{\#}_4, G^{\#}_4)$

	1	2	3	4	5	6	7
Note	$G^{\#}_4$	$D^{\#}_5$	$G^{\#}_3$	$G^{\#}_5$	$D^{\#}_4$	F_3	$C^{\#}_3$
Weight	0.78	0.53	0.53	0.41	0.32	0.30	0.26

A_3 is on the second place. Yet in seventh place in Table 3 there occurs a note which actually must be considered a root: $C\sharp_3$. Thus, in summary, we may learn from this tonal analysis of the (isolated) Tristan chord that the chord does not have much 'tonal meaning' beyond that of the chord notes as such; yet a certain functional root does exist, i.e. the $C\sharp_3$. Its estimated weight (0.26) is roughly 50% of that of the major triad's root (Fig. 5).

If the $C\sharp_3$ is actually played in addition to the original chord, it sounds quite compatible and harmonically appropriate to most musical listeners, though it may be felt that too strong an emphasis given to that note is not musically adequate. On the basis of our tonal analysis we would thus suggest the root sequence indicated in Fig. 6. (The root of the first measure is considered undefined, i.e. the Tristan chord seems to be introduced quite freely.)

CONCLUSION

Concluding our consideration of the impact of computers on music, the main results may be briefly recollected as follows.

Since there exists a high technological and commmercial potential, computers probably will in the near future take over a considerable role in music. This will enhance the positive as well as negative aspects of contemporary musical life. Thus it is timely to take the basic preconditions and implications of that development into consideration. The unique and typical prospect of computer application is that the computer will act as a system concerned with all the complex psychophysical interactions of music - as a symbolic, acoustic and auditory entity - rather than just providing another musical instrument. This evokes a strong need for solid psychophysical knowledge of musical perception, cognition and performance, and will have a strong impact on the development of music theory.

SUMMARY

Computers will soon enhance the positive as well as the negative aspects of contemporary musical life, particularly in music research, learning and teaching. realization and music therapy. From this viewpoint, basic preconditions and implications of computer applications to music are considered: the psychophysics of music realization; the realization by computer; the relationships between psychoacoustics, musical consonance, and new tonal systems; and the automatic tonal analysis of musical sounds.

The psychophysics of music realization is concerned with the interactions between three 'worlds' of musical reality: the symbolic, acoustic and auditory representations of music, respectively. Uniquely, music realization by computer aims at taking account of these interactions. As examples of tonal analysis by computer, musical chords played on a piano are analyzed. In the frame of a psychoacoustically-based concept of musical consonance, the realization of new tonal systems is considered.

ACKNOWLEDGMENTS

The author is indebted to M. Seewann and G. Stoll for their significant contributions to the tonal analysis project and the examples presented here. M. Clynes and W.D. Ward helped to improve the manuscript considerably, which is gratefully acknowledged. This research was carried out at the Sonderforschungsbereich Kybernetik, München, supported by the Deutsche Forschungsgemeinschaft.

REFERENCES

American National Standard, 1973, "Psychoacoustical Terminology," American National Standards Institute, New York.

Buxton, W.A.S., 1977, A composer's introduction to computer music, Interface, 6:57.

Eccles, J.C., 1973, "The understanding of the brain," McGraw-Hill, New York.

Fletcher, H., and Munson, W.A., 1933, Loudness, its definition, measurement and calculation, J. Acoust. Soc. Am., 5:82.

Goldstein, J.L., 1974, An optimum processor theory for the central formation of the pitch of complex tones, J. Acoust. Soc. Am., 54:1496-1516.

Helmholtz, H.L.F , 1863, "Die Lehre von den Tonempfindungen als Physiologische Grundlage für die Theorie der Musik," F. Vieweg & Sohn, Braunschweig.

Moorer, J.A., 1976, The synthesis of complex audio spectra by means of discrete summation formulas J. Audio. Eng. Soc., 24:717.

Popper, K.R., 1972, "Objective knowledge - an evolutionary approach," Clarendon Press, Oxford.

Terhardt, E., 1972, Zur Tonhöhenwahrnehmung von Klängen. I. Psychoakustische Grundlagen; II. Ein Funktionsschema, Acustica, 26:173-186.

Terhardt, E., 1976, Ein psychoakustisch begründetes Konzept der musikalischen Konsonanz, Acustica, 36:121-137.

Terhardt, E., 1978, Psychoacoustic evaluation of musical sounds, Perc. and Psychophys., 23:483-492.

Terhardt, E., 1979, Conceptual aspects of musical tones, Human. Assoc. Rev. 30(1/2):46-57.

Terhardt, E and Stoll, G., 1981, Skalierung des Wohlklangs von 17 Umweltschallen und Untersuchung der beteiligten Hörparameter, Acustica, in press.

Terhardt, E , Stoll, G., and Seewann, M., 1981, Quantitative evaluation of pitch and pitch salience for complex tonal signals, submitted to J. Acoust. Soc. Am.

Zwicker, E., 1958, Über psychologische und methodische Grundlagen der Lautheit, Acustica, 8:237.

Chapter XIX

ELECTRONIC MUSIC
A Bridge between Psychoacoustics and Music

William Hartmann

Department of Physics
Michigan State University
East Lansing, Michigan, USA

I.   INTRODUCTION

The sounds that we study in musical acoustics tend to be simple ones. For the most part we analyze the structure and production of tones of individual instruments. The sounds used by the psychoacoustician, as he tries to understand the inner workings of the auditory system, tend to be even simpler. By contrast the sounds that are normally encountered in music are complex. One may fairly ask whether the studies made by musical acousticians or psychoacousticians are really applicable in musical situations.

Lest I be misunderstood, let me quickly add that I believe that the analytical method used by musical acousticians and psychoacousticians is the right method to obtain understanding of the fundamental principles involved in music and its perception. The analytical method is at the root of all science. We can have confidence in the ultimate value of such basic research in the study of music. However, the application of the basic research to the study of actual musical situations is something of an engineering problem, one in which many basic acoustic and psychoacoustic elements are present simultaneously. One must decide which of the many elements are of primary importance in a given musical situation and which are of secondary importance. It may also happen that combinations of basic acoustic elements produce results which are different from the sum of their parts. We are then sent back to the basic research to find additional fundamental principles. Difficult though the problems are, I think that there is now opportunity for real progress to be made in the application of physical and psychological acoustics to the study of music in all its complexity.

A useful approach to the practical study of musical situations is the electronic synthesis of sounds. Electronic synthesis is useful first of all because synthesizers, digital or analog, can truly create music. Second, the

371

parameters of synthesized sounds can be known and controlled. Electronic music is a very self-conscious art. Whatever features exist in synthesized music must be deliberately put there by the musician. The discipline of creating music in a self-conscious and analytical way can lead to insights into the basic nature of music itself. I therefore propose electronic synthesis as a bridge between acoustical science and the art of music. To illustrate this point I will devote the following to examples of phenomena which occur in music which can be studied by electronic synthesis. My choice of topics is somewhat arbitrary, there are other effects which are equally important, and in all cases there is need for more work. We have just scratched the surface with these studies.

II.   MUSICAL EXPRESSION

Expression is an essential ingredient in music. In the case of wind instruments and bowed strings, where non-linear mechanisms make the tone, the instrument and the musician are so tightly coupled that it is difficult to make a physical separation between expressive devices and instrument timbre.

By contrast expression does not come naturally in electronic music. Most electronic music that we hear is deficient in expression. There are several ways that one can use electronic synthesis to give insight into the role of expression in music.

A.   Spectrally Minimal Music

The basic tools of the psychoacoustician are sine tones and noise bands. We know that music is not made up of sine tones and noise bands, but it is an instructive exercise to try to create music using only these elements. Acceptable music can be made if the composition contains voices which cover the audible range of frequencies. One notices that sine tones of different frequencies have different timbres.

With appropriate amplitude shaping the sine tones can play different musical roles. The use of spectrally minimal instruments places special demands upon the creative use of expression. Without variations in dynamics, pitch and timing there is little else of interest in the music.

B.   Synthesized Violin

The first recorded example is a synthesized violin from a portion of J.S. Bach's Great A Minor Fugue as performed by Paul Hartmann (see record enclosed with this book).

Most people regard that synthesized violin as a successful simulation. What is interesting is that the synthesizer patch which created it, shown in Fig. 1, is not particularly special electronically. The tone begins with a pulse wave which is passed through an octave band equalizer, tuned with peaks and valleys to create a broad set of fixed formants. The filter then is like a broad-band version of the Mathews-Kohut filter.

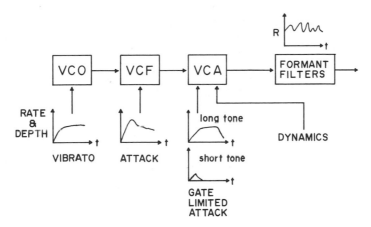

Fig. 1.   Standard synthesizer patch with notations for synthesis of violin
tone.

The most important feature contributing to the realism of this synthesized violin is the expression. The expression consists of dynamics and frequency variations. The expression is introduced electronically by control voltages from semi-automatic or manual controllers operated by the musician. In practice it is important to have a variety of manual controllers available. One can use rotary pots, or wheels, or wheels with detents, or joy sticks or foot pedals. There are applications for all of these in various musical circumstances with various artists. The point for the acoustical scientist to note is that the expression is accomplished with control voltages which can be measured. It is easy to measure the control voltages with instrumentation. More importantly one knows what to measure because the expressive possibilities have been defined by the way in which one connects the expression control voltages into the synthesizer.

Qualitative features of the synthesized violin are these. The vibrato is not constant but grows both in depth and frequency with increasing tone duration. This expressive element can be automated without injury to the illusion. The dynamics are an essential part. The dynamics have long term variations for phrasing, a shorter term part for each individual note and some microstructure. There is a tendency for notes to crescendo as they are held. In the microstructure it is important that the envelope generator which controls the voltage-controlled amplifier have a gate-limited attack. With a gate-limited attack the attack phase continues only so long as the keyboard key is depressed. (It can be contrasted with the self completing attack for which the attack phase, once initiated by a trigger from the keyboard, always completes its course, giving all notes the same attack regardless of the length of time that the keyboard is depressed.) With the gate-limited attack brief notes played on the keyboard are less intense than are notes which are fully played. The envelope generator thus plays two roles. It provides an attack for the synthesized violin note and it also simulates the duration-intensity relation. There is some conflict between these roles. To get brief notes properly reduced in intensity the analog electronic musician needs an attack time that is rather long, probably longer than the true attack time for a real violin tone.

Note also that the envelope generator has a rather rapid decay time. The rapid decay time is needed to simulate the high internal damping of string instruments. The reverberant sound field is created by a reverberation system and is not simulated by a long decay time on the synthesized violin note.

My experiments with expression have persuaded me that expression is a musically important feature which has not been given proper attention by most writers on electronic music. Most of the studies of musical instrument simulation have paid particular attention to the instrument timbre, spectrum and temporal evolution of the spectrum. I believe, however, that an important cue to musical instrument recognition by listeners is the compass of the expressive possibilities of the instrument. It is probably possible to play a sine wave with expression appropriate to a violin or appropriate to a trumpet and achieve good recognition scores from a panel of listeners on a forced-choiced task.

III. MASKING AND PARTIAL MASKING

A.   Masking and Timbre Interactions

A question of musical importance is that of mutual interactions among musical timbres. There are masking effects which, to my knowledge, have not been studied at all by psychoacousticians. One of the effects is the masking of the upper partials of bass voices by the fundamentals and lower harmonics of upper voices. As a result bass voices sound much less brilliant or less buzzy in ensemble than in solo. Figure 2 shows schematically how

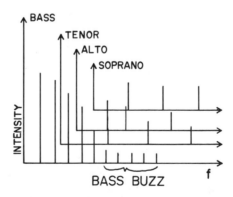

Fig. 2.   Schematic representation of the harmonics of four voices to illustrate the potential for masking of upper bass harmonics by strong harmonics of upper voices. Horizontal axes have been offset for clarity.

this happens. It shows the spectra for four voices on a common frequency axis which has been offset vertically for clarity. The high harmonics of the bass voice are closely spaced but they are weak compared with the lower harmonics of the upper voices in the same frequency region. The second recorded example is another passage from the "Great A Minor Fugue." First the passage is played with the bass voice enhanced in intensity. In the second condition the upper partials of the bass voice are not masked by the upper voices. In that condition you can hear how buzzy the bass voice really is. (Note: This demonstration is effective only when heard at low to moderate listening levels. This is a result of the non-linearity of masking.)

Masking can alter the timbres of instrument tones. Electronic synthesis offers the opportunity to study the effects because the spectra can be controlled and the relative balance among instruments can be changed in any desired way. On occasion a particular instrument tone may be completely masked.

B.   Salience in a Crowd

The composer writes an obligato part for the flute; the flute player learns the part. Will the flute obligato be prominent in the final performance? Will the flute even be heard at all? Through experience composers, orchestrators and conductors learn about relative salience for different combinations of instruments. Not infrequently, however, something goes wrong in the chain from composer to listener and instruments are not heard in proper balance. In principle, psychoacoustic models of loudness and partial masking are capable of providing the answer to questions of relative salience. Relative salience is certainly not a simple function of relative intensity alone. The spectrum matters greatly.

The entire orchestra regularly tunes to the tone of a single oboe. Though the oboe has a small fraction of the intensity of the other instruments, it can still be heard. The 'penetrating' sound of the oboe is undoubtedly due to the relatively strong upper harmonics in its tone.

I did a simple electronic experiment to try to determine the relative salience of an oboe-like tone in an orchestral context. I began with 16 low-pass filtered sawtooth waves, slightly out of tune at A 440. Within this context I compared the relative salience of a 17th low-pass filtered sawtooth wave and a high-pass filtered pulse wave, both with fundamentals at A 440. For a particular benchmark I took the 17th sawtooth wave to be as intense as all the other 16 saws put together. I found that the high-passed pulse and the 17th saw had equal salience when the pulse was 20 dB less intense that the saw, a factor of 100 in intensity. The explanation for this result can be found by comparing the spectra envelopes of the filtered saw and pulse, shown in Fig. 3. Whereas the saw has the majority of its energy in the low frequency region near 440 Hz, the pulse wave has an appreciable fraction of its energy in upper partials which rise above the spectrum for the sawtooth context in the high frequency region. The peaks in the spectral envelope of the pulse stand out like mountain peaks in a rolling landscape. The salience experiment suggests that the auditory image is similar, i.e. that frequency analysis by the auditory system plays a

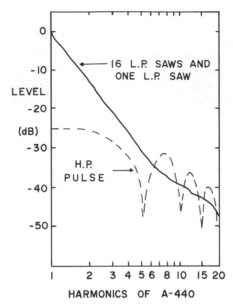

Fig. 3.   Spectral envelope for the salience experiment for low-passed saw and high-passed pulse in a context of 16 low-passed saws.

significant role in relative salience. It would be interesting to make a psychoacoustical study of this effect in terms of masking and partial masking. It is not clear whether the several peaks of the spectral envelope of a tone like the pulse contribute to salience in some simple additive way or whether a more complicated summation law is involved in the perception of salience.

C.   Salience in a Musical Context

We can expect that a study of masking effects in music will involve a number of complications. Among the complications is the tendency for the human brain to seek 'good continuation'. In a musical context it may happen that a voice is perceived when there are other sounds which, according to psychoacoustic studies, ought temporarily to mask the voice entirely. Masking may actually result in the perception of voices which are not present at all. This remarkable creative power of the human brain is the basis of the psychoacoustic method known as pulsation threshold. Plomp (1977) has constructed a dramatic musical demonstration of this 'good continuation' effect. In his demonstration the orchestral music is pulsed on and off. Then broadband noise is introduced into the silent gaps. The noise is intense enough that if the music were actually present during the noise intervals then the music would be partially masked. The brain, 'wanting' to preserve continuation of the music, fills in the gaps in the music with music segments which come entirely from within the brain.

One is tempted to incorporate the continuation effect into an artistic principle. I recall that in drawing class we were instructed to sketch with some of the lines incomplete. Apparently the human brain fills in the gaps, and comes up with an image that is more satisfactory than an image which is correct in detail on the page. A similar thing may happen in music. From studies with electronic synthesis we know that polyphonic music in which the voices have constant salience becomes monotonous. It may be an artistic advantage for voices to disappear for a while, to peek out occasionally from a masking context, and to re-emerge. Note that such a principle would suggest, other things being equal, that ducts between spectrally similar instruments (for example. two violins) would be artistically preferable to duets between spectrally dissimilar instruments (for example: violin and cello). The former duet creates a perceptual game of hide and seek, which give the listener's brain some exercise. Of course, in music, the question of the salience of a voice involves more than masking and spectral overlap. A universally used compositional technique for emphasizing a particular voice is to make it move more than the other voices in the context.

IV. ACOUSTIC SPACE

When we listen to live music we have a sensation of an acoustic space. In a realistic acoustic space we can locate the sources of the sounds in three dimensions and we have a sense of ambience, the environment for the sources. The sensation of acoustic space enhances our enjoyment of music. We use the spatial information to help separate musical lines. The significance of ambience can be gauged by noting how much is lost when we listen to music out-of-doors. In this section I want to consider the creation of the sense of acoustic space from two stereophonic recorded channels reproduced by loudspeakers. Stereo reproduction is an important topic because so much music is heard in this way and because studying it can provide insights into the perceptual processes which operate to create the sensation of acoustic space. Unfortunately we are a long way from a good understanding of what is involved in the sensation of acoustic space and we are a long way from mastery of reliable means to create it. There are a number of rather negative things that we know.

1 Stereophonic recordings made by miking acoustic instruments occasionally produce a realistic acoustic space. Much of the time they do not. One suspects that upon those occasions in which the illusion is successful it is due to a fortunate match between the recording itself, the reproducing loudspeakers and the listening room. If this is true then we cannot avoid the conclusion that the contemporary design for recording studio control rooms is quite wrong headed. In these control rooms the monitor loudspeakers are placed overhead left and right. The listener/engineer has a large mixing desk in front of him which is an effective scatterer of sound waves. The environment in which the recording is engineered bears little resemblance to the environment in which the consumer will hear it.

2.   The sense of acoustic space is unlike the other topics that I have discussed in that standard psychoacoustic models do not seem very helpful. Psychoacoustic experiments on localization are done in anechoic rooms and experiments on lateralization are done with headphones. The experiments have studied the effects of interaural phase differences and interaural intensity differences on the perception of position. There is no doubt that a listener can successfully perform localization tasks given the above interaural cues. But as Benade (1976) pointed out the localization sensations produced by these cues seem puny compared to those produced by a natural acoustic space.

3.   It is especially misleading to reinterpret the interaural headphone experimental results as interchannel effects to be expected in stereo reproduction, i.e. to assume that the interaural phase and intensity differences observed in the headphone experiments will be manifest if the headphone channels are instead routed to loudspeakers. This misconstruction greatly overestimates the effect of interchannel phase differences in the stereophonic field produced by loudspeakers.

4.   The electronic musician, intent on creating a realistic acoustic space, faces a particularly difficult task. He begins with sound sources having zero size, and all of them are located at the same point in a free field. The simplest, and most common way for the electronic musician to make a stereo recording is to pan the individual voices, more or less left or right. The result is disappointing. The voices seem to originate at the left or right speakers, or, if the listener is ideally situated, from somewhere between the speakers. This approach provides no sense of spatial extent and no sense of depth. It is common to add artificial reverberation to electronic music to provide a sense of spaciousness. However, if the reverberant signal for each voice is simply superimposed upon the original voice and panned together with it, the above deficiencies in the synthesis of an acoustic space persist. Recordings of electronic music are generally much less successful than stereo recording of acoustic instruments in producing an acoustic space. (One exception is the four channel synthesis by John Chowning, in which a great deal of attention was paid to spatial effects of moving sources.)

What acoustical elements can we identify that contribute in a positive way to an acoustic space?

There is an psychoacoustical effect which is so strong that it cannot be ignored. That is the precedence effect. The precedence effect demonstrates the mechanism whereby we suppress echoes, which would otherwise confound our ability to locate sources of sound in rooms. A simple configuration is shown in Fig 4a. The source of sound is to the left of the listener. There is a wall to the listener's right which reflects the sound and provides a potential contradictory localization cue. However, because the direct sound from the listener's left arrives first it suppresses the contradictory cue from the right.

The audio analogy to the effect is shown in Fig. 4b. Here the left loudspeaker transmits a direct sound while the right loudspeaker transmits only a reverberant sound. The third recorded example demonstrates this

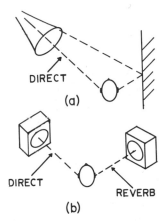

Fig. 4.   The precedence effect geometry (a) in a room (b) the audio
            analogy.

effect with a theme from Pictures at an Exhibition. One hears the direct
sound from the left loudspeaker, despite the fact that the reverberant sound
from the right loudspeaker is 10dB more intense than the direct sound! The
effect of the reverberant sound is to increase the loudness of the sound.
This can be observed from the second playing of the theme in which the
direct left channel is unaltered but the reverberant right channel is absent.

    Psychoacousticians usually consider the precedence effect in a rather
restricted way: the effect is held to be responsible for suppressing echoes
which would otherwise confuse localization and confound speech communication. It is possible, as Benade has done in his text, to turn the precedence
effect on its head, and make positive use of the echoes. The precedence
effect then appears as a part of a larger process which we may call
'Direct/Delayed Analysis'. Apparently the listener can separate the incident
sound into direct (first arriving) and delayed sounds and can compare the
two to obtain a sense of localization and ambience. Here are some of
mechanisms that may be possible.

    The delay of early echoes indicates the size of the room. The direction
of the early echoes provides information about the location of the listener
relative to walls and source. The spectrum of the echoes and reverberant
sound compared with the spectrum of the direct sound suggests the acoustical nature of the room. The ratio of reverberant to direct sound intensity
indicates the distance from the source to the listener.

    Taken one at a time these mechanisms of Direct/Delayed Analysis do
not seem very helpful. There are a multitude of geometrical configurations
which could lead to a given particular comparison between direct and
delayed sound. Hence no particular comparison result is unambiguous about
localization and ambience. We are forced to argue that the sense of
localization and of ambience are created by a compilation of many small
cues. To the psychoacoustician's traditional time-intensity trade-off experiments there could be added many other experiments to discover the potency
of localization cues, none of which, to my knowledge, have ever been done.
The suggestion is that ambience and localization cues are not only to be

found in the direct signal; highly significant cues are found in the relatively weak and subtle delayed sounds, most of which may be obscured by the direct sounds from succeeding notes in an oscillographic representation of the waveform at the listener's ear.

One of the ways that I have become convinced of the significance of the delayed sounds is by studying successful stereo pop music recordings. These recordings are made by 'tight miking' the instruments, a technique whereby a separate microphone and a separate channel of a multi-track tape recorder are devoted to each instrument. The instrument voices are balanced and stereophony is created in the mixdown process. Much can be learned about these recordings by studying the weighted sum and difference of the left and right stereo channels with an electronic configuration shown in Fig. 5.

It is easy to identify an instrument which has been tight-miked and panned because the direct sound can be cancelled in a weighted difference. Only the sound from the reverberation chamber remains. Despite the fact that the direct sound is essentially monophonic the recording may provide a good sense of localization for the instrument. The localization information must be coming from the reverberation chamber.

I should add that not all the voices in modern recordings are treated in this way. Quite generally percussion is multi-miked. Five tape channels may be dedicated to a drum kit. This also applies to massed strings, used as background or as fill (called 'sweetener' in the trade).

The multi miking technique is an example of another aspect of stereophonic recording, namely interchannel incoherence. When two stereo channels are not related by a simple amplitude proportionality factor they are to some extent incoherent. As listeners we have become familiar with the circumstance that when sound sources are close to us or surround us the direct sound from different directions is incoherent. Thus we associate interchannel incoherence with proximate sources. It may be this effect which is responsible for much of the success of stereophonic recording. Stereo reproduction provides some interchannel incoherence. (Note: This is the intention of mono to stereo converters known as 'spreaders', filters which direct part of the signal spectrum to the left and a complementary part to the right). In this way, sterephonic reproduction lends a sense of intimacy and excitement to recorded music.

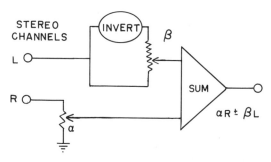

Fig. 5.   Electronic configuration for studying the weighted sum or difference of two stereo channels in recorded music.

The fourth recorded example demonstrates the effect of interchannel incoherence with a synthesized segment from Pachelbel's Canon in D. The three violin-part voices are panned left and right. In the first playing the viola and bass voices in left and right channels are incoherent. In the second playing these voices are coherent. When these two versions are compared, in a living room environment, there is a dramatic difference. The spaciousness present in the first version collapses in the second.

V.   SPECTRAL BALANCE AND THE RELATIVITY OF TIMBRE

We think of a trumpet tone as bright and piercing and of a low-register flute tone as mellow. These characteristics are properly associated with the physical spectral envelope of the tones, as measured, for example, by Luce and Clark (1967) and by Beauchamp (1974). However, the human ear has a remarkable tolerance for spectra of instruments and ensembles which are greatly skewed.

A normal spectral balance for an orchestra is characterized by a spectral envelope which decreases with increasing frequency at about -10dB per octave. But it is quite possible to accustom oneself to a spectral envelope which decreases at -5 dB per octave or at -25 dB per octave. It requires some hours of listening to these conditions of abnormal spectral balance before they sound 'right'. Once acclimated one can experience the full range of timbre sensations from grossly distorted physical cues. Within a context balanced at -5dB per octave a modest amount of energy below 200 Hz gives the impression of powerful bass. Within a context balanced at -25 dB per octave a small amount of energy in the 2 KHz region produces a sensation of a bright timbre. Thus, no timbre is intrinsically bright or dull, musical timbre depends upon context. The significance of his observation is reduced somewhat by the fact that people show a decided preference for normal spectral balance when they are given an A/B comparison without prior acclimation. This observation suggests that there is a balance which is, in a sense, absolute.

The ability to adjust to widely varying conditions of spectral balance, to suffer no information loss when the spectral envelope is skewed, is no doubt an asset to human communication in diverse environments. It is, however, a plague to recording engineers and others who process sound. The electronic musician finds himself in an especially dangerous position because of the flexibility of his instruments, instruments with no natural point of reference. As he becomes acclimated to a skewed spectral balance he can waste days generating sounds which he, and others, will find repugnant a week later. The solution to the problem is for the musician or engineer to be on his guard and to alternate sound production and sound processing work with listening to music with normal spectral balance.

VI.   ELECTRONIC MUSIC - SOME GENERAL THOUGHTS

In the above some particular aspects of human hearing and their implications for electronic music were considered. To conclude with some general comments: Two ideas have informed the development of electronic music. One might call them ABSTRACTION and UNLIMITING.

A. Abstraction

An analysis of the waveforms of solo instruments and ensembles reveals a complicated detailed structure. Are all the details important? The analog electronic artist begins with a simple palate. To recreate the sonic effect of acoustic sources he must abstract from the complexity of the natural sound those features which are psychologically significant. He dedicates his limited means to these features. The digital electronic artist has the opportunity to work in reverse. He can digitize the acoustical waveform in all its complexity and then proceed to simplify by successive elimination of details. In either case the musician constructs a sound by trial and error. In the process he develops an intuition for salient sonic features. This is the special educational value of electronic music. The concern with abstracted features immediately opens the way to caricature sounds, in which a particular feature of a natural sound is exaggerated. This approach can lead to a surrealist drama in electronic music or to humor.

B. Unlimiting

The range of acoustic parameters for musically useful sounds is limited. The range is limited ultimately by the perceptual capabilities of human listeners. Musical sounds created by the traditional instruments are limited by the mechanisms of sound production, by the dexterity of human performers. and by established norms for performance. Electronic creation of sounds is unlimiting in that acoustic paramenters can be varied over wider ranges electronically than with traditional instruments. Musicians of the 1960s expressed much enthusiasm for unlimiting, for the greater flexibility afforded by electronic synthesis. The sound of new instruments, never before experienced, or of hybrid instruments to fill the gaps between the traditional instrument sounds were eagerly expected. While it is still possible to be enthusiastic about the unlimiting possibilities in electronic music our enthusiasm is tempered by experience. In terms of listener acceptability and durability the new instruments fail more often than they succeed. It is here that we run up against the question of enjoyment in music.

There appears to be human demand for a degree of complexity in musical sounds. The sounds most easily produced on an analog synthesizer or with a computer are simple ones with fixed spectra of formants and without expression. However, with enough analog systhesizer modules or with a complicated enough computer program the electronic musician does not really have a problem in creating complexity along any physical dimension one considers. Different notes can be given different dynamics, different spectra and different temporal evolution characteristics. The electronic musician's problem does not seem to be one of mere complexity. My own view is that there also needs to be a coherence within the complexity, a unity among the details which creates in the mind of the listener the image of an identifiable sound source. Probably the image does not have to be that of one or more of the traditional musical instruments, though I find it hard to ignore the smile of recognition when a listener finds one of my synthesized sounds to be an accurate simulation of a traditional instrument. But the image ought unambiguously to point to a physical mechanism of sound production. The listener should know whether the sound is produced by striking, plucking, bowing, exploding or setting an air column into vibration by one means or another. The transient behaviour of sustained-tone sources and the response of percussive sources is not only complex. The strengths of the partials, and less importantly. their relative phases, evolve in ways which are determined by the physical nature of the source and the means of exciting it. This evolution provides potent cues to the listener about what actually is going on in the production of the tone.

The requirement for identifiable sound sources is much relaxed in dense choral passages in music. In these cases the human musical interest appears to be in the harmony and texture. (An ultimate example here is perhaps Dave Wessel's Antony, in which rich and successful textures are created with sine tones that are so closely spaced in frequency that they are essentially noise bands). It is not surprising that electronic music seems to be most successful when it produces dense tonal masses. By contrast the most marked failures in electronic music have been attempts to create long solo passages, in which the absense of coherent complexity ultimately leads to ennui. (A counter example is Brad Slocum's systhesis of Air on a G String, in which expression is so well used that this most demanding piece becomes successful.)

The coherent complexity in the sounds of acoustic instruments is the result of specific non-linear processes which are imperfectly understood at this time. The standard modules of the analog systhesizer and the digital emulations of these modules in computer music do not provide an economical means for creating coherent complexity. The non-linear networks which are created by patching together the linear modules of a synthesizer are evidently not a good approximation to the mechanisms of acoustic instruments or of most other mechanical sound sources. We can look forward to the time when our knowledge of the psychology of hearing and of musical instrument acoustics leads to an entirely new set of electronic musical instruments, and a corresponding new set of parameters for the description of musical sounds.

SUMMARY

The sonic events which are employed in psychoacoustic studies are typically simple ones. By contrast music is complex. Experiments with electronically synthesized music can help bridge the gap between psychoacoustics and music. On the one hand, electronic synthesis can be used to create real music, music which will stand up to repeated listenings by musically sophisticated listeners. On the other hand, electronic synthesis offers a degree of control of sonic parameters which approaches the precision which characterizes psychoacoustic experiments. Therefore, electronic synthesis enables one to perform well-controlled experiments within a musical context. One can perform controlled experiments on expression in performance, such as variations in frequency, intensity, timing and spectral content. Although different musical instruments are usually characterized by their timbres (time-evolving spectra), an equally important characterization may be the scope of their expressive possibilities. It appears that characteristic expressive devices may often play a more significant role in instrument identification than do the traditional elements of timbre. One can perform controlled experiments on the role of masking and partial masking in music. A number of musical experiments show timbre interaction effects which are expected on psychoacoustical grounds. For example, the upper harmonics of bass notes are masked by tones with fundamentals in the middle and upper frequency ranges, causing a dramatic change in bass tone color, and even in bass pitch salience. Other experiments show the dependence of musical instrument timbre on context, the significance of spectral balance and tolerance for imbalance. Experience with the synthesis of ambience and localization of sources in electronic music provides clues to the perceptual mechanisms involved in the sensation of an acoustic space. The well-known precedence effect can be reinterpreted as a part of Direct/Delayed Analysis, a process in which direct sound is compared with early echoes and reverberation to establish a perceptual acoustic space in detail. A stereophonic field which fails to establish an acoustic space which is self-consistent in detail, may nevertheless create a sense of proximity because of interchannel incoherence.

ACKNOWLEDGMENT

This chapter is based on work which was supported by NSF grant BNS 79-14155.

RECORDED EXAMPLES FOR THIS CHAPTER *

Example 1.   Synthesized violin

Example 2.   Masking of bass harmonics
               A. Bass in balance
               B. Bass boosted

Example 3.   Precedence effect
               A. Trumpet left with reverb. right
               B. Trumpet left only

Example 4.   Interchannel incoherence
               A. Incoherent
               B. Coherent

*   Sounds illustrating this paper are presented in the recording included with this book (See Appendix for details).

REFERENCES

Beauchamp, J.W., 1974, Time varient spectra of violin tones, J. Acoustic. Soc. Am., 56:995-1104.

Benade, A.H., 1976, "Fundamentals of Musical Acoustics," Oxford University Press, New York.

Chowning, J., 1972, "Turenas," recorded at the Stanford Center for Artificial Intelligence.

Grey, J.M., and Moorer, J.A., 1977, Perceptual evaluations of synthesized musical instrument tones, J. Acoust. Soc. Am., 62:454-462.

Houtgast, T., 1072, Psychophysical evidence for lateral inhibition in hearing, J. Acoust. Soc. Am., 51:1885-1894.

Luce, D., and Clark M., 1967, Physical correlates of brass instrument tones, J. Acoust. Soc. Am., 42:1232-1234.

Mathews, M.W., and Kohut, J., 1973, Electronic simulation of violin resonances, J. Acoust. Soc. Am., 53:1620.

Plomp, F., 1977, Demonstration at the Symposium on Musical Psychoacoustics, IRCAM, Paris.

Schroeder, M.R., 1980, Toward better acoustics for concert halls, Phyics Today, 33:24-30.

Slocum, B.A., 1977, "Sonic Sensations," BAS records. Sunnyvale, CA.

Wessel, D.L., 1977, "Antony New directions in Music," Tulsa Studios, Tulsa, Okla.

A Note

NEW MUSIC AND
NEUROBIOLOGIC RESEARCH
Can They Meet?

Richard Toop

Musicology Department
New South Wales State Conservatorium of Music
Sydney, Australia

In the popular imagination there is probably no kind of music that seems more compatible with the 'sciences', loosely understood, than radical new music. No doubt the visible impact of technology on some branches of new music (most obviously, electronic music) has helped to foster prejudices. It should be clear though that the mere use of synthesizers, computers or other electronic equipment in the production or performance of music does not necessarily make the music so produced of interest to scientific research, any more than does the use of a contact microphone in the performance of a 19th century guitar concerto (though this latter case does have obvious sociological implications).

It would be an understatement to say that examples from recent art music do not figure largely in current scientific discussion of music. In fact, dialogue between composers of 'new music' and serious researchers engaged in the study of music as a communications system, an anthropological phenomenon, or whatever, has rarely taken place to any great effect. There were some exceptions in the early 1950's particularly in relation to the early development of European tape music. The German information theory researcher Dr. Werner Meyer-Eppler* was one of the founding fathers of German electronic music (its first major exponent, Karlheinz Stockhausen, subsequently attended Meyer-Eppler's classes at Bonn University). Stockhausen (1963, 1964) makes intermittent, and often adulatory, references to Meyer-Eppler. (Stockhausen's lecture notes for the Bonn University courses have survived, and shed light on the influence of information/communications theory on Stockhausen's compositions in the mid-1950's.) Similarly, Meyer-Eppler's French counterpart Abraham Moles was much in evidence at

---

* For a brief summary of Meyer-Eppler's role in the beginnings of European electronic music, see Eimert et al., 1973.

the Parisian 'musique concrete' studios (Stockhausen, 1971). It is probably significant that both these scientists came from the field of information and communications theory, aspects of which at that time (c. 1950-1955) were in a sufficiently experimental state to embrace even the wildest irrationalities of art.

Thereafter - at least in Europe - the frost seems to have set in. One of the first broadsides was fired in the European avant-garde's own 'house journal', Die Reihe. The author was the Belgian linguist (and subsequent semiologist) Nicholas Ruwet, and the article - "Contradictions in the Serial Language" (Ruwet, 1959) - adopted what was to become a classic standpoint: the incompatability of serialism with accepted theories of linguistic construction. The line of reasoning is essentially as follows:

1)   Music is a language;
2)   Serial music appears to assert a new language;
3)   The construction of serial music is not compatible with accepted theories of language;
4)   Therefore, it is not a true language;
5)   Accordingly, serialism is not a legitimate basis for the composition of music.

Seen in retrospect (Ruwet, 1972) the article is among Ruwet's less convincing essays, not least because in his opening paragraph Ruwet sweeps the ground from underneath his own feet by conceding the worth of some products of serialism: ("Le Marteau sans Maitre" by Pierre Boulez, "Zeitmasse" and "Gruppen" by Karlheinz Stockhausen) without establishing any specific reason for exempting them from his general strictures. In effect, he ends up by tactily endorsing the thoroughly uncontroversial view that within any period of Western art music, irrespective of the current technical and aesthetic bases, the number of inept, unconvincing or uninteresting works vastly exceeds the number of what may be defined dilettantishly (since no other real basis exists) as 'significant works'.

"Quelles conclusions tirer de ces considerations? Provisoirement, aucune!" Here, certainly, one can agree with Ruwet. In 1959, when his article was published, the contacts between even orthodox musicology, ethnology and linguistics were so rudimentary as to preclude the drawing of any conclusions from preliminary interdisciplinary observations. I shall return later to the question of how far, if at all, the situation has changed.

NEW MUSIC AND LINGUISTIC ANALYSIS

At this point, I should like to draw attention to a first, essential difficulty: that of equating the procedures of new music (and by extension, those of Western art music as a whole) with those of verbal language. 'New music' is, despite its peripheral 'anti-art' ramifications, essentially 'art music'. As such, it is subject to a particular system of dialetical thinking that may well be unique to Western music. The celebrated Platonic notion of music as expounded in "The Republic" according to which "...the music and literature of a country cannot be altered without major social and political changes...", and according to which permanent moral-aesthetic criteria exist which it is the duty of every right-thinking society to establish and maintain, is one which illusory or otherwise equates pretty well with the ideological bases of the great non-Western musical traditions, such as those of India, Indonesia and Japan. However, it seems alien to virtually every phrase of Western art music history. The latter is in a continual state of flux, of re-orientation and re-definition - never more so than at present.

It may well be that linguists could accept a modest version of 'continual change' as equally applicable to verbal language. For example, there is no reason why superficial changes in vocabulary should have any effect on research into basic structural principles. But in new music, the changes of 'vocabularly' impinge directly on 'grammar', and in many cases they are neither modest nor superficial. Among other things they frequently involve a renunciation of the kind of hierarchical ordering (though not of order per se) which seems to have been the customary basis for comparison between musical and linguistic structures.

Pursuing a Hegelian notion of art one is led into the thorny field of negative dialectics, according to which each idea implicitly contains its antithesis, and is set on an inevitable course which must end in its liquidation by the latter. As far as Adorno is concerned, art has already fallen victim to this process: hence the opening lines of his last work, the "Aesthetische Theorie" (Adorno, 1969):

> Zur Selbstverständlichkeit wurde, dass nichts, was die Kunst betrifft, mehr selbstverständlich ist, weder in ihr noch in ihrem Verhältnis zum Ganzen, nicht einmal ihr Existenz-recht.*

Within a page, Adorno has moved from a questioning of art's right to exist to a funeral annoucement and prospective obituary:

> Ungewiss, ob Kunst überhaupt noch möglich sei; ob sie, nach ihrer vollkommenen Emanzipation, nicht ihre Vorausset-zungen sich abgegraben und verloren habe. Die Frage ent-zundet sich an dem, was sie einmal war.**

Clearly, not everyone is going to be in agreement with Adorno's drastic pronouncement. But agreement or otherwise is not the point at issue, in this context. The point is that Western art, uniquely, seems to be socially dynamic rather than static, and this situation is reflected in the aesthetic systems which, lately at any rate, have encrusted around it. The denial of

---

* "It has become self-evident that nothing that concerns art is self-evident any more - neither within itself, nor within its relationship to the whole - not even its right to exist..."

** "It is uncertain whether art is still possible at all; whether following its complete emancipation, it hasn't cut itself off and lost contact with its basis. The question is made burning by what it once was."

permanent criteria which lies at the heart of these systems, as well as the new art they describe, may well be at loggerheads with the strategies of scientific study of musical structures.

What is it that musico-scientific research is actually investigating? Is it music itself, or is it the cognitive response to acoustic signals which, for one reason or another, happen to be regarded as 'music'? If the former, then one must ask what music in general (let alone such provocative sub-categories as 'new music') actually is, at least in the view of the invest-igating scientist.

Since music is widely regarded as being not just sound, nor even 'organized sound' (Varese's preferred definition), but aesthetically perceived sound, conflicts between the study of music as, for example, a form of non-verbal communication based on the codification and interpretation of acoustic data, and as a potential 'art-form', are always liable to arise as soon as one moves beyond first principles. In effect, scientific study of the perception of music, or of its possible 'deep structure', at present often needs to 'de-aestheticize' the musical objects with which it operates. In such cases (e.g. Deutsch, 1977) the use of examples from Western art music is made without reference to their aesthetic ramifications; by extension, the use of music to test the recognition of, say, time-intervals might easily involve situations where not only the idea of 'art music' but even that of 'music' was of no particular importance.

THE COMPOSER AS SCIENTIST

It may be instructive to further consider material published in the periodical Die Reihe, and its critics. The very first issue of the Princeton-based Perspectives of New Music included an article by John Backus, entitled "Die Reihe: a scientific evaluation" (Backus, 1962). In essence, the article attacks the European composers (Stockhausen in particular) for imprecise use of scientific terminology, and implies, more veiledly, that this imprecision reflects poorly on the general validity of their compositions. Its primary contention, that the authors in Die Reihe habitually use terms from physics in distinctly cavalier fashion. would be hard to dispute. Backus concludes that they "obviously have a great deal to learn before their writings can begin to have any scientific validity". Clearly, this too is correct; but its relevance to the composers' real objectives is dubious, since there is no reason to suppose that the offending essays were ever intended to contribute to anything other than the literature on contemporary compositional technique.

It is true that a number of articles (e.g. Babbitt, 1962) while overtly dealing with some vital matters of serial technique, have made useful contributions to the theory of modulo 12 arithmetic. However, such cases are rare. In general, now as ever, essays on technique tend to be just that, and not disguised contributions to the literature of physics, mathematics, or any other scientific discipline. Writings on 'new music theory', for want of a better term, have sometimes been speculative, sometimes retrospective, but despite occasional proliferations of graphs and charts, in Europe at least, they have been rigorously related to actual practice. And accordingly, the scientific researcher has had no more right to expect 'assistance' from Boulez and Berio than from Bach and Beethoven.

There is one field that provides an obvious exception: that of computer music, especially in America. The early European composers of electronic music, having failed in their initial attempts to produce either novel or familiar timbres by means of superimposing sine-tones, turned to the ad hoc manipulation of electronically generated sounds (and expediently evolved the view that in tape music, all reminiscences of conventional instrumental sounds were best avoided, cf. Stockhausen, 1959). On the other hand many American composers, perhaps because of the role twelve-tone technique played in their electronic works (see for example Babbitt, 1962), persisted with attempts to duplicate the sounds of existing instruments. The synthesizer was a first step along this path; the computer is its more sophisticated successor. In this case, the requirements of composers gave rise to authentic scientific research into the nature of instrumental and other sounds which might not otherwise have taken place. This research and the subsequent evolution of computer programs for sound synthesis do involve a real collaboration between science and new music (e.g. Chowning, 1980).

On the whole, though, the scientist who wishes to incorporate new music into his studies is on his own. This had advantages and disadvantages. On the one hand, it allows him to approach the object of his research unencumbered by any but his own aesthetic superstructures. On the other, it may well restrict him to a purely phenomenological approach to works which have actually been constructed according to a complex set of 'rules'.

Post-war serialism, whether American or European, offers a fair example. Not only is each work characteristically based on particular ordering of the twelve notes of the chromatic scale; an analogous kind of ordering may also determine the rhythmic units, the intensity levels, the timbre, the octave register, the number of simultaneous pitch strands, the formal proportions, and much else. Precise analysis of even a brief piece like Stockhausen's Klavierstück VIII (1954) (cf. Toop, 1979) reveals the existence of thirteen layers of serial organisation (for the typical structuring of Babbitt's works, see Arnold and Hair, 1979).

There is relatively little likelihood of deducing such ordering patterns from the score itself (let alone from hearing) without recourse to preliminary data (the 'meta score'). Yet these ordering patterns do represent the way in which the piece is made (in certain cases, something close to the totality of what the piece is), and conclusions drawn without reference to them are of questionable validity.

HIERARCHY AND SYMMETRY IN NEW MUSIC

There appear to be certain special aspects of new music that make it unconducive to investigation by a science which, like linguistics, is itself still at a problematic stage. Linguistic research is necessarily based on the identification and analysis of basic structures, of simple relationships which can be shown to have a more or less universal validity. One fundamental assumption here is that complex structures may be understood as an elaboration of simpler ones, even though a direct reduction to simpler forms may not be possible. This notion is essentially hierarchic, and thus demands - where music is concerned - a hierarchic metalanguage such as tonality for its adequate exemplification. There is no doubt that most Western music composed between 1600 and 1830 (and much written afterwards) lends itself to such an interpretation: the 'layer analysis' of Schenker and his successors is the major triumph to date of 'reductionism', but there may well be others in the pipeline. Both semiology and transformational grammar offer potentially credible models for the interpretation of hierarchically conceived musical structures.

New music, however, is often non-hierarchic in construction. In his essay "Pour une Périodicité généralisée", the Belgian composer Henri Pousseur writes:

> La musique sérielle a été considérée pendant un certain temps comme radicalement asymétrique, comme intégralement non périodique. C'est ainsi que la ressentait son public, c'était ainsi que l'imaginaient ses auteurs, qui mettaient tout en oeuvre pour obtenir un maximum d'irrégularité. (Pousseur, 1970)*

The key word here is asymmetry. Classically, musicians have understood the term to imply a displacement of symmetry which, nonetheless, is still referential to symmetry itself (the irregular phrase lengths of much of Haydn's music exemplify this standpoint). But in new music, there are often no referential symmetries: durations of 5, 7 or 11 semiquavers are not 'distortions' of binary or ternary compounds (4, 6, 8, 12) but authentic values in their own right. The duration ♩♪ is not ∼♩ or ♪∼♩. ,
but ＞♩ or ＜♩. , just as ♩＜♩♪ and ♩. ＞♩♪ . Similarly, the fact that ♪ is the smallest unit within a given organizational system does not necessarily make it a structural basic unit (except for the musician who is trying to count his part in semiquavers). In a rhythmic sequence such as: ♪.♪♩♪♩.♩♪ the existence of a 'referential value' is frankly dubious, except in cases where the accentuation scheme imposes a superordinate metre, e.g.

$$\frac{2}{4} \quad \text{♩.♪♩} \mid \text{♫♩} \mid \text{♩♪}$$

In a typical serial situation the rhythmic values, if not tied to pitch-class or interval sets (Babbitt, 1962), are referential only to the overall set of values present. So although any value can be explained satisfactorily in relation to the system evolved for the piece, its susceptibility to broader interpretations is highly problematic. Adorno came up against this difficulty as long ago as 1951. Asked at short notice to take over a composition class at the Darmstadt Summer School from the ailing Schoenberg, he was con-

---

* "Serial music has been regarded for some time as being radically asymmetrical and totally aperiodic. This is how its audience felt it to be, and how its writers conceived of it - they took all possible measures to achieve a maximum of irregularity."

fronted by the young Belgian composer Karel Goeyvaerts and his 'off-sider', the 22-year old Karlheinz Stockhausen. Goeyvaerts was presenting his "Sonata for 2 Pianos", one of the first European examples of the kind of serialism I described above, and his 'explanations' of the piece were hard for Adorno to accept:

> Auf die Frage nach der Funktion irgendeines Phänomens darin im Sinnzusammenhang der Komposition wird mit Ableitungen aus dem System geantwortet. (Adorno 1956)*

In a sense, Adorno's objections ran parallel to those of Levi-Strauss (1964, 1976): Goeyvarets and Stockhausen retaliated by telling Adorno that he was "looking for a chicken in an abstract painting". The broad question is posed as to whether music needs 'universals' in order to 'make sense', and whether those researchers engaged in establishing relationships between musical and linguistic construction should attempt to establish criteria for music which are independent of historically and geographically determined 'styles'.

Another problematic aspect of new music, viewed as language, is its frequent avoidance of any kind of apparent repetition. If asymmetrical structures of the kind shown above were at least liable to be repeated in a consistent manner, one would have some basis for the examination of (composite) basic structures. But in practice, there is usually no more repetition between basic structures than there is within them. In effect, one is dealing with a sort of 'negative' version of tonal layer analysis: in the latter, the hierarchic structures of the overall form are reflected at every subsidiary level; in post-war serialism, the same 'rules' of non-periodicity and non-repetition tend to govern every aspect of a piece, from the local details to the total form (Toop 1979).

Of course, not all new music is serial (ever less, in fact). But whereas serial music at least has the advantage (from the researcher's standpoint) of being - by its own lights - systematic, music which is neither tonal nor serial adopts a completely ad hoc approach to the question of musical organization ('language'): its procedures are as likely to rest on psychological assumptions, on the dramatic thread of an acoustic "stream of consciousness", as on structural ones. Examples of this are as atonality itself: the early 'aphoristic' works of Webern, such as the Bagatelles for String Quartet, or more extremely, the 3 Little Pieces for Cello and Piano (1913); seem to operate on a stream-of-consciousness basis which involves an absolute minimum of repetition, and virtually defies logical structural analysis** (pace the work done in this field by Allen Forte).

Logical or not, these pieces are singularly effective as musical comm-

---

*   "Any question about the function of a particular phenomenon within the context of the composition is answered with derivations from the system."

**   For an interesting contrary view of the 3 Little Pieces, see C. Wintle (1974).

unication. The pronouncements of conservative aestheticians to the effect that atonal music is un-natural and incapable of effective emotional or intellectual communication have proved unconvincing: atonal music may have difficulties in evoking joy or complacent comfort (a provocative coupling...), but its impact and subtlety at the darker end of the emotional scale is not longer doubted.

What applies in some measure to Webern applies more drastically to the consciously 'anti-structural' works of composers like John Cage. As time goes by, more and more musicians unquestioningly accept the sounds which eventuate from Cage's later scores as 'music', even if that music doesn't happen to coincide with their own aesthetic preferences. This has considerable implications for anything as all-embracing (and, perhaps, quixotic) as a general 'theory of musical language'. For a start, it looks as though we will have to rigorously de-aestheticize our definitions - no more 'harmonious combinations of sounds'. In fact, it may be that since Cage, the only tenable basis for a definition of music is that of Pirandello's play "Right you are, if you think so" :what can be perceived as music, is music.

THE RECEPTION OF NEW MUSIC

Up to now, I have dwelt largely upon the notion of music as a 'language'. Naturally there are other viewpoints from which music, and hence also new music, may be the subject of scientific investigation. I have already referred briefly to the emotive effects of music (themselves construable as a language) which are widely though not unanimously - held to be the main reason for its almost universal practice as a human activity. Discussion of the moral and social implications of these effects are age-old: Plato's "Republic" offers a classic example of their systematisation according to mode, though the conclusions he draws are totally at odds with the way in which Western music has developed, and are moreover scarcely compatible with current political-philosophical views of individual liberty. The theory of Indian classical music, insofar as it is concerned with the raga system, takes codification of the emotive significance of scales and intervals a great deal further. In addition to the general characterisation of each raga, it assigns particular emotional connotations to each shruti within the raga (cf. Daniélou, 1968).

In Western music, the theory of emotional response to intervallic structures is still in its infancy (see Makeig, this volume). "The Language of Music" (Cooke 1959) attempted some kind of codification of emotional qualities on the basis of interval properties, in pioneering work. But Western perception of intervals is generally much less acute than that of drone-based high cultures such as the Indian one. Moreover, the emotional connotations of intervals in Western music are subject to all kinds of interferences from harmonic procedures, a fact which in itself is already sufficient to make the establishment of a comprehensive theory extremely complex. The concepts of mobile harmonic bass lines, and of vertical harmonic structures in which the lowest pitch is not necessarily 'fundamental', add further complications. The lack of even a temporary functional 'fundamental' in non-tonal music adds a final coup de grace: it is not surprising that "The Language of Modern Music", (Mitchell, 1963) clearly intended as a successor to Cooke's book, retreats for the most part into conventional non-analytical aesthetics.

Neurobiological study of music is already beginning to complement intuitive aesthetics (Clynes, 1977, 1980). One of the problems, however, is the temptation of equating observed individual responses with the music that gives rise to them. If one assumes too close an interdependence of the two, one equally assumes that what is transmitted is the same as what is received, or in semiological terms, that a signifier conveys the same signified to all subjects. But whereas the perception of color, for example, appears to be reasonably uniform in subjects without analyzable sight defects, in music, differences in individual perception seem to be the rule, rather than the exception.

Nowhere is this problem more apparent that in listeners' responses to new music. Even the apparently simple case, in which a listener declares a piece to be 'incomprehensible' is fraught with difficulties. A verbal statement which is not understood can often be reformulated in such a way that it <u>is</u> understood. Such reformulations are harder to effect in music. Indeed, even the notion of what it is that is not understood is an obscure one. Often, after all, the remark "I don't understand it" is as much a defence mechanism as a statement of fact. The common rejection of new music, even (perhaps especially) by confirmed 'music-lovers', may often reflect a distaste for what the music 'says', rather than blank incomprehension. Schoenberg's dictum, "Die Musik soll nicht schmücken, sie soll wahr sein"*, highlights a crisis in the function of a new and old music alike which is the logical outcome of the kind of cultural dynamism described earlier in relation to Hegel. If, as Levi-Strauss (1976) believes, "...when <u>I</u> hear music, <u>I listen to myself</u> through it...", then it might follow that 'new music', which - as the Adorno school would have it - metaphorically depicts the alienation of the individual in an increasingly authoritarian society, makes for disturbing listening, whereas older music serves to instill a welcome, but possibly false, sense of security.

The inability - or refusal - of many listeners to receive the 'transmissions' of new music has technical as well as aesthetic bases. Its acoustic formations are, on the whole, exceedingly complex, and presumably require decoding processes of comparable sophistication. In addition, the lack of hierarchic pitch structures and rhythmic periodicity is frequently matched at the expressive level by what one might call 'emotional aperiodicity'. Whereas tonal music generally sustains a particular expressive intention over a sufficient period of time for that intention to be clearly registered and responded to, the emotions of new music often take the form of a series of seismographic 'shocks', each demanding an instant response, and liable to be superseded or annulled at a moment's notice. It was this quality that Schoenberg noted in Webern's Bagatelles when he wrote of their capacity "to express a novel in a single gesture, a joy in a breath" (Schoenberg 1924), it is one whose emotional volatility poses problems for the researcher as well as the listener.

---

*   "Music should not be decorative - it should be truthful."

Perhaps in addition to the failure of a signifier to signify, attention should be drawn to a related - almost inverted - case, namely the invention of a signified where no signifier exists. Something of this, I would suspect, carries across into more conventional music-making. Still, it is clearly in the field of new music that the listener is most likely to invent illusory structures and connections. One of Cage's anecdotes illustrates this:

> We've now played the Winter Music quite a number of times. I haven't kept count. When we first played it, the silences seemed very long and the sounds seemed really separated in space, not obstructing one another. In Stockholm, however, when we played it at the Opera as an interlude in the dance program given by Merce Cunningham and Carolyn Brown early one October, I noticed that it had been melodic. Christian Wolff prophesised this to me years ago. He said - we were walking along Seventeenth Street talking - he said, "No matter what we do it ends by being melodic". (Cage, 1968). (The story predates the book some 10 years.)

The brain naturally imposes - or seeks to impose - order on acoustic data, even where none naturally exists. Unless the individual sounds are considerably separated in time, it requires considerable exercise of willpower to prevent the brain from making connections between them; the closer the sounds, the more impossible this becomes. On the other hand, listeners familiar with a considerable amount of highly structured new music seem able to recognize works by Berio, Babbitt, Boulez etc. with the same intuitive facility with which more conventionally-orientated listeners identify Beethoven and Brahms, and that ability also extends to previously unheard works. The latter capacity must involve some kind of 'instantaneous' analytical capacity that not only imposes some kind of order on an extremely complex set of signals, but detects an order that already exists within them. One would like to know, for example, whether Clynes' study of the inner pulse (1977) can be extended to apply to these composers?

*   *   *

I started by discussing Ruwet's objections to serialism, and doubting the existence of a purposeful dialogue between new music and linguistics in the late 1950's. Twenty years later, the literature is admittedly more extensive, but not much more helpful. The only recognition new music has received from scientific researchers (computer specialists apart) is a tacit one, evidenced in their reduced willingness to attack it.

"Quelles conclusions de tirer?" Let's attempt some. Firstly, systems of linguistic analysis, and indeed any structural systems based on the ramifications of basic structural units, seem likely to have no more success in subduing the problems posed by new music's 'language' than Achilles had in vanquishing the apocryphal tortoise. On the other hand, research into the brain's capacity to impose order on complex acoustic signals, and especially on large numbers of more or less simultaneous signals, could prove very enlightening.

Secondly, as a long term project, science needs to find some way of adsorbing aesthetics. At present, 'beauty', the key term of conventional aesthetics, is not conventionally a scientific notion, though 'well-formedness' is conditionally an aesthetic one. However, both scientific research and aesthetics <u>are</u> concerned in their various ways with the interpretation of perceptible phenomena, so there may be a possible basis for integration. If so, new music will surely have a central role to play.

SUMMARY

The developing language of New Music causes severe problems for the music analyst, who finds it difficult to keep abreast of new methods, or relate them to older ones. The musical neuropsychologist, too, is dangerously impervious to new music, except, perhaps, where certain aspects of computer music are concerned.

Specific areas are delineated where new music presents recurring challenges such as the absence of symmetry, absence of repetition, and a 'shorthand' emotional expressiveness. A neuropsychologic approach is seen to require adsorption of aesthetics, and continued study of changing means and levels of achieving creative significance.

REFERENCES

Adorno, T.W., 1956, Das Altern der Neuen Musik, <u>in</u> Dissonanzen, Vendenhoeck & Ruprecht, Göttingen (4th Ed.).

Adorno, T.W., 1970, "Aesthetische Theorie", Suhrkamp Verlag, Frankfurt-am-Main.

Arnold, S., and Hair, G., 1979, An introduction and a study: Milton Babbitt's String Quartet No. 3, <u>Persp. New Mus.</u>, 14(2)/15(1), Princeton University Press.

Babbitt, M., 162, Twelve-tone rhythmic structure and the electronic medium, <u>Persp. New Mus.</u>, 1(1):49.

Backus, J., 1962, <u>Die Reihe</u>: a scientific evaluation, <u>Persp. New Mus.</u>, 1(1):160.

Cage, J., 1968, "A Year from Monday", Calder & Boyars, London.

Chowning, J.M., 1980, Computer synthesis of the singing voice, <u>in</u> "Sound Generation in Winds Strings Computers," Royal Swedish Academy of Music Publication No. 29, Kung. Musikaliska Akademien, Stockholm.

Clynes, M., 1977, "Sentics: The Touch of Emotions," Doubleday/Anchor, New York.

Clynes, M., 1980, The communication of emotion: theory of sentics, <u>in</u> "Theories of Emotion," R. Plutchik, and H. Kellerman, eds., Academic Press, New York, pp 271-300.

Cooke, D., 1959, "The Language of Music," Oxford University Press, London.

Daniélou, A., 1968, "The Raga-s of Northern Indian Music," Barrie & Rockliff, London.

Deutsch, D., 1977, Memory and attention in music, <u>in</u> "Music and the Brain," M. Critchley and R. Henson, eds., William Heinemann, London.

Eimert, H., and Humpert, H.-U., 1973, "Das Lexikon der elektronischen Musik", Gustav Bosse Verlag, Regensburg.

Forte, A., 1973, "The Structure of Atonal Music," Yale University Press, New Haven.

Laske, O., 1973, "Introduction to a Generative Grammar of Music," State University Press, Utrecht.

Lévi-Strauss, C., 1964, "Le Cru et le Cuit," Blon, Paris.

Lévi-Strauss, C., 1976, "Structural Anthropology 2," Allen & Lane, New York.

Mitchell, D., 1963, "The Language of Modern Music," Faber, London.

Nattiex, J. -J., 1975, "Fondements d'une Sémiologie de la Musique," Union Générale d'Editions, Paris.

Pousseur, H., 1970, "Fragments théoriques I sur la Musique expérimentale," Université de Bruxelles, Brussels.

Ruwet, N., 1959, Contradictions du langage sériel, Rev. belge Musicol., 13:83-97. Also in Die Reihe, 6:65 (Eng. version).

Ruwet, N., 1972, "Langage, musique, poesie," Editions du Seuil, Paris.

Schoenberg, A., 1924, Preface to Webern's "Bagatelles for String Quartet Op. 9," Universal Edition, Vienna.

Stockhausen, K., 1959, Elektronische und instrumentale Musik, Die Reihe, 5:50 (Eng. version).

Stockhausen, K., 1963, 1964, "Texte", Vols. 1 & 2, Dumont Schauberg Verlag, Cologne.

Stockhausen, K., 1971, The origins of electronic music, Musical Times, London, 112:649.

Toop, R., 1979, Stockhausen's 'Klavierstück VIII', Miscellanea Musicologica, Adelaide, 10:93.

Wintle, C., 1974, An early version of derivation: Webern's Op.11, No. 3, Persp. New Mus. 13(2):166.

Chapter XX

A COMPUTER MODEL OF MUSIC RECOGNITION

Martin Piszczalski and Bernard A. Galler

Department of Computer and Communication Sciences
University of Michigan
Ann Arbor, Michigan, USA

INTRODUCTION

Human-like recognition of sounds by computer is an important element in the overall effort to make computers more interactive and communicative with the outside world. In a typical application sound is first converted into the required digital form for computer processing. Next, the digitized sound waves are automatically analyzed by special computer programs to identify the contents of the sounds. These analysis programs can therefore produce data suitable for later general-purpose digital computer programs that do not know or care that the input data was originally in sound form.

The recognition-of-sound stage then is the step that accepts digitized sounds as input and produces as output the contents of the sounds, akin to a human listening to and then describing the same sounds. How humans listen, consequently, becomes a major concern as we wish to instill these human-like perceptual properties in a computer system. More specifically, we wish to know: (1) what is the relevant information encoded in natural sounds; and (2) how do humans decipher the surprisingly complex and varied sounds into relatively simple messages and perceptual categories.

Quick and easy computational solutions that accurately simulate human listening have proved elusive. Work in this area instead points to the need for a deep and thorough understanding of the human hearing-comprehension system before we can hope to establish similiar broad capabilities in a machine. If sophisticated recognition capabilities could be achieved in a computer system over any substantial (but bounded) domain, then this success could suggest the general framework for developing recognition systems operation on other recognition tasks for different classes of sounds.

Research seeking the internal organization of the human hearing-comprehension system broaches a very poorly understood area of the hearing sciences; hence, this line of research could substantially contribute to that

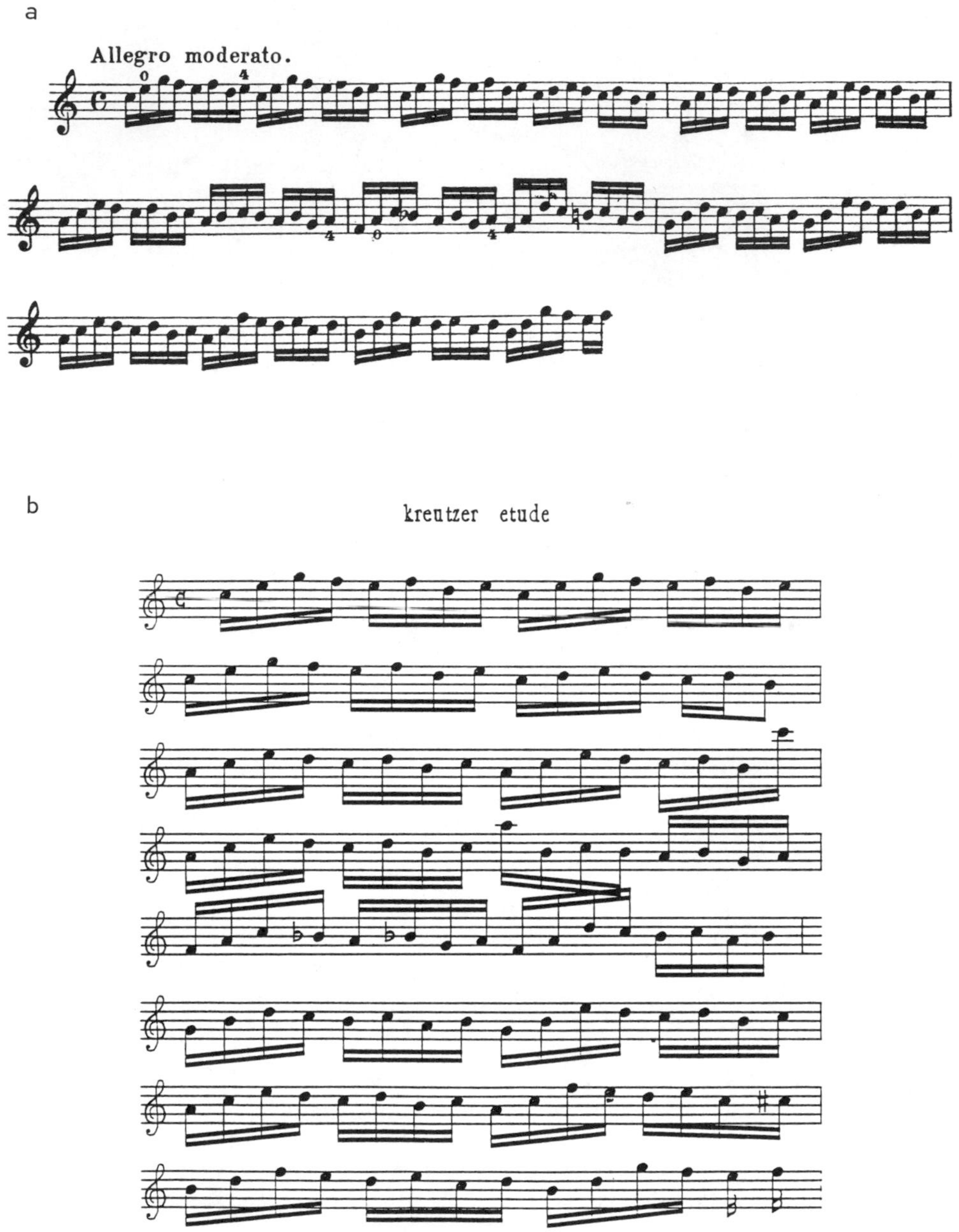

Fig. 1.   A violinist played the notation in Figure 1a, and the resulting sounds were analyzed, transcribed and plotted by computer to produce the notation in Figure 1b.

field apart from its obvious benefit to the machine-perception subfield of computer science. Most research in sound recognition has focused on the automatic speech recognition problem; in contrast, our research is centered on another subset of listening, namely what humans attend to or recognize when listening to music.

We have currently operational a computer system (Piszczalski and Galler, 1977) that automatically transcribes monophonic music played on traditional musical instruments and presents graphical output in the corresponding sheet music form, i.e., Common Music Notation (CMN). This system is roughly 85% accurate in identifying the musical note boundaries and the pitches of the notes in a played melody. The system does not need to know the musical instrument which produced the sounds (see Fig. 1).

We believe we have made a successful initial foray into the complex topic of machine perception of sounds, and further research will produce additional core knowledge about sound perception, music understanding and computer simulations of these intriguing human processes.

RESEARCH METHODOLOGY

The above stated transcription capability was achieved through the following steps:

(1) we analyze on a computer system connected music played on traditional musical instruments;

(2) we use the results of this analysis to gain insight into likely mechanisms that can produce higher-level perceptions;

(3) we then take these insights and use them to guide us in the construction of a single computer model that processes actual music and simulates human perceptions;

(4) at several intermediate stages in the computer processing we make use of powerful display aids including reconstructing new sounds from the parameterized performance (analysis-resynthesis), and generating sophisticated video graphics
(a) to check the model's performance, and
(b) to get data upon which to base further hypotheses.

(5) we also continuously check the generality and robustness of the evolving model by seeing if it can correctly handle a broad variety of performed music.

HUMAN INFORMATION PROCESSING IN THE RECOGNITION OF SOUNDS

The human hearing system processes the sensory information in some fashion that is still quite mysterious. A major objective of our research is to form a skeletal model of the human listening/comprehension apparatus, specifically for recognition of musical patterns. In our model the acoustic information is transformed through successively more abstract levels of representation; eventually the process culminates in our final concise description of the acoustic event, the music notation description (see Fig. 2). We see the application of a similar hiearchical strategy in automatic speech-understanding work (Lesser et al., 1974).

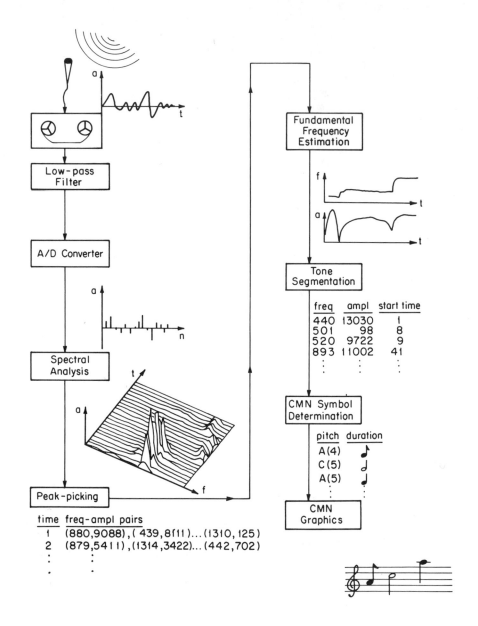

Human recognition of sounds takes the form of object identification or classification: for instance, words are being spoken or musical notes are being played. Because we categorize the acoustic events in listening, we know a good model should likewise be able to perform categorical perception on sounds (Zatorre and Halpern, 1979). If the model is really robust, it should be able to mimic human categorical responses for natural sounds such as those from our everyday listening environment. Of course one can model higher-level cognitive processes by beginning with data already categorized or digitally encoded; however, our interest is focused on how the categorization process may work on real-world sensory input, rather than artifically created data or sounds. This requires the model to "know" the internal representations of the acoustically-based information, how we may extract and encode the music information, and the functions and structure of our hearing/comprehension system.

Hearing scientists are quite certain that humans do not directly "record" the acoustic wave in listening. Instead parameters are abstracted from the sounds to form compressed representations of the acoustic event. For example, a variety of phonological units (e.g., phonemes, syllables, words) have been postulated as being significant elements in the human data structure for speech comprehension (Lesser et al., 1974). Our research is concerned with identifying and quantizing musical sounds into similar units.

As stated earlier, our strategy involves a sequence of internal representations of the acoustic event that are progressively more abstract. The original acoustic information takes on these qualitively different forms en route to the final symbolic notation. While we can discriminate several parameters among acoustic stimuli, we are most interested in those parameters which are dominant in higher-level perception. Complications occur because while loudness, pitch, and duration form the basis for some higher-level recognition tasks, they cannot be dealt with independently as disjoint perceptual elements (Zwicker et al., 1979). We often wish to know the perceptual unit that combines a known group of parameters into the

---

Fig. 2.   The principal stages for automatically transcribing musical sounds are shown. The sounds must be converted into digital form via the A/D converter. The time-varying short-time spectra are obtained via spectral analysis using the Discrete Fourier Transform. The partials in each short spectrum are identified in terms of their frequencies and amplitudes. This information is then processed to estimate one fundamental frequency for each short-time segment. Together with a pitch-related amplitude estimate, the time-varying pitch and amplitude patterns are scanned to find the musical note segments. The absolute frequencies and times of these note-like units are next evaluated to find the nearest CMN symbols on the musical pitch scale and the closest CMN duration equivalents. These CMN descriptions are then passed to the program that determines the location, type of symbol etc. to be plotted for each note in the final graphical representation.

next level of abstraction. Some speech researchers (Zwicker et al., 1979; Klatt, 1979) hypothesize that only data preprocessed by our "psychophysical filter" is used for comprehension, yet we do not know clearly what this data may be or what form it takes.

RELATED RESEARCH AND THE LISTENING MODEL

Research in neurophysiology, psychoacoustics and speech all contribute to the modelling of hearing comprehension.

The neurophysiologists probably provide the most irrefutable findings. Unfortunately, their approach is inherently slow and painstaking, not well-suited for running rapid and diverse experiments. Even so some very rudimentary neurological processes of the auditory system are not thoroughly understood, such as how frequency information is encoded and sent to the brain. The neural pathways and processes involved in the more cognitive aspects of sound recognition have been even more difficult to identify (Whitfield, 1967).

Psychoacoustic experimentation is another approach that involves testing subjects with selective low-information-content acoustic stimuli, noting their verbal responses, and using this data to draw inferences about our auditory system. While a large amount of psychoacoustic data exists from these studies, it is still uncertain how it all fits together in a unified model. Because the whole hearing system is involved in such interactions, it is difficult to establish conclusively that the key discrimination occurred in a particular hypothesized function. Higher-level cognitive studies are also afflicted with such localization problems: "What mechanism was responsible for the experimental data? Mechanical motion in the ear? Higher centers in the brain? A combination of the two?" These are thorny questions for the system modeler when looking at psychoacoustic data. In addition, these findings from low-information-content, simply-specified signals are very difficult to extend to high-information-content, complex signals like speech or music. Depending on what subset of the complex tone is considered, several, often conflicting, psychoacoustically-based predictions can be made as to what will actually be perceived when listening to the more complex sound stimuli.

For example, if several harmonics are sustained over a longer time interval, a sustained tone will be perceived; in contrast, if all the harmonics simultaneously, abruptly and sharply dip in amplitude in the middle of this time interval, then a break in the tone will be perceived (for example, as in a musical note boundary). However, what is the perception when only one harmonic follows this dip - does the listener perceive a break in the tone as in a note boundary or do the sustained harmonics overide this perception and instead create a single sustained tone effect? Relatively simple predictions of this sort cannot be made using existing psychoacoustic knowledge; many factors no doubt come into play including the absolute and relative frequencies, and the amplitudes of the components. Unfortunately, performed music is composed nearly entirely of these kinds of irregular acoustical patterns, not the neat categories of sound stimuli studied by psychoacousticians.

While many phenomena have undergone extensive psychophysical investigation, their perceptual significance in the real-world context of natural sound recognition has yet to be explored in a systematic fashion. In an isolated, controlled experiment an acoustical-perceptual relationship can be strongly demonstrated although we may never encounter these acoustical stimuli in our routine listening environments. Conversely, this same acoustical event, when embedded in complex natural sounds, may have no perceptual effect whatsoever. Consequently we seek psychoacoustic knowledge that has genuine practical importance for understanding sounds within the real-world context of our specific sound comprehension task.

In addition to neurophysiology and psychoacoustics, automatic speech-understanding research has been a third contributor to the development of a hearing model. Unfortunately, accompanying it is the mammoth problem of how natural-language understanding fits into the recognition task. For example, context cues (e.g. semantics or syntax) and the vast external knowledge sources (e.g. vocabulary) connected with speech most severely complicate the already difficult modelling problem.

Automatic Sound Pattern Recognition

Exploring automatic music recognition may also help us understand how humans recognize sound patterns in general. The music notation associated with the played music represents an idealized, prototypical sound pattern that the performer tries to produce when playing a literal interpretation of the printed music. Nevertheless, even the best performers will always deviate (sometimes intentionally) from an acoustically perfect rendering of the composition (see Fig. 3). The musically-sophisticated listener can still then map the audible performance back into the idealized CMN form. In the recognition process the listener somehow "normalizes" the perceived pattern, considering it as an acceptable match of idealized patterns internally stored in the brain.

Actual acoustical patterns may sound strikingly similar to the ears yet reveal few common elements when their underlying data are computationally analyzed or visually inspected. How such audio pattern recognition may work, therefore, is a non-trival concern of researchers in a variety of hearing-related areas. For example, Automatic Speech Recognition (ASR) research is hampered because the prototypical patterns for phoneme recognition are not precisely known or even known to exist. Hence phonemes are not now being accurately and automatically classified in ASR systems despite the heavy reliance of later processes on these preliminary identifications. (According to Robinson, ASR phoneme accuracy in 1979 was about 65%).

The authors believe that the study of music understanding provides a good bridge between the psychophysical approach and the exceedingly complex speech-understanding problem. Natural music generates complex stimuli, is representable by a concise higher-level language (music notation), and has some ideal features to be described shortly, making it well-suited for such investigations. Furthermore, a music recognition model must account for a broad cross-section of the human hearing/comprehension system and for a set of conditions rarely considered by some researchers.

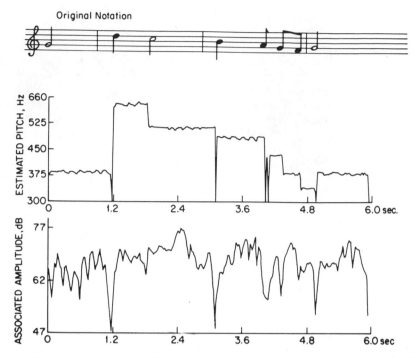

Fig. 3.   The pitch and amplitude contours from a violinist playing "Moon
           River". The original musical notes have been vertically aligned to
           indicate their approximate onset times in the two contours. The
           'wavy' segments in the pitch contour indicate the presence of
           vibrato. The amplitude or 'loudness' function is on a relative,
           uncalibrated scale. Such patterns are automatically calculated
           and analyzed to find the musical note boundaries.

ANALYTIC INVESTIGATIVE METHOD

A.   The Computer Model is the Testbed

       Our method of studying music processing centers on a computer model
capable of melody recognition. The structuring of the overall process is
done by cascaded stages (see Fig. 2). Each stage performs some function
that typically refines the data into a more compact, symbolic form. The
ordering of states is important; if some function is performed before its
input is sufficiently refined, the function will likely yield poor results.
Structuring the process and localizing functional capabilities is therefore
done in the context of an overall model; it is tested with real-world complex
input, viz., ordinary connected music played on traditional instruments.
       The accuracy of a stage in the processing can be rapidly tested on
thousands of stimuli that are inherent in a few seconds of connected music.

These natural stimuli do not have to be laboriously prepared beforehand; performed music provides them automatically. Furthermore, we can often quickly locate which section in the model failed, for we know what the final CMN melody should look like. There is no need to check the hundreds of cases where the underlying computer algorithms were apparently effective. Such procedures are ideal for focusing attention on the faults, or weak points in the system. This type of interaction gives the researcher great flexibility for testing and evaluating information-processing ideas on real-world, meaningful (analog) data.

We note that we do not attempt to model the specific mechanical/electrical activity of the human system, as Schroeder (1975) does. Our modelling concerns only the results of the auditory/perceptual processes.

B.   Graphical and Sound Feedback for Model Testing

A difficult problem in working with any complicated cognitive simulation is knowing if the processing is staying on track as it proceeds through internal cascaded computations. Is the state of the data at a particular point in the processing highly correlated with the presumed feature or is it limping along on the barest of information? We use computer graphics and sound resynthesis extensively to gain insight into this question. Obviously numeric output is also important because it shows the precise values manipulated by the computer. However, we use computer graphics to show the context of the data, and sound resynthesis, so that we may view the computer analyses as several, connected, sound modification/simplification procedures, each operating on and producing actual sounds corresponding to the state of the data at a particular processing level.

We concentrate on graphics and sound displays because: (a) within the system too much data is processed, making direct inspection of numeric data too time-consuming; (b) important broader patterns can often be buried in dense numeric data. When the data is presented in a more composite form such as graphics or sound, the more slowly varying or perceptually important patterns may emerge without being obscured by minute fluctuations in the data; (c) the human hearing "port" is a sensory channel of very high bandwidth capacity; hence, low-information-content displays of hearing-related data are inadequate for conveying a thorough picture of the information routinely handled by the human hearing sense when listening to high-information-content signals. We believe that high bandwidth displays, appropriately programmed, give the researcher a tremendous advantage in studying high-bandwidth human processes.

Audio feedback by resynthesis

Evaluation of partial results may be done by listening to synthesized sounds that represent simplified descriptions of the more complex, originally-played performance. This procedure, which may be done at several levels in the processing, helps to localize stages where vital information is lost, or patterns are being incorrectly detected.

Music is an excellent vehicle for the sound recognition problem in general because of a performance's many levels of acoustic detail (see Fig. 2). We can begin with the original performance with all its subtleties, and then progressively strip it of noise, spectral information, and minute pitch variations, all the while keeping the basic melody line. In speech analysis no such progression is possible. For example, an arbitrary word cannot be described using exceedingly simple acoustic parameters independent of an utterance, as CMN may describe a musical note independent of a particular performance or instrument.

Thus we may analyze a performance, and we may automatically extract the parameters needed to resynthesize the original performance by controlling only a small number of (software) sine-wave oscillators. This resynthesized version is found to be an excellent copy of the original sounds, capturing not only the melodic information but timbral - and phrasing-like information, and it will even suggest the lyrics for sung melodies. The music is now represented by about 500 numbers per second of music; this information describes the time-varying amplitude and frequency patterns of the partials in the performance. The resynthesized partials therefore are set to match the original analyzed partials as they were found in successive 25 msec segments representing the original time-varying spectra. Phase continuity is maintained and smoothing of the amplitudes is done to avoid abrupt changes every 25 msec in the resynthesized sounds. Looking at these numbers directly in printed form is an exceedingly cumbersome and speculative approach to understanding their significance in music perception. Recent experimentation in our laboratory shows that polyphonic music may also be automatically analyzed and resynthesized in this same way.

We note that this analysis/resynthesis capability constitutes a breakthrough in the analysis of performed music and in music perception. We know of no other case where analysis has been successful in capturing important performance nuances in performed, connected music to the point of authentically reconstructing the original sounds.

Another resynthesis program has been implemented that takes the originally digitized performance and automatically inserts a period of silence at each presumed musical note boundary. The resulting sound now has all the notes "pulled apart" in time with no two notes running together, even if they were slurred to begin with. This is the aural equivalent of the visual "exploded" diagram of the parts in a mechanical assembly. This kind of resynthesis provides a good check for note segmentation accuracy without otherwise disturbing the original recording (Piszczalski and Galler, 1979).

Other decomposition and resynthesis possibilities that we are beginning to explore include "slow-motion" and "stop-action" presentations of the sounds. In slow-motion resynthesis the connected music can be replayed with the basic spectral or pitch patterns maintained but at a slower time rate. This is an excellent way to gain insight into rapidly time-varying spectral phenomena. Spectral changes in performed music tend to be quite rapid; for example, a key short-time transitionary spectrum (25 msec duration) might set the perceived pitch direction (up or down) in a note change but be too short to be individually perceptible. The ability to slow down or even "freeze" the sound arbitrarily as in stop-action video is highly desirable for gaining insight into rapidly changing patterns.

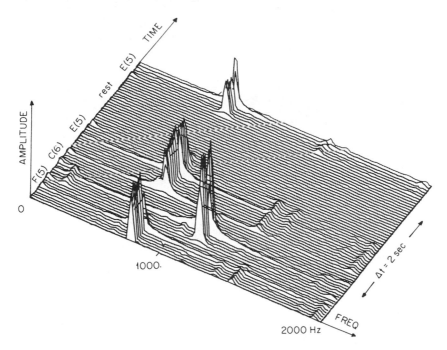

Fig. 4.   A 3-dimensional display section of sounds played on an alto recorder. The very high peaks indicate the sounded frequencies. The frequency axis is used for pitch estimation, the time axis is used for duration estimation. Computer analysis determines the tone sequence, in this case: F(5), C(6), E(5), (rest), E(5) . . .

Graphical representations of sound

To help us understand the broader patterns behind the sounds, we have developed a variety of graphical displays showing different patterns of information after partial processing. Because the time-varying spectrum is the sole basis for higher-level processing, we use a spectrographic display depicting the frequency-amplitude-time information (Fig. 4). The need for rapid display of this data also led us to develop a unique three-dimension-like color display on a computer driven display screen (Piszczalski et al., 1979) (Figs. 5 and 6).

The general search for better visual aids in our research addresses the question of cross-modal feature mapping, specifically the automatic sound-to-graphics transformation. We ask which visual forms may best suggest or accentuate in the visual form the features we so clearly hear in the sounds. Perhaps the most challenging aspect here is to try to represent visually those ambiguities in the sound that need the surrounding context for actual definition. Retaining a "fuzzy" perception in the image is desirable if multiple perceptual interpretations of the acoustic segment are possible.

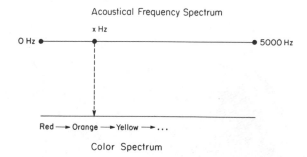

Fig. 5.   Various mappings are possible in assigning color to an acoustical
            component. In the above scheme, for example, a partial is given a
            color based only on its acoustical frequency. Changing its
            acoustical frequency slightly would then lead to a slight change in
            hue. Various mapping systems can be applied depending on the
            characteristics which are sought (for example, highlighting an
            acoustical frequency region, enhancing the musical aesthetics,
            identifying beating components, etc.).

     One area in which this occurs is in automatic speech recognition. Klatt
(1979) found that premature classification of a sound segment as being
associated with one and only one feature is a very difficult error to recover
from later. If multiple choices of varying strengths are possible, we would
like to see this array of possibilities graphically, even though only one of the
alternatives ultimately must be selected. For example, we have found that
the perceived pitch of a tone can vary by octaves depending on its context.
All the hypothetical pitches, weighted by their saliency, should be simultaneously displayed for a comprehensive picture of this event. We now do
this in a color three-dimensional display like the one used for the previously
described spectrographic data.

Moving visual images of sound

     The perceptual effect of the time dimension in music is difficult to
capture well in a static image. This led us to develop the technique of
making 16 mm motion pictures of computer-drawn images of sound in which
an animated graphical image is presented in time-synchrony with the
sounded music. In this way we may display a vast amount of information at
high rates, for example, 40 spectra per second. The full CRT screen
represents about 20,000 potential spectral values spanning the most recent
five seconds of the performance. Meanwhile, the screen is continuously
changing in synchrony (in simulated real time) with the original melody.
     The output display rate is approximately 7,000 numbers per second
(depicted in colour graphics, see Fig. 6), yet critical context-like information is immediately perceptible and understandable in this presentation.
This output medium therefore conveys an extremely broad bandwidth of

visual information about the accompanying sounds. We should note that while this display rate is exceptional for a direct-view computer output display device, it is still far from saturating the information capacity at which our eyes routinely scan and perceive the external world.

We also wish to investigate further 'smart' displays capable, for instance, of assigning an attention-getting color to a sought-after pattern or feature when it occurs in the sounds. While we use graphics for understanding music and our model's behavior, we note that this approach also has obvious implications in other contexts, such as speech aids for the deaf (Pickett, 1979), or in other situations requiring real-time comprehension by a human operator of rapidly-changing sensory data.

METHODOLOGIC ASPECTS OF ANALYSIS AND TRANSCRIPTION

Computers have been used to process naturally generated music in three principal ways:

(1) analysis of isolated tones;
(2) analysis and resynthesis of connected music for electronic music performance;

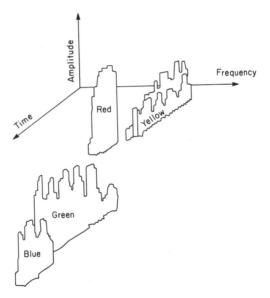

Fig. 6.   The pseudo-three-dimensional color representation allows for frequency, time and amplitude parameters to be depicted, but in addition, color may be incorporated to highlight conceptual groupings. In this case, an individual partial appears as one geometric object possessing a single color; partials differing in frequency then have different colors that aid in the visual recognition of patterns of repeating partials. (see Fig. 5 for the colour mapping technique used in the above figure.)

(3)   automatic music transcription.

J.A. Moorer (1975) gives a summary of computer methods applied to the analysis of isolated natural tones. These studies, beginning with Luce (1963), aim to parameterize natural tones and use this data for resynthesizing the original tone and timbre. Most of these efforts seek data on the partials in the tone; in resynthesis the extracted frequencies and amplitudes are varied over time following the observed patterns of the partials in the originally analyzed tones. While the methods for obtaining these parameters may differ, tones resynthesized from this data sound much like those from the natural musical instrument source (Grey and Moorer, 1977).

In the second computer application of signal processing applied to performed music (for example, Petersen, 1976; Cann, 1979), the input is an entire musical passage rather than isolated tones as above. They stop their analyses after finding some digital signal-processing parameters (such as phase and magnitude), and are primarily interested in using the parameters for resynthesizing new kinds of sounds, not for higher level perceptual analysis. Their work, therefore, is centered on the development of new sound generation techniques for electronic music synthesis.

Automatic music transcription is the third relevant area, and this is where our research lies. The goal here is to take connected music played on natural instruments and produce, soley from the sounds, the corresponding music notation. As in the analysis of speech, in a cognitive model of this complexity, the first few steps that are applied to the music signal are critically important; particularly in their efficacy in pitch identification, an early target of the processing. Data errors or erroneous assumptions in these beginning stages can cause the irrevocable loss of essential information needed for the later higher level routines.

In our analysis strategy we first transform the music signal to the frequency domain in contrast to time-domain techniques employed by three other groups which have studied the transcription problem (Moorer, 1975; Askenfeld, 1976; Tucker et al., 1977). Askenfelt and Tucker et al. both try to extract the pitch directly from the signal in the time-domain, without any attempt at first identifying the partials. Deriving the pitch (period) in this manner assumes highly periodic waveform patterns sustained throughout the music performance. Moorer's method starts with a pitch comb detector to segment the time signal into regions of constant periodicity or "harmony". The detector also directs the setting of a bank of band-pass filters to capture the harmonics of a "root" pitch. While this initial comb-filter pass does not give the pitch directly, the strategy narrows the possible pitch choices greatly since it presumes to have found where all the harmonics may lie.

In contrast with these other methods, our first signal-processing step makes no assumption that the signal at any moment is harmonic, quasi-harmonic, or even periodic. Inspecting the time-varying spectra of performed music confirms that even monophonic music is not quite this simple - grossly inharmonic components and aperiodic segments often occur in music.

We believe the human auditory system uses the spectral form of sound to identify the partials and that pitch in turn is based on the partials (see Figs. 2 & 6). Using this strategy our system is able to identify the tone-chroma pitch of 25 msec segments of connected, monophonic music with better than 95% accuracy. The instruments we have tested include trumpet, clarinet, cello, flute, recorder, trombone, oboe, bassoon, voice and piano. It is not necessary in our system to identify the instrument beforehand nor provide any specific instrument-dependent parameters (such as its pitch range). Moreover, this accuracy is maintained across widely divergent playing styles, as in classical, bluegrass and jazz music.

Second, we do not segment the waveform directly using time-domain derived information as the other three researchers do for the eventual determination of note boundaries. Reverberation and other factors due to the room or instrument inevitably blend musical notes together, making their precise note boundaries quite obscure in the time domain. We think these note-transitions are far easier to detect both visually and algorithmically from frequency-domain information. Our strategy (Piszcz-alski and Galler, 1979d) therefore bases note segmentation on higher level, frequency-based information in contrast with the approaches of others using time-domain techniques. Therefore, in our system note-segmentation decisions are made late in the overall processing, only after the continuous pitch pattern has already been extracted. The continuous pitch pattern then provides the basis for note segmentation by being the source data for pitch pattern detectors that look for note boundary patterns. This approach is in contrast with Moorer's method of first segmenting the time waveform into blocks of homogeneous segments and using this simplied information for the pitch estimater applied later in the processing. Because pitch detection and note segmentation form the backbone of any music transcription system, these distinctions in method represent fundamental differences in strategies. Still, because there is a serious lack of psychoacoustic data on this matter, no one method can now be proven to reflect most accurately the form and process used in human listening.

CONTRIBUTIONS TO THE UNDERSTANDING OF MUSIC

The decomposition and analysis approach we are developing could help suggest what acoustic parameters may play an important role in the aesthetic appreciation of a performance. For example, after a piece has been partially analyzed, accents could be added or removed, or time-varying spectral patterns could be simplified. (See Grey and Moorer, (1977), for a spectral simplification study, but only on isolated tones.)

Electronic music synthesizers combine functionally-simple signal generators and processors to produce their music. For direction synthesists rely in part on analytic information obtained from decomposition studies of natural music. Conspicuous gaps in music analysis information can cause them serious problems. For example, the acoustical basis for timbral coloring in connected music is very poorly understood. Synthesist W. Carlos (Milano, 1979) portrays today's state-of-the-art synthesizers as having available very few "colors" and only "paltry", "thin" waveforms. This often leads to thin, dull and in effect boring music, particularly if the synthesized music is to be created quite quickly. We believe that knowledge gained from the analysis of natural music should be able to suggest successful methods for testing more natural-music-based synthesis techniques. In addition, we can use iterative procedures in a computer environment to hear how several parameters relate to each other, using analyzed performances as our starting material.

CONCLUSION

Exploring performed music via computer techniques touches upon several major issues in both the sciences and the arts. In the past the acoustic complexity of musical sounds and the lack of understanding of the human sound recognition mechanism discouraged direct scientific investigation. We hypothesize that the human hearing/comprehension system contains many specialised functions, hierarchically organized, that extract significant features from sounds. We seek to define this structure through a computer model that accepts natural sound input and generates high-level, music-like descriptions of a music performance.

Only through an interactive system possessing substantial analysis software and high bandwidth interfaces to the outside world do we think it is possible to explore the acoustical and perceptual bases of music recognition. Particularly important is the availability of high bandwidth displays of data at several intermediate stages in the overall processing. These checkpoints into the processing help to convey sharply what features are being retained or discarded as the data is abstracted through the various levels of processing. The display aids can therefore guide the construction of the computer model, minimizing the guesswork in trying to understand the meaning or relevance of thousands of numbers processed by dozens of algorithms as the music is successively transformed to higher conceptual levels.

Although our computer model is to be oriented around music understanding, we believe that any successes in this area shed light on the more general human hearing-comprehension system. The human information-processing pathways no doubt diverge at some point depending on the type of recognition, but we believe many of the perceptual processes we study are fundamental to sound perception in general.

SUMMARY

Human-like recognition of sounds by computer is an important element in the overall effort by researchers to make computers more interactive and communicative with the outside world. Our research centers on a subset of the problem of hearing and comprehension by machine, namely, what humans attend to or recognize when listening to music. Our approach to this problem is through a computer model that accepts sound input from traditional musical instruments and automatically produces as output, descriptions of the sounds as a musician might present them. We explore a novel model-building technique using digital sound resynthesis and computer graphics for evaluating and improving the performance of the computer music recognition model. The larger purpose of this research is to establish a better understanding of the processes behind human perception and recognition of complex sound patterns as encountered in real-world environments.

ACKNOWLEDGMENT

This material is based upon work supported by the National Science Foundation under Grant No. MCS-7809052. Gratitude is expressed to the Bioelectrical Sciences Laboratory, The University of Michigan, for use of their facilities in this research. A major portion of this paper will also be published in the Proceedings of the Symposium on Machine Perception of the American Association for the Advancement of Science, which was held in 1980.

REFERENCES

Askenfelt, A., 1976, Automatic notation of played music (status report), Quart. Prog. and Status Rep., Speech Transmission Laboratory, Royal Inst. of Technol., Stockholm, 1-11.

Cann, R., 1979, An analysis-synthesis tutorial, Computer Mus. J., 3(4):9-13.

Grey, J.M., and Moorer, J.A., 1977, Perceptual evaluation of synthesized musical instrument tones, J. Acoust. Soc. Am., 62:454-462.

Klatt, D.H., 1979, Speech perception: a model of acoustic-phonetic analysis and lexical access, J. Phon., 7:279-312.

Lesser, V.R., Fennell, R.D., Erman L.D., and Reddy, D.R., 1974, Organization of the HEARSAY II speech understanding system, IEEE Symp. Speech Recog., 11-21, April 1974.

Luce, D.A., 1963, "Physical Correlates of Nonpercussive Musical Instrument Tones," Ph.D. Thesis, M.I.T., Cambridge, MA.

Milano, D., 1979, Wendy Carlos, Contemporary Keyboard, 5:62.

Moorer, J.A., 1975, "On-the-Segmentation and Analysis of Sound by Digital Computer," Ph.D Thesis, Stanford University, dist. as Dept. of Music Rep. Stan-M-3.

Petersen, T.L., 1976, Composing with cross-synthesis, 1st Int. Conf. on Computer Mus., M.I.T.

Pickett, J.M., 1979, Speech aids for the handicapped, J. Acoust. Soc. Am., 65.Suppl.1:s36.

Piszczalski, M.B., and Galler, B.A., 1979, Computer analysis and transcription of performed music: a project report, Computers and the Humanities: 13:195-206.

Piszczalski, M.B., and Galler, B.A., 1979, Automatic tone identification in continuously played music, J. Acoust. Soc. Am., 65. Suppl. 1:s123 (abs.).

Piszczalski, M.B., and Galler, B.A., Bossemeyer, R., Hatamian, M., and Looft, F., 1979, Performed music: analysis, synthesis and display by computer, 64th Audio Eng. Soc. Conv., November, 1979, Preprint 1536 (J-2).

Piszczalski, M.B., and Galler, B.A., 1979, Predicting musical pitch from component ratios, J. Acoust. Soc. Am., 66(3):710-720.

Robinson, A.L., 1979, More people are talking to computers as speech recognition enters the real world, Science: 16:634-638.

Schroeder, M.R., 1975, Models of hearing, Proc. IEEE: 63(9):1332-1350.

Tucker, W.H.J., et al., 1977, An interactive aid for musicians, Int. J. Man-machine Studies, 9:635-651.

Whitfield, I.C., 1967, "The Auditory Pathways," Williams & Wilkins, Baltimore.

Zatorre, R.J., and Halpern, A.R., 1979, Identification, discrimination and selective adaptation of simultaneous musical intervals, Perc. and Psychophys. 26(5):384-395.

Zwicker, E., Terhardt, E., and Paulus, E., 1979, Automatic speech recognition using psychoacoustic models, J. Acoust. Soc. Am., 65(2):487-498.

Demonstrated at the Third Workshop on Physical and Neuropsychological Foundations of Music, Ossiach, Austria, August 1980.

LIST OF SOUND EXAMPLES ON THE INCLUDED SOUNDSHEET

The Soundsheet which accompanies this book contains sound illustrations for the following chapters:

CONTENTS - Side 1

Borchgrevink

Illustration of the effects of hemispheric anaesthesia on the ability to sing a folk song. With left hemisphere anaesthesia the subject can neither sing nor count. With right hemisphere anaesthesia the subject 'sings' the melody with words, without pitch articulation but with appropriate rhythm. Pitch control is impaired but speech production and rhythm remain intact.

Clynes and Nettheim

1. Expressive sounds transformed from expressive touch. Dynamic forms were measured on the sentograph and transformed according to the transforms given in Chapter IV, in terms of frequency modulation and amplitude modulation. (The frequency contours preserve the touch form time contour on an appropriate frequency scale.) Emotions expressed are: Anger, Love, Sex, Reverence, Joy, Grief. See Table 1, p. 63 for the parameters of the transform for each emotion.

2. The expression of grief, in continuous frequency modulation, is followed by five examples of melodies derived from it (Nos. 1, 12, 18, 24, 26 from Table 3, p.75). (See graph on p. 74.) The amplitude envelope is the same for continuous and discrete frequency examples. This illustrates how a set of melodies expressing grief or sadness can be derived from the 'continuous' sound expression of grief.

Hesse

Brightness melody. Melody and counterpoint produced by appropriately varying the brightness of chromaless noise (stereo).

CONTENTS – Side 2

Clynes and Walker

Examples of ethnic and rock music (left channel) together with the sound pulse generated by the computer (right channel). During each example you may wish to vary the balance control to hear either the music channel or the pulse channel dominating. In this way you can note how they each induce rhythmic motor responses. If the pulses are correctly derived they should produce a similar rythmic motor output as the music. (See p. 202 ff)

> Bialy Mazur (Polish mazurka)
> Introduction of a Man to a Woman (Ethiopian)
> Ragupati Ragava (Indian song)
> A menyasszany szépvirag (Hungarian folk song)

> Evil Ways (Santana)
> Any Woman Blues – I'm Wild About that Thing (Bessie Smith)

Hartmann

Psychoacoustic phenomena illustrated by computer synthesis:

Ex. 1   Synthesized violin (from J.S. Bach's Great A minor fugue – by Paul and William Hartmann).

Ex. 2   Masking of bass harmonics by fundamentals and lower harmonics of the upper voices (from the same music example). Note the difference in the apparent timbre of the bass.
a) Bass in balance, harmonics masked.
b) Bass boosted allows harmonics to be heard.

Ex. 3   Precedence effect: trumpet (from Pictures at an Exhibition). The left channel transmits the direct sound while the right channel transmits a reflected sound only. Although the reverberant sound is 10dB more intense the sound is perceived as coming from the left channel, due to the precedence effect. The effect of the reflected sound is to increase the loudness of the direct sound. In the second example the reverberant sound is not present.

Ex. 4   Interchannel incoherence (from Pachelbel's Canon in D by Paul and William Hartmann). The three violin-part voices are panned left and right. In the first playing, the viola and bass voices in left and right channels are incoherent. In the second playing, these voices are coherent, and thus less distinct.

Contributors

GERALD J. BALZANO. Department of Music, University of California at San Diego, La Jolla, Cal., USA.

HANS M. BORCHGREVINK. Institute of Aviation Medicine, Blindern, Oslo, Norway.

MANFRED CLYNES. Music Research Center, New South Wales State Conservatorium of Music, Sydney, NSW, Australia.

DIANA DEUTSCH. Center for Human Information Processing, University of California at San Diego, La Jolla, Cal., USA.

ALF GABRIELSSON. Department of Psychology, Uppsala University, Uppsala, Sweden.

BERNARD A. GALLER. Department of Computer and Communication Sciences, University of Michigan, Ann Arbor, Mich., USA.

WILLIAM HARTMANN. Department of Physics, Michigan State University, East Lansing, Mich. USA.

HORST-PETER HESSE. Musicological Institute of the University of Hamburg, Hamburg, Federal Republic of Germany.

RAY JACKENDOFF. Brandeis University, Waltham, Massachusetts, USA.

FRED LERDAHL. Department of Music, Columbia University New York, N.Y., USA.

SCOTT MAKEIG. Department of Music, University of California at San Diego, La Jolla, Cal., USA.

STEPHEN McADAMS. Stanford University School of Medicine, and Center for Computer Research in Music and Acoustics, Department of Music, Stanford University, Stanford, Cal., USA.

MARVIN MINSKY. Artificial Intelligence Center, Massachusetts Institute of Technology, Cambridge, Mass., USA.

NIGEL NETTHEIM. Music Research Center, New South Wales State Conservatorium of Music, Sydney, NSW, Australia.

LEON van NOORDEN. Association for the Blind in the Netherlands, Rotterdam, Netherlands.

MARTIN PISZCZALSKI. Department of Computer and Communication Sciences, University of Michigan, Ann Arbor, Mich., USA.

KARL H. PRIBRAM. Neuropsychology Laboratories, Stanford University, Stanford, California, USA.

RUDOLF RASCH. Institute of Musicology, University of Utrecht, Utrecht, Netherlands.

JUAN G. ROEDERER. Geophysical Institute, University of Alaska, Fairbanks, Alaska, USA.

GERHARD STOLL. Institute of Electroacoustics, Technical University, Munich, Federal Republic of Germany.

JOHAN SUNDBERG. Department of Speech Communication and Music Acoustics, Royal Institute of Technology, Stockholm, Sweden.

ERNST TERHARDT. Institute of Electroacoustics, Technical University, Munich, Federal Republic of Germany.

RICHARD TOOP. Musicology Department, New South Wales State Conservatorium of Music, Sydney, NSW, Australia.

JOOS VOS. Institute of Perception, Soesterberg, Netherlands.

JANICE WALKER. Music Research Center, New South Wales State Conservatorium of Music, Sydney, NSW, Australia.

Author Index

Subject Index